Preoperative Optimization of
the Chronic Pain Patient

Preoperative Optimization of the Chronic Pain Patient

Enhanced Recovery Before Surgery

HEATH B. MCANALLY, MD, MSPH, DABA, DABPM
Medical Director, Northern Anesthesia & Pain Medicine, LLC
Eagle River, AK
Clinical Instructor, UW Anesthesia & Pain Medicine
Seattle, WA

LYNDA WELTON FREEMAN, PHD, LPC
CEO, Mind Matters Research
Director of Integrative Medicine
Alaska Regional Hospital
Anchorage, AK

BETH DARNALL, PHD
Associate Professor
Stanford University School of Medicine
Department of Anesthesiology
Stanford University
Palo Alto, CA

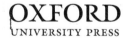

OXFORD
UNIVERSITY PRESS

OXFORD
UNIVERSITY PRESS

Oxford University Press is a department of the University of Oxford. It furthers the University's objective of excellence in research, scholarship, and education by publishing worldwide. Oxford is a registered trade mark of Oxford University Press in the UK and certain other countries.

Published in the United States of America by Oxford University Press
198 Madison Avenue, New York, NY 10016, United States of America.

CIP data is on file at the Library of Congress
ISBN 978–0–19–092014–2

1 3 5 7 9 8 6 4 2

Printed by Integrated Books International, United States of America

Contents

Preface: The Evolution of the Program

Heath B. McAnally, Lyn Freeman, and Beth Darnall

Teleology

Performing elective surgery on poorly prepared chronic pain patients is unwise, and ultimately in no one's best interest. Just as ischemic heart disease, obstructive lung disease, or diabetes can (and need to) be optimized prior to surgery, so too can (and should) chronic pain, which many believe is a disease in its own right, and which certainly jeopardizes outcome. We've come to believe that the complex dynamics of chronic pain require a priori intervention—targeting enhanced recovery *before* surgery.

In the context of growing awareness of the increasing prevalence (and financial costs of care) of postoperative pain, the International Association for the Study of Pain designated 2017 as the "Global Year Against Pain After Surgery." What has received less attention unfortunately is that elective surgery on poorly prepared patients suffering with chronic pain and comorbid substance (e.g., opioids, tobacco) dependence is increasingly shown to worsen their chronic pain state. The literature increasingly demonstrates suboptimal outcomes—both clinical and economic—when patients who are not biopsychosocially "fit for surgery" (as our forebears used to say) are directed/subjected to procedures and operations they've been told will solve their problem(s). To someone who may be worn down from months or years of suffering, and/or may not have developed sufficient resilience and self-efficacy in managing or even overcoming the issue, such an offer may be difficult to refuse. In too many cases, the incentives of the current American system function to bring desperate and passive people into the operating room much like a conveyer belt.

Incontrovertibly, the current system requires improvement and should integrate evidence-based behavioral components into perioperative pain care—especially the preoperative arena. Otherwise, and without such updating, we will continue to fail patients with chronic pain and those with substance use disorders—because we have failed to properly engage them as active stakeholders in their surgical recovery. The responsibility of course ultimately lies with the patient to implement these cognitive and behavioral lifestyle changes; however the onus is on the healthcare team to empower patients—not only with the roadmap for enhanced recovery but also with motivation, encouragement, and accountability. The conveyor belt needs to stop, the patients need to be coached into biopsychosocial-spiritual adequacy, and then they can walk into the operating room with the best fighting chance—if they even need to at that point. Fitness for surgery may just turn out to obviate the perceived need.

Holism

This book is about synthesis. The authors' medical (HM) and psychological (LF, BD) backgrounds have found common purpose and plenty of common ground in the challenge of helping people with chronic pain prepare for elective surgery. The modern emphasis on biopsychosocial-spiritual care is as important in the perioperative arena as anywhere in medicine, and the unique vulnerabilities and dangers inherent in anesthesia and surgery require comprehensive mind-body preparation if things are to go as well as they ought. As anyone who has worked even briefly with patients suffering with chronic pain knows, that most feared scourge of humanity is by no means exclusively physical/somatic. Human beings are a synthesis of matter, energy, thought, emotion, memory, and so forth, and any attempt to address so complex an issue as chronic pain via only one discipline or perspective rarely works.

In the developed world we live largely in the era of chronic disease and elective surgery, and risk factors for the former also largely dictate outcomes for the latter. These risk factors are not so much genetic or uncontrollable, but rather behavioral, and comprise toxic thoughts and toxic habits—a synthesis of pernicious (but modifiable and reversible) activities rather than attributes. As the person is complex, so is the interplay of their beliefs, conscious or subconscious thoughts, and behaviors.

Synthesis of well-established basic wellness principles/activities and personal responsibility for health with more recent learning and challenges (i.e., the opioid problem in America) constitute the meat of this work, along with support from the literature for such an effort. We live, after all, in the era of evidence-based medicine, and just because something seems like a good idea, or common sense, doesn't necessarily justify investing public or private resources toward that end.

History

Heath

I'd spent the first decade of the new millennium in the operating room primarily, with plentiful acute pain service duties but minimal chronic pain management engagement/experience. That chapter of my professional development coincided with the development of the twin "epidemics" of chronic pain and opioid dependence in the United States, and toward the latter part of this period it became apparent to me (and everyone else involved in medicine) that patients struggling with chronic pain—the majority of whom in my experience were also opioid-dependent—didn't fare so well postoperatively. It wasn't just that they required more resources in the postanesthesia care unit or on the ward; they also tended to have longer hospital stays and increased readmissions, and it seemed they more often earned the moniker "frequent flyer." I hadn't yet committed to full-time pain management (that occurred in 2012), but my awareness of a pressing community need was growing.

We began laying the groundwork for a formal "pain prehabilitation" program (which we've named VALERAS) in 2013, focusing in those early stages on prescription opioid reduction and elimination. The structure of what has evolved into our current program was a few years from systemization; we intuitively but haphazardly incorporated two guiding principles of this effort on an individually tailored basis. Those principles are that for patients whose primary source of comfort—biopsychosocially—has become opioids, *reduction and elimination of opioids requires both patient engagement and replacement with better alternatives.*

We'd learned through years of working with self-determined human beings (despite their will frequently being eroded by years of pain, psychosocial distress, and dependence on opioids) that you can't just take opioids away from someone who relies on them. The patient will go somewhere else; possibly to an illicit source. Understanding *why* a patient has become dependent on opioids is critical, and addressing that generally complex predisposition is a requisite and difficult— yet often achievable—task. That requires undermining the underlying distress— sometimes physical, always psychological, and often social and spiritual.

We also learned that a key component of such distress reduction (and the invariably accompanying opioid use reduction) is the engagement of patients as active participants in their health management, yielding symptomatic improvements that in turn further reinforce self-efficacy and motivation. These improved coping mechanisms, founded on habituation of preventive lifestyle modification are bedrock to success.

By 2015 we had formalized a program (Resume Course) for patients suffering with complex chronic pain, which we defined as those with any chronic pain issue plus comorbid opioid dependence. This program constitutes a truly biopsychosocial-spiritual and systematic approach addressing common problems contributing to chronic pain and opioid dependence, including:

- Low estimate of self-worth
- Hopelessness
- Poor nutrition/proinflammatory diet
- Poor sleep and circadian disruption
- Poor posture/alignment

- Sedentary lifestyle
- Polypharmacy
- Anxiety, PTSD, and depression
- Social isolation

A key employee-turned-colleague of mine and I created a 12-session course with each hour-long session focusing on a specific topic. I would see the patient for anywhere from 5 to 15 minutes, addressing the medical issues requiring direct physician involvement, and she would use the remaining 45+ minutes to build relationship and provide coaching. From a practical standpoint this allowed provider extension (or "force multiplication," as we used to say in the military) via nonphysician educators, increasing our impact on individual lives. We began to see unprecedented increases in successful opioid weaning and replacement with better alternatives.

Lyn

Meanwhile from the psychological side, I had spent the past two decades focusing on cultivating and harnessing perceptual change (in the form of personal imagery) to modify behavior, and also dependent health outcome variables as varied as bronchorelaxation in reactive airways disease, immunocompetence, and cancer-associated symptoms. The practical "Envision" neuroplastic brain program I developed initially for asthma patients was honed via Phase I and Phase II research funded by the National Institutes of Health and the National Cancer Institute for application in breast cancer, and showed clinically significant decreases in fatigue and sleep disturbance, with improvements in cognitive function and mood state. Of particular salience to the current project was that these improvements, when compared to a control group, showed equivalent benefit whether the interventions were delivered in person or via telemedicine.

These mind-body interventions, informed by a parallel interest in integrative medicine (along with one of the nation's first comprehensive textbooks on complementary and alternative medicine [1]), eventually found widespread application in the treatment of chronic pain, which is of course highly prevalent in a majority of chronic disease states.

Beth

In 2015 I developed a perioperative digital behavioral pain medicine treatment (My Surgical Success), an adaptation of prior work [2] focusing on developing and testing brief and scalable behavioral interventions for chronic pain based in part on a program I'd previously created (Empowered Relief), a digitized, on-demand platform providing online access to treatment.

The intervention includes three 15-minute video learning modules on pain science and pain management skills that can be applied before and after surgery to reduce distress, improve control over pain, and enhance recovery after surgery. Patients download materials to begin applying the information and tools imme-diately. We conducted our first randomized controlled clinical trial in patients receiving breast cancer surgery at Stanford Hospital. Our early results revealed that patients who received the intervention discontinued postsurgical opioids 5 days sooner than those who received a control intervention [3]. We are now conducting follow-up studies in orthopedic trauma surgery patients at Stanford Hospital, and for this next phase of research we are offering computer "tablets" on the postsurgical recovery units so patients may engage with the intervention after surgery as soon as they feel ready to engage with an electronic device.

The support of surgeons, nurses, and other hospital staff has been tremen-dous, fostering integration and setting proper expectations for the inclusion of behavioral pain medicine as a critical component of multimodal analgesia, and the standard of care.

The sustainability and scalability of the intervention—deliverable by clinicians from diverse backgrounds—lends itself to adoption in an unlimited array of settings. While the focus of this book is on preoperative optimization (and in-deed, a significant aim of My Surgical Success) the intervention is also readily accessible in the recovery period to reinforce what is hopefully previously gained education, and pain self-management principles and techniques.

Timing Is Everything

Around the midpoint of this decade we learned about the Enhanced Recovery After Surgery (ERAS) protocol addressing numerous important but largely im-mediate perioperative variables (e.g., clear fluids the day of surgery, regional and other multimodal anesthesia, early postoperative mobilization, etc.) in an effort to improve surgical outcomes and reduce hospital length of stay. While we value all of these efforts and their proven benefit, long-term improvements in postoperative pain and related outcomes have not been demonstrated with what we believe to be "too little, too late" when it comes to chronic pain that has been festering often for years if not decades. Furthermore, there lacks a focus on fostering self-efficacy/internal locus of control, which deficit lies at the root of much of the complex biopsychosocial symptomatology of chronic pain and dis-ability. This is not intended to criticize ERAS, but rather to highlight the need to supplement it with what we have come to describe as Enhanced Recovery *Before* Surgery when it comes to patients suffering with chronic pain.

Early on we performed a focus-group survey [4] of almost 60 local surgeons from different disciplines (weighted more heavily toward orthopedics and neurosurgery to match what we perceived to align with the proportionate representation of chronic pain patients in our community) asking them two questions important to the development of VALERAS. The first was "How long would you be willing to wait to optimize a chronic pain patient prior to elective surgery?" The second was "If you could change three, four, or five things about your patients prior to bringing them to the OR, what would they be in order of importance?" As we expected, the majority of surgeons (79%) favored a 2-month or longer delay, with the more seasoned ones inviting an indefinite incubation period until reasonable optimization. Also as expected, the factors most frequently voted as least desirable/most important to improve were tobacco use, opioid use, excessive BMI, anxiety/catastrophization, and unrealistic expectations, in that order, followed by other less unanimous issues. These responses provided fine-tuning to the protocol we'd been developing, and further validated our concerns that a whole lot of preemptive work that needs to occur isn't happening.

Adaptation Required

The purpose of this book is to communicate a simple and efficient outpatient preoperative optimization program for patients suffering with chronic pain. That the program is simple and efficient, however, doesn't mean that implementing such a program doesn't take a little time and effort, nor that running such a program doesn't require a hiatus in the entrenched American way of immediate gratification (to patient, surgeon, and hospital administrator alike). On the contrary, delay is deliberate and necessary if harmful habits—including such "microwave mentality" on the part of the patient—are to be undone and beneficial habits are to replace them. To expand on a key point raised by Dr. Darnall a couple years ago in the literature, such low self-efficacy/external locus of control (as well as pain catastrophizing, which she was writing about) "speed[s] the path to surgery while simultaneously undermining surgical response" [5]. To effectively combat this knee-jerk, lemming-like plunge into the sea of worsened postoperative outcome not only requires preoperative delay to change habits but also *aims* to instill a mindset of waiting until either conservative preventive care and rehabilitation either eliminate the perceived need for surgery, or at least improve the biopsychosocial-spiritual readiness of the patient for the operation.

Some of the larger, systems-level contributors to this problem alluded to earlier (e.g., physician and administrator revenue incentives based on operating room activity) are beyond the scope of this exploration and may require value-based modifications to our current productivity-based system. While such determinations are "above our pay grade," as we used to say in the military, this much should be clear to everyone:

Elective surgery on poorly prepared chronic pain patients in the United States is not smart, and ultimately in no one's best interest.

In the spirit of maximizing wise stewardship of healthcare dollars, we propose this simple systematic yet sustainable approach to preoperative optimization. My Surgical Success is eminently tailored to implementation with an absolute minimum of resources. VALERAS too requires a minimum of organizational resources—we make it work using a shared medical model combining behavioral and traditional medical practices, run largely by a nurse educator and a counselor, with oversight by a medical provider. Enough evaluation occurs, and enough intervention is usually required on a weekly basis to satisfy standard office visit evaluation and management requirements (and then some—it is a value-enriched process to the patient). From an economic perspective, there is upfront investment into the patient comprising 10 office visits, yet the cost of this program to the system is still less than that of one day's hospitalization. By focusing on a handful of readily modifiable risk factors for chronic postoperative pain, all of which have been identified in the literature as high-yield intervenable targets, significant outcome improvements may be realized with a relatively minor investment by dedicated practitioners, benefiting patients, surgeons, and the healthcare system overall.

Over the course of 10 weeks we hone in on the discrete arenas of

- tobacco cessation
- preoperative opioid reduction or elimination
- slow-wave sleep enhancement
- nutritional and exercise "prehabilitation"
- reduction of anxiety and pain catastrophization

beginning with the generally more acceptable somatic topics of toxic behaviors before exploring underlying toxic thoughts.

It cannot be overstated that this effort relies on the development and motivational enhancement of patients' inherent desire to be well, and to replace suboptimal habits with beneficial ones. As the saying goes, "people don't change until the pain of not changing outweighs the pain of change." People habituate to a behavior, injurious or otherwise, for the pragmatic reason that it brings comfort or meaning—a means of dealing with distress at some level. If we are to catalyze change, we must facilitate the attachment of emotional valence to new, self-efficacious habits that exceeds the existing affinity for suboptimal or harmful coping mechanisms.

In our experience, this is best facilitated by operant conditioning including encouragement and support from a team clearly committed to the patient's best interest. Validation of pain, followed by confident and clear education about contributors, modifiers, and an efficacious strategy for reducing it by self-determined means is rarely met with anything less than a grateful ultimately enthusiastic adoption.

References

1 Freeman LW. Mosby's Complementary and Alternative Medicine (CAM): A research based approach. 3rd ed. 2008; St Louis: Mosby.
2 Darnall BD, Sturgeon JA, Kao MC, Hah JM, Mackey SC. From catastrophizing to recovery: a pilot study of a single-session treatment for pain catastrophizing. J Pain Res. 2014;7:219–26.
3 Darnall BD, Ziadni MS, Krishnamurthy P, Mackey IG, Heathcote L, Taub CJ, Flood P, Wheeler A. "My Surgical Success": Impact of a digital behavioral pain medicine intervention on time to opioid cessation after breast cancer surgery. Pain Med. 2019 May 13. pii: pnz094. doi:10.1093/pm/pnz094. PMID: 31087093.
4 McAnally H. Rationale for and approach to preoperative opioid weaning: a preoperative optimization protocol. Periop Med. 2017;6:19.
5 Darnall BD. Pain psychology and pain catastrophizing in the perioperative setting: a review of impacts, interventions and unmet needs. Hand Clin. 2016;32:33–9.

Acknowledgments

The authors thank Dr. Jane Ballantyne, Dr. Benjamin Gardner, and Dr. Richard Ryan for their gracious reviews and edits of chapters 3, 4, and 10.

We also thank Andrea Knobloch and Ann Sanchez of Oxford University Press for their invaluable editorial assistance.

Preoperative Optimization of the Chronic Pain Patient

1

Scope of the Problem

Complications and Costs of Perioperative Chronic Pain

Heath B. McAnally

Introduction

This program and book are predicated on the relationship between chronic preoperative pain and elective surgical outcomes. Preexisting chronic pain and associated factors (e.g., anxiety and pain catastrophizing, poor physical health maintenance, toxic substance use, etc.) predict worsened outcomes including surgical complications and failures, increased hospital length of stay (LOS) and unplanned admissions/readmissions, chronic postsurgical pain (CPSP), chronic postoperative opioid use and dependence, and chronic disability. As discussed in what follows, the literature indicates that preoperative comorbidities may actually be more predictive of postoperative outcome than are intraoperative factors such as surgical skill or happenstance, or postoperative factors.

Included in the discussion are brief economic analyses of the potential costs of nonoptimized preoperative chronic pain in the context of these various suboptimal outcome measures. While constituting only crude estimates, the order of magnitude of these projections highlights the critical importance of cost-effective preoperative optimization efforts. The key question behind the remainder of the book and indeed the entire effort is whether or not such preoperative intervention on chronic pain and associated risk factors works and is worthwhile. We address that question in subsequent chapters.

The Importance of Being Optimized

Surgery and anesthesia have become exponentially safer over this past century, and this in concert with advances in technology and resources in the developed world have led to a massive procedural industry that provides the bulk of healthcare revenues/expenditures [1, 2] depending on which side of the coin one views. The costs of surgery, however, comprise far more than those accrued within the operating room itself.

In the previous decade, Davenport et al published data [3] from an investigation of nearly 6,000 operations at the University of Kentucky comprising 50% orthopedic and neurosurgical cases, 34% general surgical cases, and the remainder from the thoracic, vascular, and plastic specialties. While complexity of the operation was the most important factor by far influencing date-of-surgery costs, regression models showed that preoperative risk factors (of which pulmonary and renal issues were the greatest contributors) significantly outweighed both surgical complexity and even the development of postoperative complications in terms of predicting overall perioperative expenditures. While not necessarily intuitive at first consideration, the findings were interpreted by the authors as suggesting that both the cost of treating preoperative comorbidities independent of complications, and also the cost of subthreshold complications not registering in the database outweighed those of obvious major complications (Figure 1.1).

More recently, an investigation of over 22,500 patients undergoing surgery (primarily thoracoabdominal; no elective orthopedic or neurosurgical operations) at Johns Hopkins University between 2009 and 2013 [4] revealed similar findings. The authors reported after a complex analysis that 86% of the variability of perioperative costs at their institution "was attributable to the level of the

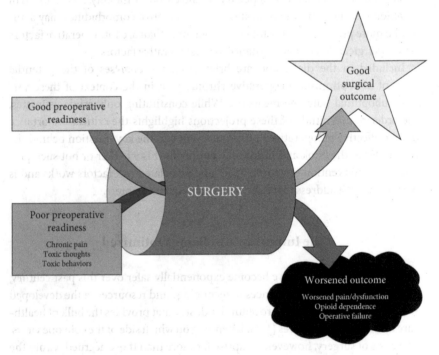

Figure 1.1. Preoperative Readiness Predicts Surgical Outcomes

individual patient." In this investigation postoperative complications predicted a greater share of overall cost than did preoperative comorbidities, but the latter were not insignificant, contributing a little over half the variance in cost seen from complications.

In reviewing some of these data, Snowden and Anderson [5] have come to the conclusion (as have many others, witness the recent proliferation of Enhanced Recovery After Surgery protocols) that "targeting preoperative optimization towards the prevention of postoperative morbidity as a primary outcome . . . is likely to be the most cost-effective strategy." This chapter is a brief exploration of the evidence in support of focusing efforts on preoperative optimization of chronic pain and its associated modern comorbidities prior to elective surgery.

Surgery and Chronic Pain Statistics

Pain is perhaps the most common factor leading to surgery, certainly occurring with greater frequency than nonelective drivers such as resectable cancer or other urgent pathology such as high-grade coronary atherosclerosis or cerebral aneurysms.

In 2010, 48 million outpatient/same-day operations occurred in the United States in 2010 [6], which were roughly distributed evenly between hospital-based and freestanding surgery centers. In comparison, eight million inpatient operations occurred in the United States in 2012 [7]. We can assume that essentially all of the ambulatory procedures were elective. While a breakdown of elective versus urgent/emergent nature is not available for the inpatient operations, four of the top five most common inpatient operative procedures in 2012 involved the musculoskeletal system (e.g., knee and hip arthroplasties, lumbar and cervical laminectomies and fusions [7]) as shown in Figure 1.2. While neurologic and other functional deficits undoubtedly underlay a significant proportion of these procedures, it is also a safe bet that the vast majority of these musculoskeletal procedures were both elective and associated with preoperative chronic pain. From the ambulatory side, in 2010, 24% were performed on the musculoskeletal and neurologic systems, totaling 11.3 million procedures [6]. Again, it is likely that the vast majority of these procedures were both elective and associated with preoperative chronic pain.

Besides these more obvious chronic pain-related operations, numerous typically less noxious procedures from other surgical disciplines are performed every day on patients suffering with chronic pain, given the very high prevalence of this condition in our society, as discussed in what follows.

According to an often-cited report from the Institute of Medicine in 2011, one in three Americans suffer with some form of chronic pain [8]. This figure

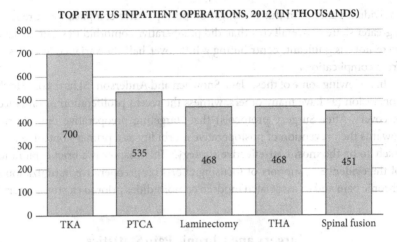

Figure 1.2. Most Common Inpatient Operations

undoubtedly exceeds the prevalence of chronic pain leading to significant biopsychosocial dysfunction. Nonetheless applying this 1:3 factor to the more than 50 million operative procedures expected 2019 (as well as the logic that patients with chronic noncancer pain [CNCP] more frequently self-select for operative intervention) yields an estimate of somewhere around 20 million operations occurring in the context of CNCP.

Chronic Pain and Associated Comorbidities as Predictors of Postoperative Complications

A surprisingly small body of literature to date has shown that chronic pain in and of itself is an independent risk factor for postoperative complications. This is undoubtedly due in no small part to the fact that, as discussed previously, many elective operations, and certainly most major ones (e.g., joint arthroplasty, spinal operations), essentially occur for the purpose of addressing preoperative pain and as such the denominator approaches 100%. Adding to the difficulties in establishing a clear causal link is the subjective and considerably heterogeneous nature of pain, and how it is coped with. The classical Cartesian stimulus–response schema and subsequent development of our understanding of nociceptive biology over the past century has increasingly been shown insufficient to explain the tremendous variance in pain experiences. Monozygotic twins frequently show widely divergent responses to identical stimuli [9, 10] and systematic reviews have shown that anatomic pathology doesn't correlate well at all with chronic pain syndromes [11, 12].

There is increasing appreciation that personal resilience, pain coping mechanisms (and their consequences), and numerous other psychological factors are more predictive of the chronic pain experience. Along those lines, the literature does consistently show that many comorbidities associated with certain pain phenotypes confer worsened outcomes in terms of immediate post-operative complications and intensity of care (LOS, unplanned admissions, and readmissions), surgical outcomes, chronic postoperative pain, and dysfunction. (See Table 1.1.)

One of the most consistent risk factors investigated recently (no doubt in the context of the American opioid epidemic) is chronic opioid use. Chronic opioid use will almost always occur in the context of chronic pain when considering the surgical patient population; opioid dependence outside of the context of chronic pain does not motivate people to seek surgery. Having said that, it may not be accurate to assume one variable as a surrogate for the other, as both conditions are complex and multifactorial. Nonetheless, the association between the two (and other kindred factors such as tobacco use, sedentary lifestyle and poor diet, anxiety and pain catastrophizing, and low self-efficacy) render consideration of shared predictive relationship reasonable.

Table 1.1. Postoperative Complications of Chronic Pain and Associated Comorbidities

---

- Worsened acute postoperative pain

- Increased postoperative opioid use, with increased opioid-related adverse drug effects (ORADE)

- Increased hospital length of stay

- Unplanned postoperative admissions

- Increased readmissions

- Increased surgical site infection rate

- Increased wound dehiscence

- Increased arthroplasty failure with need for revision

- Increased spinal fusion failure

- Increased rate of chronic postsurgical pain

Effect of Preoperative Chronic Pain (and Chronic Opioid Use) on Immediate Postoperative Nonsurgical Complications

Preexisting chronic pain has been shown to predict worsened/more severe acute postoperative pain [13–16]. Confounding factors such as chronic opioid use, poor general health, and anxiety/pain catastrophizing abound and render what is already a multifactorial puzzle (including type of surgery and other postoperative variables) somewhat ambiguous. Nonetheless, consensus statements [17, 18] and clinical practice guidelines including recent enhanced recovery pathways [19, 20] recognize the importance of screening for preexisting chronic pain syndromes to facilitate more intensive/targeted and multimodal approaches in attempts to more effectively prevent and treat severe postoperative pain.

Heightened acute postoperative pain is certainly an outcome worthy of attention in its own right, but adding to the significance of this problem are the issues of increased perioperative complications associated with increased opioid analgesic use, and also the clear evidence of progression of uncontrolled acute postoperative pain to a chronic postsurgical pain state. Opioid-related adverse drug effects (ORADE) of significance include nausea and vomiting severe enough to compromise discharge, ileus, altered mental status and falls, and severe respiratory depression/apnea.

A large analysis of over 300,000 operations from 380 hospitals between 2008 and 2010 showed a 12% incidence of postoperative ORADE (defined as new codes from the International Classification of Diseases 9 [ICD-9] pertaining to central nervous system, respiratory, gastrointestinal, urologic, or other major events in the context of opioid therapy) with an average cost increase of $4,700 and LOS increase of 3.3 days [21]. Another recent investigation into postoperative ORADE among a sample of 37,000 surgical patients from 26 hospitals showed a 13.6% incidence, with an average cost increase of $6,700, LOS increase of 3.4 days, a 36% higher readmission rate, and a 3.4-fold increase in mortality [22]. Of note, preoperative risk factors for developing ORADE were analyzed, and preoperative opioid use conferred a statistically significant 34% increased risk of ORADE, nearly double the risk conferred from other comorbidities (Charlson Comorbidity Index) and more than triple the risk conferred from obesity. Other studies [23, 24] have confirmed preoperative opioid use as a risk factor for postoperative ORADE.

The association between severity of acute pain and the likelihood of chronification has been shown in multiple nonsurgical scenarios, such as shingles/post-herpetic neuralgia and lumbago [25], and also in the postoperative setting. Heightened acute postoperative pain (more common among patients suffering with preexisting chronic pain and also preoperative opioid use) is also associated with pain chronification [26–30]—not unlike a positive feedback loop. As Dr. Joel Katz puts it, "pain begets pain" [31].

Effect of Preoperative Chronic Pain (and Chronic Opioid Use) on Postoperative Length of Stay

To date, few studies specifically demonstrate that preoperative chronic pain is associated with increased postoperative hospital LOS, possibly because of significantly heterogeneous LOS categories. Recent trends toward "fast-track" discharge after historically more painful orthopedic operations, and so forth, may provide opportunity for greater sensitivity of analysis. Halawi et al [32] have published the only report to date demonstrating specific and statistically significant association between reported preoperative pain levels and LOS; while their study was not set up to investigate duration/chronicity of pain or other discriminant psychosocial variables, they did note a correlation between reported preoperative pain levels and chronic opioid use.

Multiple recent investigations [33–38], however, have shown clear association between chronic preoperative opioid use and increased LOS. Increased postoperative pain requiring parenteral opioid administration certainly contributes to this phenomenon, however, other related problems such as ORADE, discussed earlier, all delay discharge.

Most of these studies show increased LOS between one and two days. While this difference may not sound significant at first take, when considering the increased prevalence of chronic preoperative opioid use among the surgical patient population [39] and the fact that the 2015 cost for one day's hospitalization in the United States ranged between $1,800 and $2,400 (depending on the type of hospital), the magnitude of these costs becomes a little more apparent. With an average $2,100/day cost and an average extra 1.5 days' hospitalization applied to what is likely a conservative estimate of 15% opioid-tolerant patients among the 8 million inpatient operations that occurred in 2012 [7], a staggering $3.8 billion per year from LOS increases alone may be attributable to suboptimally managed preoperative chronic pain.

While a few studies [34, 36, 40–44] hint at a link between preexisting chronic pain and associated comorbidities, and increased residential care requirements post-hospitalization, that is, transfer to skilled nursing facilities (SNFs) upon hospital discharge, there is not a clear nor consistent association. Many other large-scale investigations into SNF transfer correlate sociodemographic factors, increased age, and physical deconditioning measures such as the Risk

Assessment and Prediction Tool (RAPT) score [45–50]. This is not surprising considering the specialized purpose and function of such facilities, which does not include comfort care, and the more stringent admission and reimbursement criteria with recent strong economic disincentives, and so forth, pressuring against such discharge disposition [51].

Effect of Preoperative Chronic Pain (and Chronic Opioid Use) on Unplanned Postoperative Admissions and Readmissions

A recent analysis of nearly 1.3 million ambulatory surgical procedures performed at nearly 500 hospitals revealed roughly a 4% rate of unplanned hospital admission [52]. Uncontrolled postoperative pain—correlating strongly with preoperative chronic pain—has been shown (beginning three decades ago) to be one of, if not the leading cause (ranging from 10% to 20%) of these unplanned admissions [53–55]. Applying these figures (4% unplanned admission rate, 15% of which are due to uncontrollable pain) to an outpatient surgical volume of 50 million cases per year, it is possible that 300,000 postoperative pain-control admissions occur annually.

With an average hospital admission cost of over $10,000 [56], it is conceivable that a significant proportion of this potential $3-billion expenditure on unplanned admissions may be attributable to suboptimal management of preoperative pain.

The literature similarly demonstrates uncontrolled postoperative pain among the top two or three factors for postsurgical readmission [57–60]. A large VA series of over 200,000 patients stratified by reported postoperative pain levels showed a 14.4% readmission rate in the highest pain stratum compared to an overall rate of 10.8% [61]. In addition, unlike the situation of unplanned admissions after ambulatory surgery, available data show an association of preoperative chronic pain and chronic opioid therapy (COT) or dependence with readmission [35, 36, 38, 62, 63].

A recent report from the University of Michigan [35] comparing outcomes between patients receiving COT (21% of the study populace) versus opioid-naive patients undergoing elective abdominopelvic operations over a 6-year period (total $n = 2,413$) showed significant increases in readmission rate in the COT group. After adjusting for other covariates (including age, socioeconomic status, tobacco use, BMI, and American Society of Anesthesiologists [ASA] score), COT conferred an odds ratio of 1.57 for overall 30-day readmission ($p < 0.02$). The same group also examined a larger sample, from multiple states ($n > 200,000$), also undergoing elective abdominopelvic operations [36]. In this investigation, the prevalence of COT was 8.8%; those patients had a readmission rate of 4.5% compared to 3.6% among the opioid-naive ($p < 0.001$). Chronic opioid therapy was also stratified by dose in this study, and correlation was seen between increased opioid dose and readmission rate. Another nationwide study [62] focused on COT dose as a risk factor for readmission among kidney donors ($n > 14,000$ with a COT prevalence of 11%). Doses were stratified into <130 morphine milligram equivalents (MME), 130–305 MME, and >305 MME. Patients from the lowest MME stratum did not show a statistically significant increase in readmission, however there was a marked increase in readmission conferred by COT in the middle stratum (5.2% readmission rate compared to 2.6% in the opioid-naive) and even greater risk in the highest stratum (6.8%). These data are not dissimilar to the important findings published recently by Nguyen et al [64] and reviewed in greater detail in chapter 10, showing marked postoperative functional improvements seen in opioid-dependent individuals who weaned their preoperative opioid dose by at least 50% prior to surgery.

From the spine surgery population, nearly 25,000 posterior lumbar fusion patients from the Humana database (from 2007–2015) were recently analyzed for complication rates based on preoperative COT [63]. Of this sample, 55% used opioids preoperatively, with 22% ($n = 5,500$) of the overall sample receiving COT for greater than 6 months. After adjusting for covariates, COT conferred an overall readmission odds ratio of 1.15 ($p = 0.02$), but when stratifying by readmission reasons, conferred an odds ratio of 1.8 ($p = 0.001$) for pain-related readmission.

Finally, Gupta et al [38] used the National Readmission Database to examine whether opioid-dependent patients underwent postoperative readmission more frequently than their opioid-naive counterparts during the years 2013–2014. The nearly 95,000 opioid-dependent patients had a readmission rate of 14.3% compared to a rate of 8.8% among the 15.9 million patients without that diagnosis (odds ratio 1.72; odds ratio 1.26 after adjusting for relevant covariates, $p < 0.0001$.)

While readmission-specific costs were not provided in the studies discussed previously, applying average 2013 US national readmission costs ($8,600–$15,700 depending on payer) [65] to the recent National Readmissions Database analysis [38] covering the majority of readmissions during 22 months of 2013–2014 yields significant figures. As discussed earlier, a 5.5% greater postoperative readmission rate was seen in the opioid-dependent cohort ($n = 94,903$ compared to 15.9 million without that diagnosis) which would comprise 5,200 readmissions in that group over that time period (averaging 2,800 per year when considering that only 22 months were captured). Applying a lower-end cost estimate ($10,000) to that number yields annual readmission costs associated with opioid dependence of $28 million; a substantially higher figure would result from considering the prevalence of chronic pain and chronic opioid use in surgical patients who do not have an official diagnosis of opioid dependence in their medical record.

Effect of Preoperative Chronic Pain (and Chronic Opioid Use) on Surgical Outcomes

As discussed previously, few investigations have specifically addressed the question of whether chronic preoperative pain predicts worsened surgical outcomes, likely owing to the fact that much elective surgery (and especially musculoskeletal system operations) occurs in the context of chronic pain by default. Numerous comorbid/pathologic states occurring in the context of chronic pain however (e.g., dysregulation of cortisol and hypothalamic-pituitary-adrenal axis, sleep deprivation, deconditioning, kinesiophobia, depression, etc.) are associated with worsened surgical outcomes and form the subject matter of subsequent chapters.

Perhaps the majority of recent research in this arena has been focused on the association of chronic preoperative opioid use (COT) and worsened surgical outcomes. Jain et al's recent large (n = 24,610 patients) study of lumbar spinal fusion patients found a nearly 20% higher rate of wound complications not otherwise specified among the 5,500 patients receiving COT.

Several studies have shown that COT is associated with surgical site (and other) infections. Menendez et al [66] examined the National Inpatient Sample for 2002–2011 looking specifically at elective orthopedic operations and found that the nearly 16,000 patients among this dataset with a diagnosis of opioid dependence or abuse experienced a 2.5-fold higher incidence of surgical site infection compared to the 9.3 million patients without a diagnosis of opioid dependence or abuse. Among general surgery patients, Cron et al [35] showed that patients with preoperative COT (n = 502) had a surgical site infection rate of 14.9% compared to 8.3% in the control group of 1,900 patients (p < 0.001). In the living kidney donor study discussed earlier [62], patients receiving moderate- to high-dose COT preoperatively had markedly higher rates of readmission due to infection (as well as hernia).

In vitro and animal studies have shown for some time that chronic opioid use impairs angiogenesis, fibroblast, and other repair cell function, delaying wound healing [67–70]. More recently, Shanmugam et al [71] found that 786 patients (from a sample of 25,636 abdominopelvic surgical patients) experiencing postoperative wound dehiscence were more likely to have used COT postsurgically.

Several recent orthopedic publications have highlighted increases in arthroplasty complications including arthrofibrosis and periprosthetic failures [33, 34, 72]. A particularly large study of over 12,700 total knee arthroplasty patients using COT required significantly higher revision rates than nearly 20,000 controls [73].

Effect of Preoperative Chronic Pain (and Chronic Opioid Use) on the Development of CPSP

Estimates of the incidence of CPSP vary widely, likely owing to the operative procedures represented in the series (i.e., thoracotomies, mastectomies, and limb amputations reliably confer greater postoperative pain than do laparoscopic cholecystectomies or knee arthroscopies), with the literature reporting anywhere from a 1:10 to 1:2 figure [74, 75, 76]. Approaching the issue retrospectively rather than prospectively, in a series of over 5,100 patients at a UK pain clinic, 23% attributed their chronic pain to surgery [77]. This alleged etiology ranked ahead of trauma (19%) and second only to "degenerative factors" (34%).

The economic cost of CPSP is impossible to measure accurately, but has been estimated at hundreds of billions of dollars globally [78] and at over $40,000 per incident case in the United States [79]. Again, by rough calculation, if 10% of 50 million operations in the United States will result in CPSP at that incident cost, a staggering figure of $200 billion is generated. These figures correlates loosely with application of Crombie et al's data [77] of chronic pain etiology introduced earlier to an often-cited overall $635 billion annual cost of chronic pain in the United States [80] (see Table 1.2).

Investigations over the past two decades have shown that CPSP is certainly a multifactorial issue involving patient factors and surgical ones (most notably type of operation), with increasing recognition of biopsychosocial complexities [15, 81, 82]. While numerous psychosocial factors have been shown in several studies to hold the highest predictive value for the development of CPSP [15, 83], most notably anxiety and pain catastrophizing [84, 85], other studies suggest that CPSP may be most strongly predicted by preoperative chronic pain [26, 74, 86–89]. Chronic preoperative opioid use has also been shown in numerous investigations to be a risk factor for CPSP [28, 33–34, 81, 90–93]. Nonetheless, the interwoven nature of psychosocial variables such as anxiety/catastrophization, PTSD, substance dependence, and depression and CNCP is such that isolating the specific effect of a solitary (and poorly defined) covariate is challenging at best. Furthermore, CNCP does not generally exist without multiple underlying biological comorbidities as well, including obesity, pro-inflammatory diet, malnutrition, sleep deprivation, sedentary lifestyle, and so forth. Specific data on these associations, and data implicating these conditions (either directly or as confounders) with poor operative outcomes, are presented in subsequent chapters.

Table 1.2. Estimated US Costs of Chronic Pain–Related Postoperative Complications

Complication	Rate or rate increase attributable to chronic preoperative pain/ associated comorbidities	Estimated cost per complication	Estimated total annual cost attributable to chronic preoperative pain/associated comorbidities
[a]Opioid-related adverse drug effects (ORADE)	34% relative increase in ORADE with chronic preoperative opioid therapy (COT) (Overall ORADE rate 12%–13.6%)	$4,700–6,700 per ORADE	*$2 billion (60 million operations x 15% COT rate × 4% increased absolute rate)
Increased postoperative length of stay (LOS)	Average increase of 1–2 days with COT	$2,100 per day	$3.8 billion (8 million inpatient operations × 15% COT rate 1.5 days)
Unplanned admissions	0.6% rate of admissions for uncontrollable pain	>$10,000 per admission	$3 billion (50 million outpatient operations × 0.6%)
Readmissions	15%–63% relative increase in readmission rate from preoperative pain or COT	>$10,000 per readmission	>$28 million (95,000 surgical patients with diagnosis of opioid dependence × 5.5% increased absolute rate)
Chronic postsurgical pain (CPSP)	Cannot estimate due to continuous nature of variables and lack of data	$40,000 per incident case	Cannot calculate from available data, but likely on the order of $20 billion

[a]ORADE costs comprise part of LOS, unplanned admission, and readmission costs.

When considering the interdependence of these chronic problems (most of which are rooted in the tenacious soil of low self-efficacy and in many cases low self-esteem), it seems intuitive that any realistic attempt at optimizing the chronic pain syndrome preoperatively will require not only a concerted biopsychosocial-spiritual and ideally multidisciplinary approach but also adequate time. Changes, let alone sustained changes in health behaviors, require time to cultivate, and investigations into some of the more obvious intervenable risk factors such as tobacco, alcohol and opioid use, deconditioning, obesity, and so forth, not surprisingly show greater success and better postoperative outcomes with an adequate intervention window, as discussed in greater detail later in the book. While current (immediate) perioperative approaches highlighting multimodal anesthesia and analgesia are laudable, in the context of so complicated an issue as chronic pain they are "too little, too late."

References

1 Resnick AS, Corrigan D, Mullen JL, Kaiser LR. Surgeon contribution to hospital bottom line: not all are created equal. Annals Surg. 2005;242:530–9.
2 Merritt Hawkins. 2016 Physician inpatient/outpatient revenue survey. https://www.merritthawkins.com/uploadedFiles/MerrittHawkins/Content/Pdf/Merritt_Hawkins-2016_RevSurvey.pdf. Accessed March 14, 2018.
3 Davenport DL, Henderson WG, Khuri SF, Mentzer RM Jr. Preoperative risk factors and surgical complexity are more predictive of costs than postoperative complications: a case study using the National Surgical Quality Improvement Program (NSQIP) database. Ann Surg. 2005;242:463–8; discussion 468–71.
4 Gani F, Hundt J, Daniel M, Efron JE, Makary MA, Pawlik TM. Variations in hospitals costs for surgical procedures: inefficient care or sick patients? Am J Surg. 2017; 213:1–9.
5 Snowden CP, Anderson H. Preoperative optimization: rationale and process: is it economic sense? Curr Opin Anaesthesiol. 2012; 25:210–16.
6 Hall MJ, Schwartzman A, Zhang J, Liu X. Ambulatory Surgery Data from Hospitals and Ambulatory Surgery Centers: United States, 2010. National Health Statistics Report Number 102. February 28, 2017.
7 Fingar KR, Stocks C, Weiss AJ, Steiner CA. Most Frequent Operating Room Procedures Performed in U.S. Hospitals 2003–2012. HCUP Statistical Brief #186. December 2014. Agency for Healthcare Research and Quality, Rockville, MD.
8 Institute of Medicine (US) Committee on Advancing Pain Research, Care, and Education. Relieving Pain in America: A Blueprint for Transforming Prevention, Care, Education, and Research. Washington DC: National Academies Press; 2011.
9 Mogil JS. Pain genetics: past, present and future. Trends Genet. 2012; 28:258–66.
10 Nielsen CS, Knudsen GP, Steingrímsdóttir ÓA. Twin studies of pain. Clin Genet. 2012;82:331–40.
11 Bedson J, Croft PR. The discordance between clinical and radiographic knee osteoarthritis: a systematic search and summary of the literature. BMC Musculoskelet Disord. 2008;9:116. doi: 10.1186/1471-2474-9-116. Review. PubMed PMID: 18764949; PubMed Central PMCID: PMC2542996.
12 Brinjikji W, Luetmer PH, Comstock B, et al. Systematic literature review of imaging features of spinal degeneration in asymptomatic populations. Am J Neurorad. 2015; 36:811–16.
13 Thomas T, Robinson C, Champion D, McKell M, Pell M. Prediction and assessment of the severity of post-operative pain and of satisfaction with management. Pain. 1998;75:177–85.

14 Kalkman CJ, Visser K, Moen J, Bonsel GJ, Grobbee DE, Moons KGM. Preoperative prediction of severe postoperative pain. Pain. 2003;105:415–23.
15 Ip HY, Abrishami A, Peng PW, Wong J, Chung F. Predictors of postoperative pain and analgesic consumption: a qualitative systematic review. Anesthesiology. 2009;111:657–77.
16 Gan TJ. Poorly controlled postoperative pain: prevalence, consequences, and prevention. J Pain Res. 2017;10:2287–98.
17 Vickers A, Bali S, Baxter A, et al. Consensus statement on the anticipation and prevention of acute postoperative pain: multidisciplinary RADAR approach. Curr Med Res Opin. 2009;25:2557–69.
18 Kaye AD, Helander EM, Vadivelu N, et al. Consensus statement for clinical pathway development for perioperative pain management and care transitions. Pain Ther. 2017;6:129–41.
19 American Society of Anesthesiologists Task Force on Acute Pain Management. Practice guidelines for acute pain management in the perioperative setting: an updated report by the American Society of Anesthesiologists Task Force on Acute Pain Management. Anesthesiology. 2012;116:248–73.
20 Katz J, Weinrib A, Fashler SR, et al. The Toronto General Hospital Transitional Pain Service: development and implementation of a multidisciplinary program to prevent chronic postsurgical pain. J Pain Res. 2015;8:695–702.
21 Oderda GM, Gan TJ, Johnson BH, Robinson SB. Effect of opioid-related adverse events on outcomes in selected surgical patients. J Pain Palliat Care Pharmacother. 2013;27:62–70.
22 Kessler ER, Shah M, Gruschkus SK, Raju A. Cost and quality implications of opioid-based postsurgical pain control using administrative claims data from a large health system: opioid-related adverse events and their impact on clinical and economic outcomes. Pharmacotherapy. 2013;33:383–91.
23 Minkowitz HS, Gruschkus SK, Shah M, Raju A. Adverse drug events among patients receiving postsurgical opioids in a large health system: risk factors and outcomes. Am J Health Syst Pharm. 2014;71:1556–65.
24 Minkowitz HS, Scranton R, Gruschkus SK, Nipper-Johnson K, Menditto L, Dandappanavar A. Development and validation of a risk score to identify patients at high risk for opioid-related adverse drug events. J Manag Care Spec Pharm. 2014;20:948–58.
25 Dworkin RH. Which individuals with acute pain are most likely to develop a chronic pain syndrome? Pain Forum. 1997;6:127–36.
26 Perkins F, Kehlet H. Chronic pain as an outcome of surgery—a review of predictive factors. Anesthesiology. 2000;93:1123–33.
27 Joshi GP, Ogunnaike BO. Consequences of inadequate postoperative pain relief and chronic persistent postoperative pain. Anesthesiol Clin North Am. 2005;23:21–36.
28 VanDenKerkhof EG, Hopman WM, Goldstein DH, et al. Impact of perioperative pain intensity, pain qualities, and opioid use on chronic pain after surgery: a prospective cohort study. Reg Anesth Pain Med. 2012;37:19–27.
29 Steyaert A, De Kock M. Chronic postsurgical pain. Curr Opin Anaesthesiol. 2012;25:584–8.
30 de Leon-Casasola O. A review of the literature on multiple factors involved in postoperative pain course and duration. Postgrad Med. 2014;126:42–52.

31   Katz J. Pain begets pain: Predictors of long-term phantom limb pain and post-thoracotomy pain. Pain Forum. 1997;6:140–144.

32   Halawi MJ, Vovos TJ, Green CL, Wellman SS, Attarian DE, Bolognesi MP. Preoperative pain level and patient expectation predict hospital length of stay after total hip arthroplasty. J Arthroplasty. 2015;30:555–8.

33   Pivec R, Issa K, Naziri Q, Kapadia BH, Bonutti PM, Mont MA. Opioid use prior to total hip arthroplasty leads to worse clinical outcomes. Int Orthop. 2014;38:1159–65.

34   Sing DC, Barry JJ, Cheah JW, Vail TP, Hansen EN. Long-acting opioid use independently predicts perioperative complication in total joint arthroplasty. J Arthroplast. 2016;31(9 Suppl):170–4.

35   Cron DC, Englesbe MJ, Bolton CJ, et al. Preoperative opioid use is independently associated with increased costs and worse outcomes after major abdominal surgery. Ann Surg. 2017;265:695–701.

36   Waljee JF, Cron DC, Steiger RM, Zhong L, Englesbe MJ, Brummett CM. Effect of preoperative opioid exposure on healthcare utilization and expenditures following elective abdominal surgery. Ann Surg. 2017;265:715–21.

37   Raad M, Jain A, Neuman BJ, et al. International Spine Study Group. Association of patient-reported narcotic use with short- and long-term outcomes after adult spinal deformity surgery: multicenter study of 425 patients with 2-year follow-up. Spine (Phila Pa 1976). 2018 Oct 1;43(19):1340–6. doi:10.1097/BRS.0000000000002631

38   Gupta A, Nizamuddin J, Elmofty D, et al. Opioid abuse or dependence increases 30-day readmission rates after major operating room procedures: a national readmissions database study. Anesthesiology. 2018 May;128(5):880–90. doi:10.1097/ALN.0000000000002136

39   Wilson JL, Poulin PA, Sikorski R, Nathan HJ, Taljaard M, Smyth C. Opioid use among same-day surgery patients: prevalence, management and outcomes. Pain Res Manag. 2015;20:300–4.

40   Sharareh B, Le NB, Hoang MT, Schwarzkopf R. Factors determining discharge destination for patients undergoing total joint arthroplasty. J Arthroplasty. 2014;29:1355–58.

41   Halawi MJ, Vovos TJ, Green CL, Wellman SS, Attarian DE, Bolognesi MP. Opioid-based analgesia: impact on total joint arthroplasty. J Arthroplasty. 2015;30:2360–3.

42   Zarling BJ, Yokhana SS, Herzog DT, Markel DC. Preoperative and postoperative opiate use by the arthroplasty patient. J Arthroplast. 2016;31:2081–4.

43   Ayala AE, Lawson KA, Gruessner AC, Dohm MP; Western Slope Study Group. Preoperative patient-recorded outcome measures predict patient discharge location following unicondylar knee arthroplasty. J Arthroplasty. 2017;32:386–9.

44   Rondon AJ, Tan TL, Greenky MR, et al. Who goes to inpatient rehabilitation or skilled nursing facilities unexpectedly following total knee arthroplasty? J Arthroplasty. December 21, 2017. pii: S0883-5403(17)31121-X. doi: 10.1016/j.arth.2017.12.015.

45   Lin JJ, Kaplan RJ. Multivariate analysis of the factors affecting duration of acute in-patient rehabilitation after hip and knee arthroplasty. Am J Phys Med Rehabil. 2004;83:344–52.

46   Bozic KJ, Wagie A, Naessens JM, Berry DJ, Rubash HE. Predictors of discharge to an inpatient extended care facility after total hip or knee arthroplasty. J Arthroplasty. 2006;21(6 Suppl 2):151–6.

47 Hansen VJ, Gromov K, Lebrun LM, Rubash HE, Malchau H, Freiberg AA. Does the Risk Assessment and Prediction Tool predict discharge disposition after joint replacement? Clin Orthop Relat Res. 2015;473:597–601.

48 Inneh IA, Clair AJ, Slover JD, Iorio R. Disparities in discharge destination after lower extremity joint arthroplasty: analysis of 7924 patients in an urban setting. J Arthroplasty. 2016;31:2700–4.

49 Keswani A, Tasi MC, Fields A, Lovy AJ, Moucha CS, Bozic KJ. Discharge destination after total joint arthroplasty: an analysis of postdischarge outcomes, placement risk factors, and recent trends. J Arthroplasty 2016;31:1155–62.

50 Gholson JJ, Pugely AJ, Bedard NA, Duchman KR, Anthony CA, Callaghan JJ. Can we predict discharge status after total joint arthroplasty? A calculator to predict home discharge. J Arthroplasty 2016;31:2705–9.

51 Bozic KJ, Ward L, Vail TP, Maze M. Bundled payments in total joint arthroplasty: targeting opportunities for quality improvement and cost reduction. Clin Orthop. 2014;472:188–93.

52 Bongiovanni T, Ross J, Krumholz HM, et al. Unplanned hospital admissions after same-day surgery. J Am Coll Surg. 2016;223:S121. ISSN 1072-7515 https://doi.org/10.1016/j.jamcollsurg.2016.06.251.

53 Gold BS, Kitz DS, Lecky JH, Neuhaus JM. Unanticipated admission to the hospital following ambulatory surgery. JAMA. 1989;262:3008–10.

54 Greenburg AG, Greenburg JP, Tewel A, Breen C, Machin O, McRae S. Hospital admission following ambulatory surgery. Am J Surg. 1996;172:21–3.

55 Rosero EB, Joshi GP. Hospital readmission after ambulatory laparoscopic cholecystectomy: incidence and predictors. J Surg Res. 2017;219:108–15.

56 Weiss AJ, Elixhauser A. Overview of Hospital Stays in the United States, 2012. HCUP Statistical Brief #180. October 2014. Agency for Healthcare Research and Quality, Rockville, MD. http://www.hcup-us.ahrq.gov/reports/statbriefs/sb180-Hospitalizations-United-States2012.pdf.

57 Clement RC, Derman PB, Graham DS, et al. Risk factors, causes, and the economic implications of unplanned readmissions following total hip arthroplasty. J Arthroplasty. 2013;28(8 Suppl):7–10.

58 Garcia RM, Choy W, DiDomenico JD, et al. Thirty-day readmission rate and risk factors for patients undergoing single level elective anterior lumbar interbody fusion (ALIF). J Clin Neurosci. 2016;32:104–8.

59 Garcia RM, Khanna R, Dahdaleh NS, Cybulski G, Lam S, Smith ZA. Thirty-day readmission risk factors following single-level transforaminal lumbar interbody fusion (TLIF) for 4992 patients from the ACS-NSQIP database. Global Spine J. 2017;7:220–6.

60 Webb ML, Nelson SJ, Save AV, et al. Of 20,376 lumbar discectomies, 2.6% of patients readmitted within 30 days: surgical site infection, pain, and thromboembolic events are the most common reasons for readmission. Spine (Phila Pa 1976). 2017;42:1267–73.

61 Hernandez-Boussard T, Graham LA, Desai K, et al. The fifth vital sign: postoperative pain predicts 30-day readmissions and subsequent emergency department visits. Ann Surg. 2017; 266:516–24.

62 Lentine KL, Lam NN, Schnitzler MA, et al. Predonation prescription opioid use: a novel risk factor for readmission after living kidney donation. Am J Transplant. 2017;17:744–53.

63 Jain N, Phillips FM, Weaver T, Khan SN. Pre-operative chronic opioid therapy: a risk factor for complications, readmission, continued opioid use and increased costs after one- and two-level posterior lumbar fusion. Spine (Phila Pa 1976). March 20, 2018. doi: 10.1097/BRS.0000000000002609. [Epub ahead of print] PubMed PMID: 29561298.

64 Nguyen LC, Sing DC, Bozic KJ. Preoperative reduction of opioid use before total joint arthroplasty. J Arthroplasty. 2016;31(9 Suppl):282–7.

65 Barrett ML, Wier LM, Jiang HJ, Steiner CA. All-Cause Readmissions by Payer and Age, 2009–2013. HCUP Statistical Brief #199. December 2015. Agency for Healthcare Research and Quality, Rockville, MD. http://www.hcup-us.ahrq.gov/reports/statbriefs/sb199-Readmissions-Payer-Age.pdf.

66 Menendez ME, Ring D, Bateman BT. Preoperative opioid misuse is associated with increased morbidity and mortality after elective orthopaedic surgery. Clin Orthop Relat Res 2015;473:2402–12.

67 Lam CF, Chang PJ, Huang YS, et al. Prolonged use of high-dose morphine impairs angiogenesis and mobilization of endothelial progenitor cells in mice. Anesth Analg. 2008;107:686–92.

68 Rook JM, Hasan W, Mccarson KE. Morphine-induced early delays in wound closure: involvement of sensory neuropeptides and modification of neurokinin receptor expression. Biochem Pharmacol. 2009;77:1747–55.

69 Martin JL, Koodie L, Krishnan AG, Charboneau R, Barke RA, Roy S. Chronic morphine administration delays wound healing by inhibiting immune cell recruitment to the wound site. Am J Pathol. 2010;176:786–99.

70 Martin JL, Charboneau R, Barke RA, Roy S. Chronic morphine treatment inhibits LPS induced angiogenesis: implications in wound healing. Cell Immunol. 2010;265:139–45.

71 Shanmugam VK, Fernandez S, Evans KK, et al. Postoperative wound dehiscence: predictors and associations. Wound Repair Regen. 2015;23:184–90.

72 Zywiel MG, Stroh DA, Lee SY, Bonutti PM, Mont MA. Chronic opioid use prior to total knee arthroplasty. J Bone Joint Surg Am. 2011;93:1988–93.

73 Ben-Ari A, Chansky H, Rozet I. Preoperative opioid use is associated with early revision after total knee arthroplasty: a study of male patients treated in the veterans affairs system. J Bone Joint Surg Am. 2017;99:1–9.

74 Kehlet H, Jensen TS, Woolf CJ. Persistent postsurgical pain: Risk factors and prevention. Lancet. 2006; 367:1618–25.

75 Macrae WA. Chronic post-surgical pain: 10 years on. Br J Anaesth 2008;101:77–86.

76 Correll D. Chronic postoperative pain: recent findings in understanding and management. F1000Research. 2017;6:1054. doi:10.12688/f1000research.11101.1.

77 Crombie IK, Davies HTO, Macrae WA. Cut and thrust: antecedent surgery and trauma among patients attending a chronic pain clinic. Pain 1998;76:167–71.

78 Weiser TG, Regenbogen SE, Thompson KD, et al. An estimation of the global volume of surgery: a modelling strategy based on available data. Lancet. 2008;372:139–44.

79 Parsons B, Schaefer C, Mann R, et al. Economic and humanistic burden of post-trauma and post-surgical neuropathic pain among adults in the United States. J Pain Res. 2013; 6:459–69.

80 Gaskin DJ, Richard P. The economic costs of pain in the United States. J Pain. 2012;13:715–24.

81 Chapman CR, Vierck CJ. The transition of acute postoperative pain to chronic pain: an integrative overview of research on mechanisms. J Pain. 2017;18(4):359. e1–359.e38. doi: 10.1016/j.jpain.2016.11.004. Epub 2016 Nov 28. Review. PubMed PMID: 27908839.

82 Schug SA, Bruce J. Risk stratification for the development of chronic postsurgical pain. Pain Reports. 2017;2(6):e627. doi:10.1097/PR9.0000000000000627.

83 Hinrichs-Rocker A, Schulz K, Järvinen I, Lefering R, Simanski C, Neugebauer EA. Psychosocial predictors and correlates for chronic post-surgical pain (CPSP): a systematic review. Eur J Pain. 2009;13:719–30.

84 Khan RS, Ahmed K, Blakeway E, et al. Catastrophizing: a predictive factor for postoperative pain. Am J Surg. 2011;201:122–31.

85 Theunissen M, Peters ML, Bruce J, Gramke HF, Marcus MA. Preoperative anxiety and catastrophizing: a systematic review and meta-analysis of the association with chronic postsurgical pain. Clin J Pain. 2012;28:819–41.

86 Katz J, Seltzer Z. Transition from acute to chronic postsurgical pain: risk factors and protective factors. Expert Rev Neurother. 2009;9:723–44.

87 Tsirline VB, Colavita PD, Belyansky I, Zemlyak AY, Lincourt AE, Heniford BT. Preoperative pain is the strongest predictor of postoperative pain and diminished quality of life after ventral hernia repair. Am Surg. 2013;79:829–36.

88 VanDenKerkhof EG, Peters ML, Bruce J. Chronic pain after surgery: time for standardization? A framework to establish core risk factor and outcome domains for epidemiological studies. Clin J Pain. 2013; 29:2–8.

89 Clark AJ, Spanswick CC. Why anesthesiologists need to care about the way chronic pain is managed. Can J Anesth. 2014; 61:95–100.

90 Lawrence JT, London N, Bohlman HH, Chin KR. Preoperative narcotic use as a predictor of clinical outcome: results following anterior cervical arthrodesis. Spine (Phila Pa 1976). 2008;33:2074–8.

91 Hoofwijk DM, Fiddelers AA, Peters ML, et al. Prevalence and predictive factors of chronic postsurgical pain and poor global recovery 1 year after outpatient surgery. Clin J Pain. 2015;31:1017–25.

92 Martinez V, Üçeyler N, Ben Ammar S, et al. Clinical, histological, and biochemical predictors of postsurgical neuropathic pain. Pain. 2015;156:2390–8.

93 Cheah JW, Sing DC, McLaughlin D, Feeley BT, Ma CB, Zhang AL. The perioperative effects of chronic preoperative opioid use on shoulder arthroplasty outcomes. J Shoulder Elb Surg. 2017 Nov;26(11):1908–14. doi:10.1016/j.jse.2017.05.016. Epub 2017 Jul 20.

2

Rationale and Process Overview for Preoperative Optimization of Chronic Pain

Heath B. McAnally

Introduction: Should We Be Focusing on a Priori Intervention?

We begin this chapter by summarizing the development of preoperative risk assessment in general over the past half-century, with more recent efforts (such as the American Society of Anesthesiologists' Perioperative Surgical Home, and the Toronto General Hospital Transitional Pain Service) specifically geared toward risk stratification for the development of significant postoperative pain syndromes. While these programs and protocols are a welcome start, we also propose that a more comprehensive approach with a strong behavioral health component that also emphasizes preventive lifestyle modifications—recently termed "prehabilitation"—will be required to yield meaningful benefit for patients suffering with chronic pain, from both an individual and a public health/macroeconomic vantage.

We then transition to a brief discussion of current evidence of benefit for these efforts, both clinical and economic. Principles of evidence-based standards of care and wise allocation of resources/fiscal responsibility require that in high-impact and high-prevalence conditions such as chronic pain, benefits clearly outweigh risks and justify the costs. The federal government is increasingly implementing drastic overhaul to the reimbursement system, and one of those changes particularly relevant to the perioperative arena is the advent of bundled and capitated payments, which further incentivizes quality care with minimization of both postoperative complications and costs involved in preventing and treating them.

Finally we briefly introduce the preoperative optimization program we have developed for patients struggling with chronic pain; the remainder of the book unpackages that in greater detail.

Evolution of Preoperative Optimization

From Bedside Assessment to the Perioperative Surgical Home

Elective surgery is a modern development unique to the developed world with its technologic advances, affluence, increased life expectancy and quality-of-life expectations, and also chronic disease burden. Prior to the latter part of the 20th century, for the past half-millennium the operating room was not something people sought out of their own volition, but rather an undesirable destination reserved for salvaging life in the context of very limited operable pathology. In stark contrast, as pointed out in the introductory section of the previous chapter, today the vast majority of surgery in the developed world comprises elective operations dealing increasingly with issues of functionality, comfort, and even aesthetics.

In keeping with the urgent/emergent roots of surgery, preoperative preparation was of necessity limited by constraints of time, and also more primitive means. The decision to operate was essentially a unilateral one made by the surgeon, with reactive preparation efforts [1] generally made on an inpatient basis and essentially limited to basic vital system interventions. Typically the anesthesiologist would assess the patient the night before nonemergent surgery to formulate a more nuanced anesthetic and monitoring plan, attend to premedication requirements, and possibly provide brief education.

With the increase in elective operations, more opportunity arose to weigh the risks versus benefits of proceeding to the operating room (OR) "as is," without delay for correcting morbid conditions. Paralleling the ascendancy of outpatient or "day surgery" over the past few decades [2], the vast majority of which again is elective, a move toward preemptive assessment and optimization of modifiable risk factors began to occur, and more and more outpatient-based preoperative testing began—partially fueled by "defensive medicine" [3]. This growth in indiscriminate preoperative laboratory and other testing (e.g., electrocardiography, chest X-rays, cardiac stress testing, etc.) especially in low-risk patients or those undergoing low-risk procedures has recently been identified as a major source of needless expenditure [4] and has recently come under fire from the US Department of Health and Human Services as well, resulting in initiatives such as the "Choosing Wisely Campaign" [5].

As early as the 1950s, the development of preoperative assessment or preadmission clinics (PACs) within hospitals began. Part of the rationale for these centers is to more appropriately direct preoperative testing based on standardized protocols for risk stratification and targeted ordering of tests. While the role and complexity of these centers has diversified beyond their initial focus on identification, risk-stratification, and attempts to intervene on high-morbidity conditions (e.g., occult coronary vascular disease, severe hypertension, and the like) to now include coordination of care and patient and family education, they remain reactive entities for the most part with "linear" decision-making algorithms [1] dictating progression along the pathway to the operating room. Lack of accessible and interdigitating computerized health data, integrative and multidisciplinary assessment, efficient preoperative testing, and postoperative care planning have all been criticized as gaps in these more traditional PAC models [6–8].

Nonetheless, some valuable process improvements and improvements from these more protocol-driven and standardized assessment models have been realized as discussed in what follows, and many lessons such as the efficacy and in many cases even superiority of non-physician-led systems (with specialists such as anesthesiologists and cardiologists serving in a consultant role) have been learned [9].

The latest advancement in the evolution of preoperative optimization efforts has been the development and implementation of multidisciplinary and integrated care processes with a strong focus on communication between all stakeholders (patient, surgeon, anesthesia care team, and other perioperative care personnel) to facilitate both effective and efficient identification of patients who will require more intensive workup and treatment throughout the phases of care (preoperative, intraoperative, and postoperative) [1]. Increasing efficiency (via reduction of needless expenditures) is in and of itself a worthwhile goal in the era of dwindling reimbursement, but when coupled with the mounting economic pressures of quality-based or bundled payments, which dramatically reduce revenue in the context of suboptimal outcomes, there is burgeoning interest in the development of more agile and resource-conservative approaches that can demonstrate both margin and outcomes improvements. Such improvements are of interest not only to operating room managers and hospital administrators but also to most accountable care organizations (ACOs) [10] and to an increasing number of physicians and their respective professional societies [6, 7, 11, 12].

One such care model that has been proposed and implemented at a growing number of academic institutions is the perioperative surgical home (PSH) model, introduced by the American Society of Anesthesiologists (ASA) as "a patient-centered and physician-led multidisciplinary and team-based system of coordinated care that guides the patient throughout the entire surgical experience" [6]. In keeping with published practice guidelines such as the Enhanced Recovery After Surgery (ERAS) protocols discussed later, this model attempts to address some of the aforementioned perceived weaknesses (erratic, insufficient, or excessive preoperative testing, lack of coordination of care across phases) in traditional PACs with a standardized framework addressing common problems in each phase as shown in Figure 2.1. It envisions an "integrated" entity, namely,

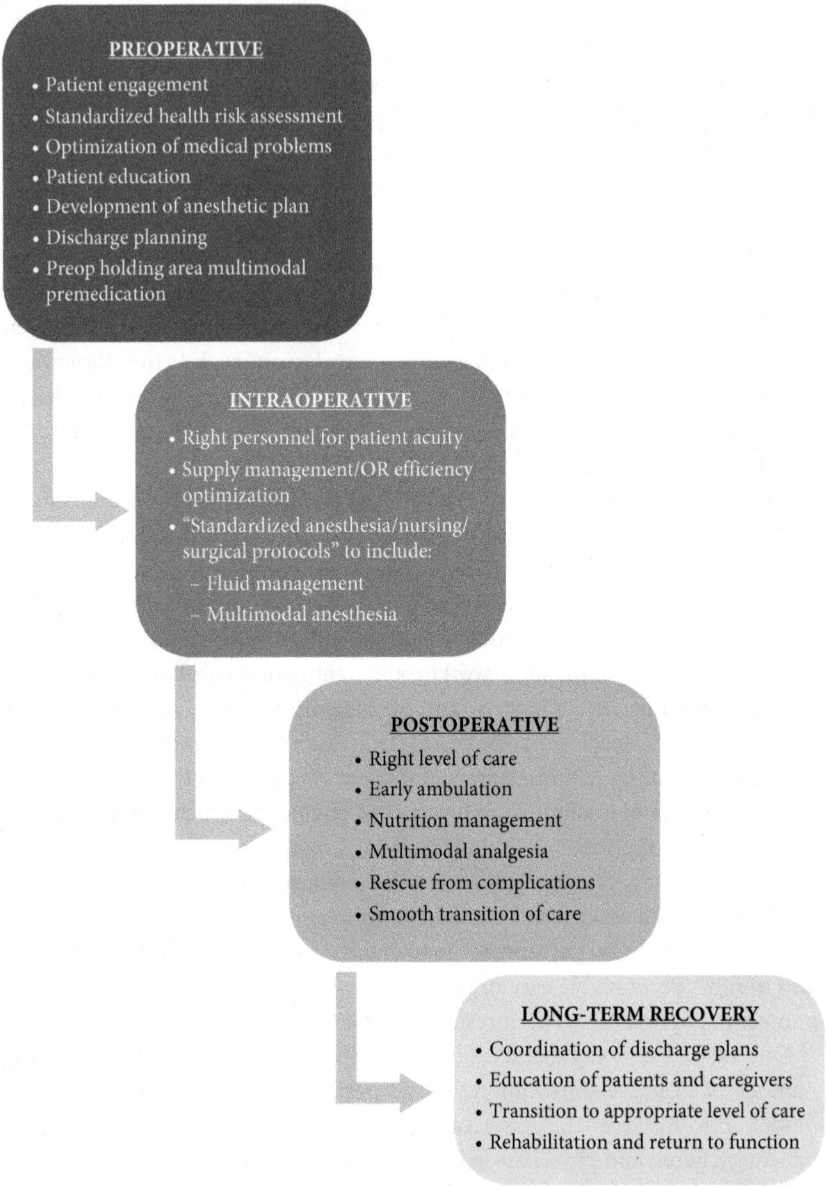

PREOPERATIVE

- Patient engagement
- Standardized health risk assessment
- Optimization of medical problems
- Patient education
- Development of anesthetic plan
- Discharge planning
- Preop holding area multimodal premedication

INTRAOPERATIVE

- Right personnel for patient acuity
- Supply management/OR efficiency optimization
- "Standardized anesthesia/nursing/surgical protocols" to include:
  - Fluid management
  - Multimodal anesthesia

POSTOPERATIVE

- Right level of care
- Early ambulation
- Nutrition management
- Multimodal analgesia
- Rescue from complications
- Smooth transition of care

LONG-TERM RECOVERY

- Coordination of discharge plans
- Education of patients and caregivers
- Transition to appropriate level of care
- Rehabilitation and return to function

Figure 2.1. The American Society of Anesthesiologists' Perioperative Surgical Home Model

the PSH, as responsible for the processes of development, implementation, analysis, and improvement of the local perioperative care system, versus a "modular" or "siloed" system (where "Surgeons, anesthesiologists, nurses, hospitalists, administrators, physical and respiratory therapists, and information technology experts are really just a loose assemblage of components asked to work together to deliver care") [13].

The effort has been developed with considerable influence from Lean Six Sigma (LSS) quality improvement methodology, which focuses on reducing waste (both material and time) and needless expenditures, and standardizing processes and competencies. While the LSS managerial concept has been touted as revitalizing productivity and competitiveness for many major business entities and has been widely adopted into numerous industries, it has also fallen under criticism from various angles, one of which is stifling creativity and exploration [14, 15]. While these qualities are not generally advocated in the context of clinical medicine, flexibility is required when such heterogeneous entities as human beings (and systems designed to care for them) are the subjects. The PSH concept appears to recognize the tension between the need for decreasing process variability while at the same time championing "tailored optimization" and "personal recovery pathways." We also contend that both predetermined care plans and flexibility and "patient-centricity" (another PSH core tenet) are prerequisite in attempting to address the complex, multifactorial milieu of chronic pain.

Enhanced Recovery Pathways

The PSH model has also been heavily influenced by recent perioperative care innovations such as the ERAS protocols. These pathways have evolved over the past decade owing to increasing awareness of the benefits of standardization of certain key preoperative, intraoperative, and postoperative processes based on evidence-based interventions. Several such ERAS protocols exist and have been tailored to fit certain surgical disciplines, but the majority have in common key features such as optimizing fluids and nutrition, infection and deep venous thrombosis prophylaxis, adequate and opioid-sparing analgesia, and removal of drains and catheters as soon as possible, as shown in Figure 2.2.

While these protocols laudably address several key aspects of perioperative pain management (e.g., preoperative education, multimodal analgesia, opioid-sparing efforts) we argue that in the case of chronic pain they are still "too little, too late." The neuroadaptations in the central nervous system associated with chronic pain [16–18] and frequently associated with entrenched maladaptive coping behaviors are indeed reversible [19, 20] but require considerably more time and effort in most cases than the administration of a handful of pills in the

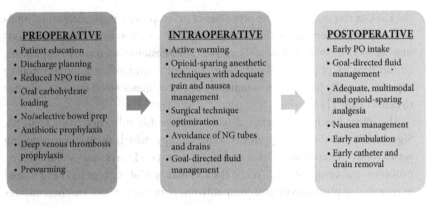

PREOPERATIVE
- Patient education
- Discharge planning
- Reduced NPO time
- Oral carbohydrate loading
- No/selective bowel prep
- Antibiotic prophylaxis
- Deep venous thrombosis prophylaxis
- Prewarming

INTRAOPERATIVE
- Active warming
- Opioid-sparing anesthetic techniques with adequate pain and nausea management
- Surgical technique optimization
- Avoidance of NG tubes and drains
- Goal-directed fluid management

POSTOPERATIVE
- Early PO intake
- Goal-directed fluid management
- Adequate, multimodal and opioid-sparing analgesia
- Nausea management
- Early ambulation
- Early catheter and drain removal

Figure 2.2. Typical Enhanced Recovery After Surgery (ERAS) Protocol

preoperative holding area and a few minutes of education. Along those lines, perhaps the biggest deficit of these protocols in the context of chronic pain is the lack of accommodation/intent regarding behavioral health, which is increasingly recognized as essential in addressing that condition [21–23].

Put another way, these approaches are entirely reactive when it comes to chronic disease states, including chronic pain. This is understandable, given the limited scope of perioperative medicine in general; however, we contend that in the context of elective surgery, chronic pain requires an expansion of both time allotted and efforts made to proactively replace unhealthy cognitive and lifestyle patterns (which invariably accompany and contribute) with healthy ones.

Transitional Pain Services

Another recent advancement specifically targeting perioperative management of chronic pain is the transitional pain service (TPS) model developed at Toronto General Hospital and the University of Toronto to fulfill the recognized need for "a multidisciplinary preventive approach that involves intensive, perioperative psychological, medical, physical therapy, and pharmacological management interventions aimed at preventing and treating the factors that increase the risk of CPSP [chronic postsurgical pain] and associated disability" [24]. While the Toronto TPS was formulated with a specific mission to identify patients at risk of developing CPSP and preventing that outcome, its principles of practice are broadly applicable to preoperative optimization of chronic pain as well. Those include risk stratification based on preexisting chronic pain, opioid use, and behavioral pathology including post-traumatic stress disorder, anxiety, and pain catastrophizing; patients at risk are then offered coordinated and comprehensive preoperative and postoperative multidisciplinary care including psychological consultation and therapy (acceptance and commitment therapy). Preoperative opioid reduction is implemented when possible.

Prehabilitation

While what is currently known as "prehabilitation" does not constitute a care pathway in its own right nor specifically address chronic pain, we include a very brief introduction to it here, in part owing to its increasing representation in ERAS protocols but also, more importantly from our perspective, to its importance in treating chronic pain. The term "prehabilitation" was coined in the 1980s as "a proactive, preventive approach to exercise, diet and lifestyle changes, designed to maximize health and wellness" [25]. More recently it has been defined as "the process of enhancing one's functional and mental capacity to buffer against potential deleterious effects of a significant stressor" [26].

Engaging patients in active self-management of pain and related symptoms is the essence of behavioral chronic pain management, and improvements in conditioning and physical distress tolerance invariably seem to increase psychological reserves as well. This cultivation of self-efficacy and an internal locus of control are of vital importance in overcoming learned helplessness, fear-avoidant behaviors, and periprocedural anxiety that may accompany chronic pain [27–30]. Numerous studies discussed in greater detail in chapter 7 corroborate that increasing physical activity correlates not only with increasing pain resilience but also with a decrease in pain perception itself [31–33], likely through a host of complementary mechanisms including restoration/enhancement of central modulation [34] and neural plasticity [35, 36].

Finally, the intent and major perceived benefit of prehabilitation in the literature is the improvement of physical fitness and nutritional status, both of which are important in the context of facing the catabolic state of controlled trauma that is surgery. Physical activity also supports improved mood and sleep, two factors that dramatically impact pain and recovery from surgery. The current literature (discussed in chapter 7) seems to favor a trimodal approach [37–39] featuring supervised exercise programs, nutritional counseling, and stress management/psychological support not otherwise specified.

For most patients struggling with chronic pain (and in some cases their surgeons) the focus will have to change to one of long-term goals as well as short-term, antecedent improvements in health rather than immediate objectives of relief as quickly as possible.

Rationale for Preoperative Optimization

Justification: Clinical Outcomes Benefits

The fact that preoperative risk factors (including chronic pain) are associated with poor outcomes (and economic drain) as discussed at some length in the previous chapter, however, does not necessarily indicate or justify targeted investigation and intervention. Evidence of benefit should be demonstrated as well as evidence that benefit outweighs potential risk as well as cost (discussed at greater length later).

The literature on efficacy (improved clinical outcomes) from general preoperative assessment has been mixed without convincing benefit from indiscriminate testing on outcomes or operating room efficiency [40, 41]. These data in concert with increasing recognition of significant costs associated with such traditional "shotgun" approaches (e.g., routine laboratory assessments, electrocardiography, cardiac stress testing, etc.) have in fact led to more streamlined clinical practice guidelines such as the American Heart Association/American College of Cardiologists' preoperative cardiac evaluation guideline [42] and numerous guidelines from the American Society of Anesthesiologists. Traditional/ routine screening and intervention protocols have been modified over the past couple decades to take into account the fact that while certainly prevalent and potentially devastating, moderate or in some cases even severe atherosclerosis in the context of many low-risk procedures does not require workup let alone optimization.

A recent review examining diverse preoperative initiatives such as targeted evaluations, general preoperative education, smoking cessation programs, exercise programs and others reviewed 117 investigations and found that of those reporting clinical outcomes, 82% of these studies demonstrated significantly positive results [10].

Few investigations to date have examined the clinical efficacy of the PSH model; an initial study by Garson et al presenting outcomes data from their total joint-focused PSH at the University of California Irvine reported what they felt to be significant improvements in outcomes of transfusion (9.8%), length of stay (LOS, 2.7 days), and readmissions (1.1%) compared to national pooled data for those same outcomes (21%, 4 days, and 4.5% respectively) [43]. The same group reported that the following year they found further statistically significant improvements in LOS but not in other indices [44]. In the California Kaiser Permanente system, implementation of a PSH program for total knee arthroplasty also showed significant reduction in LOS and skilled nursing facility admissions (2.4 days and 80%, respectively) for that care pathway compared to a group of patients that preceded them just prior to initiation of the PSH program

(3.4 days and 94%, respectively) with no differences in readmission rates [45]. At the University of Alabama, implementation of a total joint arthroplasty program resulted in a significantly reduced rate of admission and LOS in the intensive care unit, but significant impact on overall LOS or readmission rates were not seen [46].

There are multiple investigations and reviews aimed at elucidating evidence of clinical benefit from ERAS protocols. The majority of these publications come from the colorectal surgical discipline, which is the subspecialty that started the initiative. Many other publications stem from the oncologic surgical discipline. Most of these operations are not elective and likely also occur in a populace with significantly poorer physiologic status, more frequently perturb vital systems, and require postoperative critical care; results thus may not fully "translate" to more commonly performed neuromusculoskeletal procedures. Nonetheless, good evidence exists that these protocols are beneficial, showing reduced complications and length of stay [47–49]. While most studies and reviews do not contain sufficient methodologic or outcomes detail to analyze effects on specific complications (and the heterogeneity of protocols is vast) a recent meta-analysis focusing on ERAS effects on postoperative infection did show significant benefit [50]. The one systematic review of ERAS protocols in orthopedics [51] reported reduced lengths of stay and no decrement in quality of life indicators or patient satisfaction up to 12 months following surgery.

No studies reporting the efficacy of TPS have been published at the time of this writing.

In terms of outcomes justification for specific preoperative optimization of chronic pain and associated comorbidities, evidence that improvements in postoperative outcomes are associated with reductions in pain catastrophizing [52], preoperative opioid use [53], tobacco use [54–56], malnourishment [57, 58], and physical deconditioning [59–62] exists, and these data are discussed at greater length in subsequent chapters.

Justification: Cost-Effectiveness Benefits

Evidence of clinical outcomes benefit alone, however, is also not enough to indicate or justify targeted intervention. While the ethical justice principle of appropriate resource allocation demands reduction and if possible elimination of needless expenditures stemming from preventable complications, the magnitude of which has been highlighted in the previous chapter, in an era of increasingly limited per capita healthcare monies, that same principle also demands fiscal data to back up good ideas.

From a pragmatic standpoint, surgical reimbursements, just like their medical counterparts are now also increasingly subject to reductions for substandard outcome as discussed briefly earlier. Operating room revenue is shifting from a simple volume-based "fee-for-service" model to one of quality or outcomes-based reimbursement with both penalties and incentives being rendered by both governmental and private payers. There is as such ample incentive for understanding and intervening on areas and processes with substandard value.

There has been realization for some time that preoperative optimization is not only economically feasible but also mandatory in this new era [63]. This understanding is supported by well-documented findings showing that of all of the contributors to perioperative costs, patient risk factors by far outweigh surgical variability and even postoperative complications [64].

In keeping with those data, identification and modification of preventable risk factors for elective surgery has been performed for a few decades now with quality and economic outcome data generally supporting more targeted efforts. As discussed previously, plentiful data exist showing that indiscriminate preoperative testing is not beneficial financially (in addition to not influencing outcomes) [3, 4, 65]; conversely the implementation of PACs has been shown to result in cost savings via a more streamlined and targeted approach based on standardized risk assessment and testing protocols [41, 66–68].

More recent integrated perioperative care processes such as the PSH model have been reviewed recently [10] in terms of cost:benefit ratio, and of the 117 studies reviewed, 23 of them included financial outcomes. Of these studies, 82% are reported to have shown positive financial outcomes although there is so much heterogeneity among interventions that drawing firm conclusions is difficult at best. One financial study of the PSH model applied to orthopedics (total knee and hip arthroplasties) posited a roughly $7,000 savings per patient [69] comparing their costs to national benchmark data. Of note, the authors did not even account for cost-savings owing to reduced complication rates, which likely results in underestimation of benefit.

Again, while limited by significant heterogeneity in protocols/methodology, surgical populations, and outcome measures, investigations of financial benefit from ERAS protocols applied to abdominopelvic and vascular surgical populations show predominantly positive cost savings not infrequently in the range of several thousand dollars per patient [49, 70, 71].

At the time of this writing, no studies have been published showing financial benefit from TPS. It is perhaps worth mentioning that American thought leader advocates of this practice model recognize that even with a somewhat pared-down version of the original Toronto roster, with a "multidisciplinary team . . . optimally comprised of a pain medicine specialist, internal medicine hospitalist, addiction medicine specialist, pain psychologist, licensed social worker, and advanced practice registered nurse. . . . A small community hospital may be hard-pressed to mobilize the comprehensive services and personnel required to successfully implement a full-scale perioperative Transitional Pain Service." [72].

A paucity of data likewise exists for financial benefit from current prehabilitation efforts; one early study showed reduced health services use postoperatively for arthroplasty patients undergoing prehabilitation [73], while another report on lumbar spine fusion patients showed significant cost savings for patients randomized to prehabilitation versus standard rehabilitation [74]. More recent systematic reviews and meta-analyses [75–77] have not shown cost benefit from prehabilitation programs in the context of arthroplasty. Negative results have been challenged on the basis of questionable therapeutic validity, and positive results have been challenged based on heterogeneity of intervention and outcome measures.

In terms of financial justification for specific preoperative optimization of chronic pain and associated comorbidities, it seems clear that at the very least, improving our identification and risk stratification (e.g., via measurable factors such as opioid use or pain catastrophizing) of patients suffering with complex chronic pain syndromes is a reasonable endeavor—this is not resource-intensive. Unlike many conditions, chronic pain and its associated comorbidities of opioid dependence, tobacco use, obesity, and so forth, don't generally require expensive diagnostic excursions as the data are manifest.

Furthermore, interventions for these comorbidities are generally not only low-cost and virtually zero-risk but also may serve to reduce the incidence of other complications (e.g., respiratory, cardiovascular, and cerebrovascular events) that constitute an ongoing tremendous source of postoperative morbidity and mortality and healthcare costs.

Finally, it should be considered that preoperative improvements in chronic pain and its associated comorbidities may in fact in many cases obviate the perception of need for surgical intervention, and correspondingly reduce the incidence of unnecessary elective operations. We see this not infrequently in the setting of low back pain with or without radiculopathy.

Process Overview

Establishing Surgeon and System Buy-In

The surgeon remains the "Captain of the Ship" within perioperative medicine; without their expert clinical judgment and operative skills there would be no operation. While different systems confer differing levels of autonomy and authority to the surgeon in terms of scheduling, protocol adherence, and so forth, the bottom line is that establishing surgeon buy-in is essential to successful and smooth program implementation. They must recognize the importance of the issues associated with operating on patients suffering with chronic pain (and it is the rare surgeon that does not these days) and shape the culture of their practice to align with the vision and process of a preoperative optimization program (POP).

Communication between the surgical office and the POP begins frequently with education and marketing efforts; while most surgeons again are well aware of the problems of worsened surgical outcomes, and increased postoperative distress for all parties involved when chronic pain is not optimized prior to elective surgery, specific tactful dissemination of data regarding current POP existence, function, and outcomes will likely be required. Ongoing communication including requests for feedback from the surgical office is also obviously beneficial if not vital. Before launching our program we spent a few weeks surveying and interviewing the majority of our local surgeons not only to assess their perceived need for the program and things they deemed important to intervene on but also to advise them of the establishment of the program. Such communication with other referral sources such as the primary care community, and also the anesthesia community, PAC or PSH if applicable, and hospital administration is also highly beneficial.

It cannot be overstated that while more pragmatic concerns such as identification and early referral are necessary for any such program, perhaps the most fundamental issue in terms of establishing *patient* buy-in (not to mention truly fulfilling ethical principles of autonomy and beneficence) is the establishment of a culture of nonjudgment, respect, and compassion for those suffering with chronic pain, regardless of the presence of other afflictions such as mental illness and substance abuse. It is incumbent on the chronic pain care team to model and communicate these values to all parties involved, including the surgical office.

Patient Identification and Risk Stratification

Early identification of candidates for the POP program will likely most often occur within the surgical office (although the primary care office and even existing chronic pain clinics also serve as sources.) As discussed earlier, unlike more potentially occult conditions (undiagnosed coronary vascular disease or hypothyroidism) chronic pain is rarely hidden and in many cases is the reason for surgical consultation in the first place. Comorbid conditions with high risk for poor outcomes (e.g., opioid dependence) are much more readily discerned these days as well with the advent of electronic records and prescription drug monitoring programs, which may yield clues as to high-dose opioid prescriptions and multiple prescribers/pharmacies, and so forth. All that to say, identification should not be a difficult thing; establishing patterns of recognition and early referral to the POP, however, may take some time and repetitive inquiry.

Risk stratification is of the essence for cost-effectiveness and for highlighting specific arenas that require intensive focus such as pain catastrophizing or posttraumatic stress disorder, polysubstance dependence or abuse, and poor sleep and diet.

While any patient may develop any complication including severe acute and also chronic postsurgical pain (CPSP) and its associated problems, certain risk factors have been shown consistently to confer increased risk and are shown in Table 2.1. Many of these form the subject matter of subsequent chapters. Individual risk factors are not for the most part considered or discussed in this chapter other than to draw attention to the fact that while numerous studies have implicated female gender as a risk factor for increased CPSP, the largest systematic review to date ($n > 23,000$ patients) did not find it to be a risk factor and in fact found an equal amount of studies indicating female gender to be protective (i.e., male gender to be predictive) [78].

Risk assessment or prediction tools have been developed [79, 80] but have not been widely adopted; they tend to be somewhat cumbersome. Given that the literature seems to be very consistent in showing anxiety, preexisting chronic pain, and chronic opioid use to be significant risk factors for poor postsurgical pain outcomes we advise that a simple risk stratification into moderate or high-risk categories occur on the basis of these three readily identifiable factors and

Table 2.1. Risk Factors for Increased Postsurgical Pain and Associated Complications

Sociodemographic	Cognitive/Emotional	Behavioral	Surgical	Other
• Younger age • Isolation/poor social support	• Anxiety • Pain catastrophization • Post-Traumatic Stress Disorder	• Chronic opioid use • Tobacco use • Sleep deprivation? • Sedentary lifestyle?	• Increased surgical duration • Low-volume Surgical unit/team • Open vs. laparoscopic technique • Intraoperative nerve damage • Certain operations (e.g., amputation, mastectomy, thoracotomy, total knee arthroplasty)	• Preexisting chronic pain

their combination. Given the prevalence of these factors and what appears from the literature to be strong association with the outcome, we posit a high likelihood ratio.

More issue-specific instruments may be used either at the level of the referral source or certainly within the POP itself not only for purposes of patient identification but also for assessment of arenas deserving greater focus of attention; these include validated psychological assessment tools, opioid risk stratification tools, and physical function assessments such as the 6-minute walk test. These and more are described in greater detail in subsequent chapters. Assessment of readiness to change (discussed more in the next chapter) is also part of risk stratification.

Introduction to the 10-Week Program

Our VALERAS POP in its current iteration (see Figure 2.3) comprises a 10-session weekly program with joint behavioral and clinical medicine teams participating in a templated but tailored process addressing what we feel to be fundamental cognitive and behavioral issues conferring poor postoperative prognosis and that constitute the subject matter of sections 2 and 3 of this book. We chose a 10-week timeframe for numerous reasons including plentiful evidence for a minimum requirement of 2 to 3 months for effective habit change as discussed in greater detail in the next chapter, as well as literature evidence of increasing benefit with longer-term discontinuation of toxic habits such as tobacco and opioid consumption and incorporation of beneficial habits such as improved diet and exercise. Furthermore, the waiting period for many elective operations in this country and abroad is frequently at least 2 months, and with the current trend of increasing preoperative authorization burdens from insurance carriers, there is generally a built-in 2- to 3-month approval process anyhow.

While the cost of 10 outpatient visits may seem formidable at initial glance, it is generally exceeded by the cost of one extra day's hospitalization or those associated with postoperative complications.

In addition, our (HM, LF) POP includes more traditional preoperative assessment functions including cardiac, pulmonary, and endocrine screening and workup given my (HM) background as an anesthesiologist. In smaller communities without a dedicated PSH we recommend this practice to increase value to the patient and system.

Other important considerations include how to navigate inpatient perioperative management and also postdischarge management/aftercare; these are addressed in a subsequent chapter.

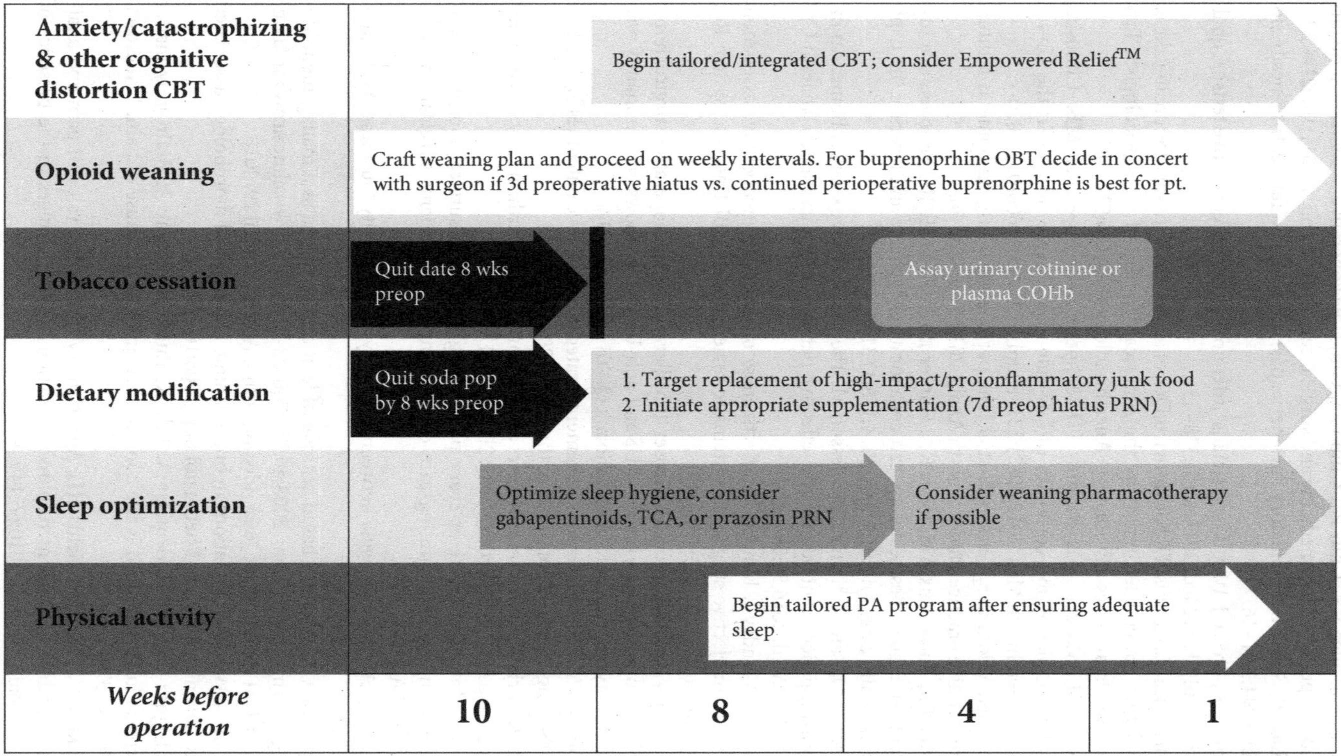

	10	8	4	1
Anxiety/catastrophizing & other cognitive distortion CBT	Begin tailored/integrated CBT; consider Empowered Relief™			
Opioid weaning	Craft weaning plan and proceed on weekly intervals. For buprenorphine OBT decide in concert with surgeon if 3d preoperative hiatus vs. continued perioperative buprenorphine is best for pt.			
Tobacco cessation	Quit date 8 wks preop		Assay urinary cotinine or plasma COHb	
Dietary modification	Quit soda pop by 8 wks preop	1. Target replacement of high-impact/proionflammatory junk food 2. Initiate appropriate supplementation (7d preop hiatus PRN)		
Sleep optimization	Optimize sleep hygiene, consider gabapentinoids, TCA, or prazosin PRN		Consider weaning pharmacotherapy if possible	
Physical activity		Begin tailored PA program after ensuring adequate sleep		
Weeks before operation	10	8	4	1

Figure 2.3. VALERAS Model of Preoperative Optimization of the Chronic Pain Patient

References

1 Lee A, Kerridge RK, Chui PT, Chiu CH, Gin T. Perioperative Systems as a quality model of perioperative medicine and surgical care. Health Policy. 2011;102:214–22.

2 White PF Smith I. Ambulatory anesthesia: past, present, and future. Int Anesthesiol Clin. 1994;32:1–16.

3 Brown SR, Brown J. Why do physicians order unnecessary preoperative tests? A qualitative study. Fam Med. 2011;43(5):338–43.

4 Apfelbaum JL, Connis RT, Nickinovich DG, et al. Practice advisory for preanesthesia evaluation: an updated report by the American Society of Anesthesiologists Task Force on Preanesthesia Evaluation. Anesthesiology 2012;116:522–38.

5 Colla CH, Morden NE, Sequist TD, Schpero WL, Rosenthal MB. Choosing wisely: prevalence and correlates of low-value health care services in the United States. J Gen Intern Med. 2015;30(2):221–8. doi:10.1007/s11606-014-3070-z.

6 Kain ZN, Vakharia S, Garson L, et al. The perioperative surgical home as a future perioperative practice model. Anesth Analg. 2014;118:1126–30.

7 Vetter TR, Boudreaux AM, Jones KA, Hunter JM Jr, Pittet JF. The perioperative surgical home: how anesthesiology can collaboratively achieve and leverage the triple aim in health care. Anesth Analg. 2014;118:1131–6.

8 Desebbe O, Lanz T, Kain Z, Cannesson M. The perioperative surgical home: An innovative, patient-centred and cost-effective perioperative care model. Anaesth Crit Care Pain Med. 2016;35:59–66.

9 Hines S, Munday J, Kynoch K. Effectiveness of nurse-led preoperative assessment services for elective surgery: a systematic review update. JBI Database System Rev Implement Rep. 2015;13:279–317.

10 Kash BA, Zhang Y, Cline KM, Menser T, Miller TR. The perioperative surgical home (PSH): a comprehensive review of US and non-US studies shows predominantly positive quality and cost outcomes. Milbank Q. 2014;92:796–821.

11 Froimson M. Perioperative management strategies to improve outcomes and reduce cost during an episode of care. J Arthroplasty. 2015;30:346–8.

12 Kim K, Iorio R. The 5 clinical pillars of value for total joint arthroplasty in a bundled payment paradigm. J Arthroplasty. 2017;32:1712–16.

13 Kain Z. Integrating care at every point along a patient's surgical journey. http://drzeevkain.health/integrating-care-every-point-along-apatients-surgical-journey/. Accessed April 29, 2018.

14 Hindo B. At 3M, a struggle between efficiency and creativity. Business Week. June 6, 2007.

15 Paparone CR. A values-based critique of lean and six sigma as a management ideology. Army Logistician. 2008;40:PB 700-08-01. http://www.almc.army.mil/alog/issues/JanFeb08/critique_6sig_ideology.html. Accessed April 29, 2018.

16 Schmidt-Wilcke T. Variations in brain volume and regional morphology associated with chronic pain. Curr Rheumatol Rep. 2008;10:467–74.

17 Rodriguez-Raecke R, Niemeier A, Ihle K, Ruether W, May A. Brain gray matter decrease in chronic pain is the consequence and not the cause of pain. J Neurosci. 2009;29:13746–50.

18 Baliki MN, Geha PY, Fields HL, Apkarian AV. Predicting value of pain and analgesia: nucleus accumbens response to noxious stimuli changes in the presence of chronic pain. Neuron. 2010;66:149–60.

19 Seminowicz DA, Wideman TH, Naso L, et al. Effective treatment of chronic low back pain in humans reverses abnormal brain anatomy and function. J Neurosci. 2011;31:7540–50.

20 Rodriguez-Raecke R, Niemeier A, Ihle K, Ruether W, May A. Structural brain changes in chronic pain reflect probably neither damage nor atrophy. Langguth B, ed. PLoS ONE. 2013;8(2):e54475. doi:10.1371/journal.pone.0054475.

21 Kress HG, Aldington D, Alon E, et al. A holistic approach to chronic pain management that involves all stakeholders: change is needed. Curr Med Res Opin. 2015;31:1743–54.

22 Darnall BD, Scheman J, Davin S, et al. Pain psychology: a global needs assessment and national call to action. Pain Med. 2016;17:250–63.

23 Interagency Pain Research Coordinating Committee. National pain strategy: a comprehensive population health-level strategy for pain. https://iprcc.nih.gov/sites/default/files/HHSNational_Pain_Strategy_508C.pdf. Accessed April 29, 2018.

24 Katz J, Weinrib A, Fashler SR, et al. The Toronto General Hospital Transitional Pain Service: development and implementation of a multidisciplinary program to prevent chronic postsurgical pain. J Pain Res. 2015;8:695–702.

25 Spain J. Prehabilitation. Clinics Sports Med. 1985;4:575–85.

26 Carli F, Zavorsky GS. Optimizing functional exercise capacity in the elderly surgical population. Curr Opin Clin Nutr Metab Care. 2005;8:23–32.

27 Smeets RJ, Vlaeyen JW, Kester AD, Knottnerus JA. Reduction of pain catastrophizing mediates the outcome of both physical and cognitive-behavioral treatment in chronic low back pain. J Pain. 2006;7:261–71.

28 Sullivan AB, Scheman J, Venesy D, Davin S. The role of exercise and types of exercise in the rehabilitation of chronic pain: specific or nonspecific benefits. Curr Pain Headache Rep. 2012;16(2):153–61.

29 Ambrose KR, Golightly YM. Physical exercise as non-pharmacological treatment of chronic pain: Why and when. Best Pract Res Clin Rheumatol. 2015;29(1):120–30. doi:10.1016/j.berh.2015.04.022.

30 Mihalko SL, Cox P, Beavers DP, et al. Effect of intensive diet and exercise on self-efficacy in overweight and obese adults with knee osteoarthritis: The IDEA randomized clinical trial. Transl Behav Med. April 4, 2018. doi: 10.1093/tbm/iby037. [Epub ahead of print] PubMed PMID: 29635402.

31 Hayden JA, van Tulder MW, Malmivaara A, Koes BW. Exercise therapy for treatment of non-specific low back pain. Cochrane Database Syst. 2005;Rev. 3:CD000335. doi: 10.1002/14651858.CD000335.pub2.

32 Busch AJ, Barber KA, Overend TJ, Peloso PM, Schacter CL. Exercise for treating fibromyalgia syndrome. Cochrane Database Syst. 2007;Rev. 17:CD003786. doi: 10.1002/14651858.CD003786.pub2

33 Fransen M, McConnell S, Harmer AR, Van der Esch M, Simic M, Bennell KL. Exercise for osteoarthritis of the knee. Cochrane Database Syst. 2015;Rev.1:CD004376. doi: 10.1002/14651858.CD004376.pub3

34 Ellingson LD, Stegner AJ, Schwabacher IJ, Koltyn KF, Cook DB. Exercise strengthens central nervous system modulation of pain in fibromyalgia. Stroman PW, ed. Brain Sciences. 2016;6(1):8. doi:10.3390/brainsci6010008.

35 Nijs J, Meeus M, Versijpt J, et al. Brain-derived neurotrophic factor as a driving force behind neuroplasticity in neuropathic and central sensitization pain: a new therapeutic target? Expert Opin Ther Targets. 2015;19:565–76.

36 Tajerian M, Clark JD. Nonpharmacological interventions in targeting pain-related brain plasticity. Neural Plasticity. 2017;2017:2038573. doi:10.1155/2017/2038573.

37 Li C, Carli F, Lee L, et al. Impact of a trimodal prehabilitation program on functional recovery after colorectal cancer surgery: a pilot study. Surg Endosc. 2013;27:1072–82.

38 Santa Mina D, Scheede-Bergdahl C, Gillis C, Carli F. Optimization of surgical outcomes with prehabilitation. Appl Physiol Nutr Metab. 2015;40:966–9.

39 Minnella EM, Bousquet-Dion G, Awasthi R, et al. Multimodal prehabilitation improves functional capacity before and after colorectal surgery for cancer: a five-year research experience. Acta Oncol. 2017;56:295–300.

40 Benarroch-Gampel J, Sheffield KM, Duncan CB, et al. Preoperative laboratory testing in patients undergoing elective, low-risk ambulatory surgery. Ann Surg. 2012;256:518–28.

41 Kash BA, Cline KM, Timmons S, Roopani R, Miller TR. International comparison of preoperative testing and assessment protocols and best practices to reduce surgical care costs: a systematic literature review. Adv Health Care Manag. 2015;17:161–94.

42 Fleisher LA, Fleischmann KE, Auerbach AD, et al. 2014 ACC/AHA guideline on perioperative cardiovascular evaluation and management of patients undergoing noncardiac surgery: executive summary: a report of the American College of Cardiology/American Heart Association Task Force on practice guidelines. Developed in collaboration with the American College of Surgeons, American Society of Anesthesiologists, American Society of Echocardiography, American Society of Nuclear Cardiology, Heart Rhythm Society, Society for Cardiovascular Angiography and Interventions, Society of Cardiovascular Anesthesiologists, and Society of Vascular Medicine Endorsed by the Society of Hospital Medicine. J Nucl Cardiol. 2015;22:162–215.

43 Garson L, Schwarzkopf R, Vakharia S, et al. Implementation of a total joint replacement-focused perioperative surgical home: a management case report. Anesth Analg. 2014;118:1081–9.

44 Cyriac J, Garson L, Schwarzkopf R, et al. Total joint replacement perioperative surgical home program: 2-year follow-up. Anesth Analg. 2016;123:51–62.

45 Qiu C, Cannesson M, Morkos A, et al. Practice and outcomes of the perioperative surgical home in a California integrated delivery system. Anesth Analg. 2016;123:597–606.

46 Vetter TR, Barman J, Hunter JM Jr, Jones KA, Pittet JF. The effect of implementation of preoperative and postoperative care elements of a perioperative surgical home model on outcomes in patients undergoing hip arthroplasty or knee arthroplasty. Anesth Analg. 2017;124:1450–8.

47 Nicholson A, Lowe MC, Parker J, Lewis SR, Alderson P, Smith AF. Systematic review and meta-analysis of enhanced recovery programmes in surgical patients. Br J Surg. 2014;101:172–88.

48 Lau CS, Chamberlain RS. Enhanced recovery after surgery programs improve patient outcomes and recovery: a meta-analysis. World J Surg. 2017;41:899–913.

49 Visioni A, Shah R, Gabriel E, Attwood K, Kukar M, Nurkin S. Enhanced recovery after surgery for noncolorectal surgery?: A systematic review and meta-analysis of major abdominal surgery. Ann Surg. 2018;267:57–65.

50 Grant MC, Yang D, Wu CL, Makary MA, Wick EC. Impact of enhanced recovery after surgery and fast track surgery pathways on healthcare-associated infections: results from a systematic review and meta-analysis. Ann Surg. 2017;265:68–79.

51 Jones EL, Wainwright TW, Foster JD, Smith JR, Middleton RG, Francis NK. A systematic review of patient reported outcomes and patient experience in enhanced recovery after orthopaedic surgery. Ann R Coll Surg Engl. 2014;96:89–94.

52 Darnall B. My Surgical Success: A perioperative psychological intervention. PAIN Reports. 2017;2(4):e604.

53 Nguyen LC, Sing DC, Bozic KJ. Preoperative reduction of opioid use before total joint arthroplasty. J Arthroplast. 2016;31(9 Suppl):282–7.

54 Møller AM, Villebro N, Pedersen T, Tønnesen H. Effect of preoperative smoking intervention on postoperative complications: a randomised clinical trial. Lancet. 2002;359:114–17.

55 Theadom A, Cropley M. Effects of preoperative smoking cessation on the incidence and risk of intraoperative and postoperative complications in adult smokers: a systematic review. Tob Control. 2006;15:352–8.

56 Thomsen T, Villebro N, Møller AM. Interventions for preoperative smoking cessation. Cochrane Database Syst Rev. 2014;(3):CD002294. doi: 10.1002/14651858. CD002294.pub4.

57 Braga M, Wischmeyer PE, Drover J, et al. Clinical evidence for pharmaconutrition in major elective surgery. J Parenter Enteral Nutr. 2013;37(5 Suppl):66S–72S.

58 Hegazi RA, Hustead DS, Evans DC. Preoperative standard oral nutrition supplements vs immunonutrition: results of a systematic review and meta-analysis. J Am Coll Surg. 2014;219:1078–87.

59 Santa Mina D, Clarke H, Ritvo P, et al. Effect of total-body prehabilitation on postoperative outcomes: a systematic review and meta-analysis. Physiotherapy. 2014;100:196–207.

60 Moran J, Guinan E, McCormick P, et al. The ability of prehabilitation to influence postoperative outcome after intra-abdominal operation: a systematic review and meta-analysis. Surgery. 2016;160:1189–1201.

61 Pouwels S, Hageman D, Gommans LN, et al. Preoperative exercise therapy in surgical care: a scoping review. J Clin Anesth. 2016;33:476–90.

62 Moyer R, Ikert K, Long K, Marsh J. The value of preoperative exercise and education for patients undergoing total hip and knee arthroplasty: a systematic review and meta-analysis. JBJS Rev. 2017;5(12):e2. doi:10.2106/JBJS.RVW.17.00015. PubMed PMID: 29232265.

63 Snowden CP, Anderson H. Preoperative optimization: rationale and process: is it economic sense? Curr Opin Anaesthesiol. 2012;25:210–16.

64 Davenport DL, Henderson WG, Khuri SF, et al. Preoperative risk factors and surgical complexity are more predictive of costs than postoperative complications: a case study using the National Surgical Quality Improvement Program (NSQIP) Database. Ann Surg. 2005;242:463–71.

65 Pasternak L. Preoperative testing: moving from individual testing to risk management. Anes Analg. 2009;108:393–4.

66 Fischer S. Development and effectiveness of an anesthesia preoperative evaluation clinic in a teaching hospital. Anesthesiology. 1996;85:196–206.

67 Finegan BA, Rashiq S, McAlister FA, O'Connor P. Selective ordering of preoperative investigations by anesthesiologists reduces the number and cost of tests. Can J Anaesth. 2005;52:575–80.

68 Correll DJ, Bader AM, Hull MW, Hsu C, Tsen LC, Hepner DL. Value of preoperative clinic visits in identifying issues with potential impact on operating room efficiency. Anesthesiology. 2006;105:1254–9.

69 Raphael DR, Cannesson M, Schwarzkopf R, et al. Total joint perioperative surgical home: an observational financial review. Periop Med (Lond). 2014;3:6. doi: 10.1186/2047-0525-3-6.

70 Lemanu DP, Singh PP, Stowers MD, Hill AG. A systematic review to assess cost effectiveness of enhanced recovery after surgery programmes in colorectal surgery. Colorectal Dis. 2014;16:338–46.

71 Stowers MD, Lemanu DP, Hill AG. Health economics in Enhanced Recovery After Surgery programs. Can J Anaesth. 2015;62:219–30.

72 Vetter TR, Kain ZN. Role of the perioperative surgical home in optimizing the perioperative use of opioids. Anesth Analg. 2017;125:1653–57.

73 Beaupre LA, Lier D, Davies DM, Johnston DB. The effect of a preoperative exercise and education program on functional recovery, health related quality of life, and health service utilization following primary total knee arthroplasty. J Rheumatol. 2004;31:1166–73.

74 Nielsen PR, Andreasen J, Asmussen M, Tønnesen H. Costs and quality of life for prehabilitation and early rehabilitation after surgery of the lumbar spine. BMC Health Serv Res. 2008;8:209. doi: 10.1186/1472-6963-8-209. PubMed PMID: 18842157;PubMed Central PMCID: PMC2586633.

75 Jordan RW, Smith NA, Chahal GS, Casson C, Reed MR, Sprowson AP. Enhanced education and physiotherapy before knee replacement: is it worth it? A systematic review. Physiotherapy. 2014;100:305–12.

76 Cabilan CJ, Hines S, Munday J. The effectiveness of prehabilitation or preoperative exercise for surgical patients: a systematic review. JBI Database System Rev Implement Rep. 2015;13:146–87.

77 Wang L, Lee M, Zhang Z, Moodie J, Cheng D, Martin J. Does preoperative rehabilitation for patients planning to undergo joint replacement surgery improve outcomes? A systematic review and meta-analysis of randomised controlled trials. BMJ Open. 2016;6(2):e009857. doi: 10.1136/bmjopen-2015-009857. Review. PubMed PMID: 26839013;PubMed Central PMCID: PMC4746481.

78 Ip HY, Abrishami A, Peng PW, Wong J, Chung F. Predictors of postoperative pain and analgesic consumption: a qualitative systematic review. Anesthesiology. 2009;111:657–77.

79 Janssen KJ, Kalkman CJ, Grobbee DE, Bonsel GJ, Moons KG, Vergouwe Y. The risk of severe postoperative pain: Modification and validation of a clinical prediction rule. Anesth Analg. 2008;107:1330–9.

80 Althaus A, Hinrichs-Rocker A, Chapman R, et al. Development of a risk index for the prediction of chronic post-surgical pain. Eur J Pain. 2012;16:901–10.

3

The Primacy of Motivation in Preoperative Optimization

Heath B. McAnally and Beth Darnall

Introduction

Human disease etiologies often involve a complex interplay of genetic, environmental, psychological, and sociocultural factors. In recent decades, the developed world has entered the era of chronic self-inflicted disease. In terms of morbidity and mortality, infectious and traumatic insults have yielded first place to accelerated degenerative, inflammatory, and metabolic pathologies associated with neglect of basic health maintenance as well as overindulgence/excess. Cardiovascular disease, diabetes, cancer, and chronic pulmonary disease constitute the major causes of disability and death in the United States, and as the Centers for Disease Control has put it, "Much of the chronic disease burden results from a small number of key risk factors that include high blood pressure, tobacco smoking and second-hand smoke exposure, high BMI, physical inactivity, alcohol use, and diets low in fruits and vegetables and high in sodium and saturated fats." [1] Such risk factors are largely behaviorally mediated.

Whether or not chronic pain is to be considered a disease in its own right, that highly prevalent and dysfunctional condition is largely influenced if not mediated by omission of healthy biopsychosocial-spiritual behaviors, and commission of unhealthy ones [2–8]. Many of these factors—both biological and cognitive-behavioral—appear to be even more prevalent in the elective surgical population than in the general population [9, 10] and via their association with pain likely fuel the demand for elective surgery for pain while simultaneously undermining its efficacy [11] in part by increasing postsurgical pain and opioid use as discussed in the previous chapter.

This effort and book are ultimately about replacing such harmful psychobehavioral patterns with beneficial ones. Our belief is that effective preoperative optimization of patients suffering with chronic pain requires recognition of the primacy of behavior therein. It is our desire to entrain physicians and other healthcare providers and staff in the paradigm that behavioral choices and patterns which may arise from conscious or subconscious motivators (e.g., comfort and distress modification) and habits underlie and sustain the majority of chronic pain conditions, and furthermore are key to mitigating pain's impact if not even eliminating it.

The arrangement of the book chapters reflects that valuation, with chapters on "pure" psychological issues (motivation, habit, anxiety, and catastrophic thinking) preceding those issues more often/traditionally viewed through a biological lens (toxic substances and toxic physical habits.) Within the chapters on "biological" issues, following a brief introduction comprising descriptive epidemiology and pathophysiology for the subject, each chapter is arranged according to a cognitive-behavioral construct as outlined in greater detail at the beginning of chapter 6.

In this chapter we begin from a pragmatic and therapeutic (to the extent that term may be applied) perspective with a brief overview of what is commonly called motivational interviewing today and its crucial role in facilitating the behavioral changes/lifestyle modifications that are foundational to this program. This chapter is not a "how-to" manual; for deeper understanding and techniques/ tactics the reader is referred to Miller and Rollnick's seminal text [12] and the many targeted monographs in their Applications series [13–15]. From there we proceed to a brief elaboration of relevant and applicable constructs from both current and past theories of motivation, understanding of which we believe to be fundamental to any work with autonomous beings. This chapter also serves as the natural introduction to the subject of the next, which constitutes the greatest obstacle to, and conversely what is potentially the greatest tool for shaping behavior: habit. It is our belief that as healthcare professionals become more accustomed to considering these common chronic pain and illness contributors via this biobehavioral perspective, and correspondingly more familiar and facile with truly biopsychosocial-spiritual treatment approaches we will see a significant decline in perioperative chronic pain—both antecedent and consequent.

Motivational Interviewing in Perioperative Medicine

Colloquial understanding of the adjective "motivational" today often involves the idea or context of trying to get people to do what we want them to do/what we think they should be doing. This viewpoint is not confined to managerial seminars and the business world, but more recently has infiltrated healthcare as we've gravitated from the traditional paternalistic model to a more participatory and shared decision-making one, and yet still operate in a directive manner most of the time. While the traditional authoritative style, with passivity on the part of the patient, will always be required in many acute situations (e.g., myocardial infarction or a ruptured appendix) for the most part effective management of chronic conditions requires a far more indirect and empowering approach—something not easy for seasoned healthcare providers and caregivers who are invested with valid information on what is best for people and in particular their patients. It's a subtle shift from seeking to align the patient with what we want them to do, to seeking their empowerment to improve their own lot, but this change of focus to a supportive and even "hands-off" role may in fact be critical in most cases for eliciting and maintaining healthy efforts. Recognition and respect of the autonomy of competent individuals is more likely not only to engender cooperation in achieving short-term goals, such as improving their nutrition or activity level, but also to facilitate sustained change. While there is and will always be a need for health experts to provide information and guidance, *how* we go about it is undoubtedly far more tied to outcome than is what we actually share.

Motivational interviewing (MI) has become one of the most familiar and widely adopted counseling styles over the past two decades with application in addiction treatment, general counseling, and in medical practice of all disciplines involving any element of chronic condition management and continuity of care. It is defined by the authors as

> a collaborative conversation style . . . a person-centered counseling style for addressing the common problem of ambivalence about change . . . designed to strengthen personal motivation and commitment to a specific goal by eliciting and exploring the person's own reason for change within an atmosphere of acceptance and compassion. [12]

Motivational interviewing was designed for, and finds its utility in, working with people who are (generally) aware of the need for behavioral change, but who at the same time experience significant obstacles to changing. Both of these "vectors" in the mathematical sense exist on a highly dynamic spectrum, and the tension or ambivalence between them does as well. There may be no desire or even personal acknowledgment of the need for change, or the person may be desperate. More often than not they are somewhere in between, and assessment of "readiness to change" is an essential component of the process, both at the outset and throughout. Obstacles may include pragmatic barriers to change such as limited resources (of time, energy, support, money, etc.) or conflicting motives that favor sustaining the status quo/behavior in question; typically at least some degree of both factors coexist.

Typically, a simple assessment of readiness to change (e.g., a direct question with or without visual aid such as a 0 to 10 scale) is used to determine a person's status. Often considered in conjunction with MI is a behavioral change model (and readiness assessment) so well accepted and discussed in the literature that we will briefly introduce it here. The transtheoretical model (TTM) of behavioral change, also frequently referred to as the stages of change model developed by Prochaska and DiClemente [16] is undoubtedly the most widely recognized and used construct over the past few decades to conceptualize and represent where an individual is in their process of implementing change. The TTM describes six stages of change:

- Precontemplation. In this stage people are essentially unwilling to change, generally not perceiving any reason to/benefit. They may not even perceive their current behavioral state to be a problem.
- Contemplation. In this stage people have begun the process of weighing pros and cons of changing versus not changing.
- Preparation. In this stage people have begun to exercise some degree of will toward change and are planning on such, even making introductory/preparatory action. Note that this stage (and subsequent ones) do not preclude coexisting ambivalent motives, nor struggle.
- Action. This stage is arbitrarily defined as the first six months of significant change behavior.
- Maintenance. This stage is arbitrarily defined as ongoing change behavior beyond the initial six months.
- Termination. This stage essentially represents total transformation, where the prechange state no longer is desired/exerts any pull.

Figure 3.1 portrays a linear adaptation of the TTM we (HM) use clinically to discuss these concepts with patients; the model is generally portrayed as a cycle with exit and entry points at every stage. (While we recognize that change, or any behavior for that matter, is generally not a linear process as depicted here, we've come to believe that reinforcement of relapse is in essence "setting the bar low" and counterproductive to motivation.) The TTM itself does not prescribe interventions; however, a considerable body of work has been performed over the past few decades linking different approaches and tactics supporting the person's efforts to the stage they are in [17]. A discussion of these methods is outside the scope of this chapter.

Miller and Rollnick place supreme weight of importance on "the spirit of MI," and it bears reproducing here (and is also shown in what follows). The first core value is that of acceptance of the individual unconditionally, with sincere valuation of their inherent worth. This includes and extends beyond simply respecting their autonomy; active appreciation of their unique strengths and ongoing achievements is required. Second is compassion, which is defined in this context as a dedication to pursuing and promoting the individual's best interest and prioritizing their needs. Third is evocation, which is a deliberate and skilled

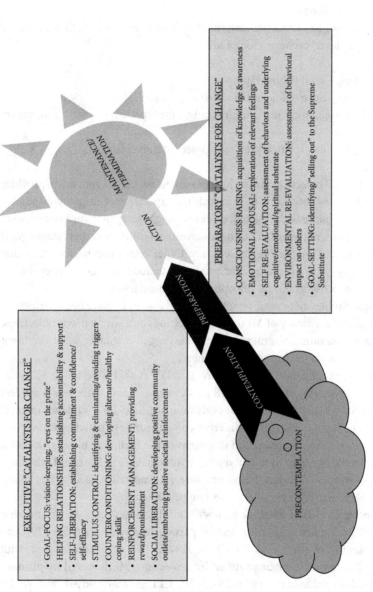

EXECUTIVE "CATALYSTS FOR CHANGE"

- GOAL-FOCUS: vision-keeping; "eyes on the prize"
- HELPING RELATIONSHIPS: establishing accountability & support
- SELF-LIBERATION: establishing commitment & confidence/ self-efficacy
- STIMULUS CONTROL: identifying & eliminating/avoiding triggers
- COUNTERCONDITIONING: developing alternate/healthy coping skills
- REINFORCEMENT MANAGEMENT: providing reward/punishment
- SOCIAL LIBERATION: developing positive community outlets/embracing positive societal reinforcement

PREPARATORY "CATALYSTS FOR CHANGE"

- CONSCIOUSNESS RAISING: acquisition of knowledge & awareness
- EMOTIONAL AROUSAL: exploration of relevant feelings
- SELF RE-EVALUATION: assessment of behaviors and underlying cognitive/emotional/spiritual substrate
- ENVIRONMENTAL RE-EVALUATION: assessment of behavioral impact on others
- GOAL-SETTING: identifying/"selling out" to the Supreme Substitute

MAINTENANCE/ TERMINATION

ACTION

PREPARATION

CONTEMPLATION

PRECONTEMPLATION

Adapted from Prochaska, Diclemente & Norcross 1992; Diclemente & Scott, 1997

Figure 3.1. Transtheoretical/Stages of Change Model

By AKgaspasser [CC BY-SA 4.0 (https://creativecommons.org/licenses/by-sa/4.0)], from Wikimedia Commons process of eliciting the individual's own expert capacity at understanding and helping themselves. Finally, MI relies on the principle of collaboration, perhaps best communicated by the authors' metaphor comparing the process to "dancing rather than wrestling."

There are four key processes described by Miller and Rollnick that constitute the "strategic-level" orchestration of MI:

- Engaging—establishing rapport
- Focusing—developing and maintaining the goal
- Evoking—eliciting/nurturing/refining the patient's own motivation for change
- Planning—helping to crystallize a practical game plan

Different tactical objectives and techniques on the part of the counselor/provider facilitate these key processes. They include the expression of empathy, avoidance of argument, "rolling with resistance," developing discrepancy (helping patients recognize their ambivalence and the inconsistencies between their stated goals and actions), and supporting self-efficacy. Other core interviewing skills that support all of these objectives and processes include the use of open-ended questions, reflective listening, affirming, and summarizing.

Multiple studies, systematic reviews, and meta-analyses have been performed to investigate the efficacy of MI in various settings and with various objectives. There have been numerous mixed reviews and negative studies; some pertinent positive ones, however, are summarized here.

In the context of general medical care, Lundahl et al [18] performed a meta-analysis of 48 studies including 9,618 participants; overall there was a modest and statistically significant omnibus odds ratio of 1.55 (95% confidence interval [CI] 1.41–1.71, $p < 0.001$) for 51 different comparisons evaluated. Specific positive effects were seen on reduction of substance use including tobacco, alcohol, and marijuana; decrease in sedentary behavior; decrease in BMI; and other significant outcomes including blood pressure and mortality rate. In this meta-analysis, there was not a beneficial effect on healthy eating.

In a recent Cochrane database review examining the effect of MI on smoking cessation, 28 studies with over 16,000 participants were analyzed [19] and showed significant effect (risk ratio 1.26; 95% CI 1.16–1.36) toward successful quitting. Interestingly, when stratified by profession, MI delivered by primary care physicians yielded a risk ratio of 3.49 (95% CI 1.53–7.94) and MI delivered by counselors showed a more modest effect with risk ratio 1.25 (95% CI 1.15–1.63), however only two trials with $n = 736$ were reviewed for physicians compared to 22 trials with $n > 13,500$ for counselors.

O'Halloran et al [20] investigated the benefit of MI in improving phys-ical activity in people with various chronic health conditions; 10 randomized controlled trials incorporating varying degrees and means of MI, and targeting various (self-reported) physical activity adherence measures were reviewed, with data from eight of these trials pooled for meta-analysis. A standard mean difference of 0.19 (95% CI 0.06–0.32) was seen during immediate follow-up.

Armstrong et al [21] performed a systematic review of MI in weight loss in the obese; 11 studies ($n = 1,448$) were included in a meta-analysis, and a nonstatistically significant effect (standard mean difference -0.51; 95% CI -1.04–0.01) was seen with MI compared to other interventions.

Alperstein and Sharpe [22] provided an interesting meta-analysis of MI's ef-fect on treatment adherence in the chronic pain setting, with secondary analyses of self-reported pain intensity, and physical functioning. As far as adherence to treatment and reduction in pain intensity, short-term follow-up data (dura-tion not specified) suggests small but significant improvements on both of these outcomes. Five studies ($n = 631$ participants) showed an overall effect of MI on adherence to treatment (Hedges g statistic = 0.441; 95% CI 0.08–0.8) and four studies ($n = 449$) showed an overall effect of MI on pain intensity reduction (Hedges g statistic = 0.27; 95% CI 0.4–0.5). However, while retaining a positive trend, both associations lost statistical significance when follow-up was specifi-cally evaluated at 6 months in studies with that variable clearly defined. Pooled data from five studies ($n = 779$) showed a weekly positive but statistically insig-nificant effect of MI on physical functioning. While it was not discussed specif-ically within this review, one potential (and optimistic) source of effect dilution over time is that attrition of participants in the intervention groups may have occurred due to improvement in symptoms.

Most of these reviews admit to considerable heterogeneity among the outcome variables (not unusual when attempting to measure behavior.) Furthermore, es-sentially all note that interpretation is challenged by what is essentially no stand-ardization of the MI process by its very nature, nor in the experience and skill of the individuals delivering it.

Having said that, the primacy of therapeutic alliance is well recognized by vir-tually all experts in the field including Rollnick and Miller [23–25], and investi-gation of MI processes and specific components suggests that strict adherence to protocols, and so forth, is of far less importance than counselor interpersonal skills. In a relatively early investigation of causal mechanisms of MI, it was noted by the authors (including Dr. Miller) that "therapist behaviors that have tradi-tionally been viewed as inconsistent with the spirit of MI are in fact compat-ible with this method if clinicians convey them with the requisite interpersonal skills" [26]. In this study, the authors note that directive and even confrontational interchanges may be well-received and result in change behavior if patients perceive "a genuine and authentic stance . . . honesty and transparency."

Nonetheless, MI continues to maintain its elevated status especially among those disciplines more obviously aligned with behavioral and lifestyle change such as substance abuse rehabilitation, and nutrition and dietary fields. Incorporating its basic principles into preoperative optimization counseling holds great face validity given the preponderance of self-change objectives inherent therein, especially in the chronic pain population. For those unfamiliar with MI, there is no better way of grasping its principles than to be exposed to hypothetical and real-world scenarios demonstrating its application. Toward that end, hypothetical examples of contrasting directive versus MI approaches to each of the preoperative issues that form the subjects of chapters 6 through 10 is provided; the reader is referred to Miller and Rollnick's textbook [12] and other volumes in their Applications series [13–15] for further examples and for exposure to the fundamental principles of the method.

Health, Motivation, and the Enigma of Behavior

"Why Ask Why?"

Motivational interviewing is a powerful and validated method of assisting people in making the choices they generally know they should (and on occasion gently providing that knowledge) by overcoming ambivalence and facilitating self-efficacy. As the creators of the technique put it—its purpose is to "help people change," which process must be carried out by the individual's initiative if it is to be successful and sustained.

However, applying MI without a basic framework for understanding human motivation is a little like performing a rotator cuff repair without understanding the anatomy and kinesiology of the shoulder joint, or like placing a ureteral stent without understanding and attending to why the patient is making stones. The patient almost certainly doesn't want shoulder pain and decreased strength/range of motion, and undoubtedly would prefer resolution of their ureteropelvic obstruction and colic. While the analogies are imperfect of course—the procedural interventions are passive on the part of the patient—like MI, they will presumably assist the patient with at least transient improvement possibly even approaching restoration of normal function and empower them in that sense to resume active management (rehabilitative physiotherapy with decreased pain and limitation, increased hydration without fear of glomerular filtration.) However, without addressing the underlying pathologic diatheses (*why is he sitting hunched over his computer all day, and why is she drinking 2 liters of cola every day?*) maximal benefit is unlikely to occur and the patient remains at risk for recurrence or progression of disease.

The Relationship Between Motivation and Health Behaviors

Motivation is a fairly intuitive concept in our modern era, and as such when we ask:

- "Why are some people motivated to pursue a healthy biopsychosocial-spiritual lifestyle while so many others are not?"

Or,

- "Why doesn't pain serve as the ultimate motivator for more people to improve their lifestyle?"

the meaning and intent of the questions don't require explanation. What does require exploration and clarification is the complexity of human behavior (as relates to motivation and health behaviors given the context of this chapter and this book)—a task obviously beyond the capability of these authors!

Motivation, discussed at some length throughout the rest of this chapter is but one determinant of any human behavior including health behavior. As noted in a recent systematic review of health behavior theories, many other factors including habit (the subject of the next chapter), cues, available resources, and other contextual issues such as opportunities and costs all exert simultaneous influence on behavior at any given moment [27].

A full survey of the development of concepts and theories on motivation from Western academic thought is also beyond the scope of this book and our expertise. Rather, we will attempt to present key salient principles and theories proposed and supported by research in the context of the two questions asked previously. Those questions (which encompass the behavioral challenges and choices so prevalent in our society today responsible for this entire effort) provide scenarios wherein most of the fundamental theoretical and practical issues related to health behavior may be explored. In doing so we will attempt to weave a cogent and pragmatic framework within which MI techniques can be more intuitively accessed and applied.

What Is Health?

Defining health is obviously foundational at the outset of such a discussion, but not as simple as it may seem on first consideration. The World Health Organization in 1984 refined its previously idealistic definition ("a state of complete physical, mental and social well-being") to the less ambitious "extent to which an individual or group is able to realize aspirations and satisfy needs and to change or cope with the environment. Health is a resource for everyday life, not the objective of living; it is a positive concept, emphasizing social and personal resources, as well as physical capacities" [28]. From a more practical and succinct standpoint the US Healthy People 2020 proposes a goal of "high-quality, longer lives free of preventable disease, disability, injury and premature death" [29] toward which recommended efforts targeting environmental, social, and individual lifestyle modifications can be directed. Both documents from which these statements are quoted are referenced to highlight the expert consensus recognition of the requirements of a holistic biopsychosocial scope and also active effort in achieving and maintaining health.

What Is Motivation?

Motivation from a behavioral science standpoint has been defined as "the process whereby goal-directed activities are energized, directed, and sustained" [30]. A more nuanced and pragmatic definition is that motivation is that which tries to explain "why a person in a given situation selects one response over another or makes a given response with great energization or frequency" [31].

Basic to an understanding of human motivation is the recognition that it has to do with achieving goals. We will make the assumption at least for the purposes of this endeavor that all human behavior is purposeful or goal-directed (and therefore motivated); the null hypothesis that some human behavior is without goal or purpose cannot be proven. Goals may be conscious or unconscious, clear or obscure, fixed/constant or dynamic, and despite some basic uniformity across populations and among individuals (e.g., survival goals) they certainly vary perhaps as much as they align. For example, in some societies the well-being of the family or group supersedes that of the individual whereas in others the opposite is true. Moral, religious, and spiritual goals range from primary to background to nonexistent among peoples of the world. This variety stems from both personal factors and cultural ones; an appreciation of biopsychosocial-spiritual diversity is thus paramount to understanding human motivation, and certainly motivation as applied toward unidimensional arenas such as physical, or mental, or relational well-being.

Considerable tension within an individual or relationship may exist as a result of competing or conflicting goals and motivations, sometimes overt but often "under the radar." Consider the following lighthearted example: you are enjoying a thrilling new movie in a packed theater on opening weekend with a group of friends that includes an attractive individual you hope to impress and possibly even pursue a romantic relationship with. Unfortunately you drank three large cups of coffee throughout the day due to fatigue from not sleeping well the night before (due to your anxiety over the outing) and then without thinking also consumed a 32-oz caffeinated soda pop during the first half of the movie. It's now two-thirds of the way through the film and you begin to notice mounting motivation to excuse yourself (biologic drive). *Do I stay or do I go now?* You'd rather not miss what appears to be a pivotal scene approaching, certainly considering the price of admission (curiosity and justice motives). Being of a somewhat reserved and self-conscious personality, you fear the shame of revealing your vulnerability and disrupting your friends and hopeful significant other (embarrassment-avoidance motive). And since you chose seats in the middle of one of the fore aisles, you worry about disrupting strangers on your way out and back in (conflict avoidance motive). *Why doesn't someone else get up and go? Are they all in renal failure?* (social comparison motivation). You figure there's at least 40 more minutes of "high-adrenaline" footage ahead that from personal experience you know will increase your glomerular filtration even more, increasing intravesicular pressure and mercilessly assaulting your fortitude. *I don't think I can do this* (crisis of self-efficacy).

On a more serious note, another example not unfamiliar to many clinicians is the situation where an individual with a chronically painful and functionally limiting ailment (e.g., severe degenerative arthritis of the hip with avascular necrosis of the femoral head) refuses conservative and surgical recommendations owing to a multitude of competing and conflicting motives. The pain is severe and interfering with most axes of life, but fear of both known and unknown risks of the operation—possibly amplified by previous surgical experience or the stories of others—is overwhelming. Refusal to engage in physical therapy due to a combination of pain-avoidance and ignorance of symptomatic (and overall health) benefit sabotage improvement. Neglect of lifestyle modifications (dietary improvement/weight loss and regular exercise, counseling for moderate depression) stem from inertia or laziness, lack of self-efficacy, or a habit of defeatism. Secondary gain motives may cloud the picture as well; physical improvement might result in loss of disability status and welfare subsidization, or cessation of opioid prescriptions that the patient is dependent on personally, or which may be undergoing diversion for economic or dysfunctional/abusive relationship preservation reasons. *My doctor told me that my alcohol consumption is worsening the condition, but it's the only stress relief I have.*

In light of this complexity then, the two questions we are considering in this discussion (why isn't the pursuit of health a universally primary goal, and why doesn't the experience of pain drive more people to improve their health) become less apropos human existence though they remain pertinent to the purpose of this effort, namely preoperative optimization as demonstrated through the remainder of the book.

Core Elements of Motivation

Despite the tremendous variability of human motivation and the factors that influence it, which we touch on briefly in the section that follows, there are some underlying fundamental elements that serve as a logical starting point for an exploration of principles and theories of goal-directed behavior. The distinction between the two headings is somewhat nebulous; one of the most consistent and universal features of human motivation is its heterogeneity. The categorization of topics is accordingly somewhat arbitrary; the hierarchy of needs—all about plurality of motives—is presented in this section on commonalities, while self-efficacy, held by many to be a cardinal feature of goal-directed activity, appears in the following section on variability. Nonetheless, they are presented in an arrangement hoped to optimally inform our efforts to assist our patients in choosing a course of action that reflects their best interest, respecting their autonomy while increasing their knowledge, competence, and hopefully motivation.

Motivation as Drive Reduction

Motivation science began in earnest in the early 1900s within the behaviorist tradition, investigating learning and reinforcement phenomena in animal models. Prior to this, motivational analysis lay predominantly within the province of philosophy and religion, both largely dismissed and forgotten over the past century in the modern quest for objectively verifiable explanations—arguably to our detriment both in terms of understanding and application. The behaviorists, both classical and Skinnerian looked at all animate behavior as a conditioned response to either reward or punishment, disregarding psychosocial and spiritual dimensions in their attempt to explain and even predict human actions.

The behaviorist camp held sway over at least academic views on motivation for roughly three decades during the middle part of the 20th century. Representative of this approach, eminent research psychologists Hull and his protégé Spence elaborated a drive reduction theory proposing that responses to stimuli were programmed when they satisfied a basic biologic need perception or drive (e.g., hunger, thirst, sexual arousal) [32]. Originally formulated as an explanation for learning, it was subsequently expanded to propose universal prediction of motivation and behavior. Its ultimate failure to achieve unifying theory status is retrospectively obvious given its disregard for higher cognitive, emotional, social, and spiritual factors [33]. Overwhelming evidence and new theories grounded in the "Cognitive Revolution" beginning in the 1960s led for the most part to the abandonment of this overly simplistic and reductionist model. Curiosity

[34], vicarious learning (learning and alteration of behavior by hearing from or observing others, as opposed to enactive or experiential learning) [35], and social and spiritual modulation of behavior [36], among other phenomena, are unexplainable by the programming paradigm of the behaviorists.

Nonetheless, some useful insights (especially as pertains to habit, the subject of the next chapter) may be gleaned from this camp, and an expansion of the basic concept of drive reduction theory beyond the simple biologic arena increases its applicability and utility. For example, the reduction of anxiety, whether situational or existential seems to demand or at least motivate an increasingly prominent allocation of personal resources in our modern developed society. While seemingly extraneous at first glance, the relief of boredom may be construed as an attempt to mitigate *angst* [37] and in and of itself may thus be considered a primary driver for many [38]. Transcending death and meaninglessness is argued to underlie a host of otherwise seemingly disparate motives [39, 40] and to that end entertainment, achievement, socialization, or isolation, and chemical coping, to name a few, have become preeminent goals for many—frequently trumping the pursuit of health and wellness.

And so drive reduction, at least in its larger context including psychosocial needs, provides many possible avenues of addressing our two questions (Why isn't the pursuit of health a universal drive, and Why doesn't the experience of pain drive more people to improve their health?) While it seems cardinal to those of us in healthcare and human services that health and its multifaceted benefits should theoretically result in numerous drive reductions—including the mitigation of pain, and anxiolysis—it is increasingly neglected. This may be due to simple ignorance, lack of absolute or relative incentive salience, and fatigue among other issues—especially in the face of multiple goals competing for our limited resources and energy. "Delay discounting"—a phenomenon discussed in greater detail later—posits that for most humans, motivation is stronger when tied to a proximal goal, and unfortunately the long-term (or even short-term) benefits of health are often overshadowed by more pressing drives.

Neurobiology and Motivation

Recent advances in the biological sciences have yielded insights into the interface between the functions of various brain regions and some of the more universal basic aspects of goal pursuit. Motivation requires an incentive with some degree of benefit (no matter how proximate or abstract) that may be instinctive or learned. The desirability (not necessarily equivalent to likability) [41] of a goal and the reinforcement of activities designed to achieve it seem to be associated with several interactions between midbrain (e.g., ventral tegmental area, substantia nigra), deep forebrain (e.g., striatum, nucleus accumbens, amygdala, hypothalamus) and neocortical (e.g., anterior cingulate and prefrontal cortices) structures [42] as well as the hormonal/endocrine system [43]. The neurotransmitter dopamine has been viewed as central to the processes of assigning valence and salience to both innate goals (satisfaction of biologic drives) and acquired ones (psychosocial satisfaction, drug use). Its exact role is contentious, and no longer held to be the final reward currency in the hedonic/mesolimbic pathway, but rather a marker registering learning traces in the striatum (and other areas such as the nucleus accumbens) in response to differences between predicted and experienced reward [44, 45]. While complex beyond the scope of this book, suffice it to say that the role of dopamine in motivation seems to involve the reinforcement of processes that increase the congruence between anticipated and received reward, and encourage adaptation of behavior to maximize the likelihood of a desired outcome.

Again, many phenomena (e.g., curiosity and interest, abstract intellectual or self-development goals, delayed gratification capacity) are not explained by what we can discern about neurotransmission and synaptic plasticity. Nonetheless, recognition of the biologic within the biopsychosocial-spiritual is certainly important (albeit not likely to be overlooked in our modern scientific climate) both philosophically and practically, as methods of harnessing and directing cognitive and behavioral improvement efforts may be better informed by our advancing knowledge in this arena.

Plurality of Motives

Even within early drive theory and other behavioral learning paradigms, the existence of multiple cooperative, competing, or conflicting goals was recognized. The clearest and most persistent explication, however, of this diversity was proposed as a response by Abraham Maslow to what he deemed an overly simplistic and animal-based conditioning view of motivation and behavior. His enduring hierarchy of needs theory [46] outlines a progression of successive tiers of needs or motivators portrayed as a pyramid, with more basic/primal needs and goals occupying lower levels and more advanced and abstract ones occupying higher levels (Figure 3.2). At the base are what he labeled physiological needs, which if unmet will "dominate the organism" to the exclusion of higher-tier needs until they are met, in which case the individual then turns their conscious or subconscious attention sequentially to safety, love, esteem, and finally self-actualization pursuits.

Maslow allows that the ordering of tiers is not inviolable but rather a generalization. Obvious and striking examples of exceptions to his hierarchy

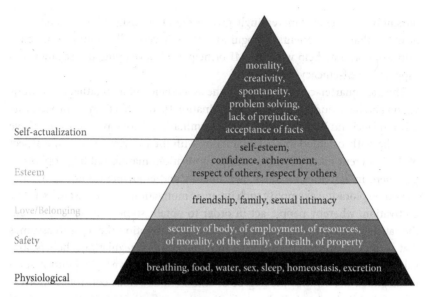

morality,
creativity,
spontaneity,
problem solving,
lack of prejudice,
acceptance of facts

self-esteem,
confidence, achievement,
respect of others, respect by others

friendship, family, sexual intimacy

security of body, of employment, of resources,
of morality, of the family, of health, of property

breathing, food, water, sex, sleep, homeostasis, excretion

Self-actualization

Esteem

Love/Belonging

Safety

Physiological

Figure 3.2. Maslow's Hierarchy of Needs
By J. Finkelstein—CC BY-SA 3.0, https://commons.wikimedia.org/w/index.php?curid=1315147

include martyrs, prisoners of war, or individuals choosing to remain in abusive relationships subjugating safety or physiological needs to higher psychosocial or spiritual ones. The theory is not all-encompassing, and as he recognizes, there are other behavioral determinants, a dramatic example of which he does not discuss being the compulsion engendered by addiction to engage in behaviors clearly harmful in all five tiers.

Nonetheless, his construct provides considerable insight into the indisputable phenomenon of multiple goals that may be complementary, competing in a "prepotent" hierarchy, or in some cases flat-out contradictory. The evident answers to the two questions at the heart of this discussion (Why don't more people prioritize their health, and Why doesn't the experience of pain lead more people to improve their health?) are better understood in view of the fact that for many the relative salience of health falls below that of comfort and convenience, or other pursuits (e.g., job promotion, diversion).

Of particular interest to these authors is the fact that Maslow does not address reduction or elimination of pain as a need or motivator; this notable absence (contrasted to today's priorities) may serve as either an indicator of increasing prevalence or diagnosis in this country over the past several decades, or a sociological shift in the importance assigned to pain. One also wonders if he would have assigned pain avoidance to the category of physiological need or a higher tier. At any rate, culturally today the importance assigned to the short-term pursuit of pain relief is increasingly greater than that assigned to the pursuit of health; enhancing patients' recognition of such generally counterproductive prioritization may help with the MI principles of developing discrepancy and supporting self-efficacy.

The past quarter-century has seen the ascendancy of a metatheory of motivation and behavior termed self-determination theory (SDT) by its progenitors Edward Deci and Richard Ryan. Self-determination theory assumes that people are inherently oriented toward interacting with their environment. One aspect of this inherent motivation is intrinsic motivation, manifested by people's engagement in activities for their own interest and enjoyment. Play, sport, and curious exploration exemplify such intrinsic motivation, in contrast to extrinsic motivation, whereby people act in order to obtain some end separable from the satisfactions of acting per se [47]. Self-determination theory also assumes that people are inherently prone to internalize social regulations, beliefs, and values into their own schema, and the extent to which this external information is integrated determines the degree of autonomous versus controlled motivation of their behavior. Self-determination theory further posits three cardinal psychological needs of autonomy, competence, and relatedness, which serve as the ultimate goals that underlie human activity. Autonomy and competence are self-explanatory, and refer to the willingness and capability of decisions and actions performed by an individual, respectively. People who are *autonomously* motivated are more likely to enjoy that behavior and persist in the absence of direct external motivators, whereas when the latter serves as the only driver, individuals are likely to persist at a behavior only as long as the external reinforcement continues, and holds sway. Relatedness refers to the complex social motive of positive feedback from others that enhances both self-esteem and connectedness, which serves as a goal unto itself. People are more likely to internalize goals and values transmitted by people with whom they experience relatedness.

Research has shown that these three needs (autonomy, competence, relatedness) are universally important for motivation and wellness across ages, cultures, and socioeconomic strata [48–50] and that humans are most likely to volitionally engage in (and sustain) behaviors that satisfy these three needs. In the context of health behavior, tailoring interventions to enhancement of these needs has been shown in multiple contexts to result in a greater degree of sustained positive change including smoking cessation, dietary improvement, increased physical activity, adherence to medical treatment, and so forth [50–52].

There is a great deal of obvious overlap between the theoretical framework of SDT and the practical process of MI, and the literature increasingly supports the association and alliance of these two recent constructs [53, 54]. It appears that successful enhancement of patients' sense of autonomy, empowering them to decide and maintain a course of action they feel to be in their best interest is the most effective means of helping people change behaviors [55]. Cultivation of such an atmosphere respecting (and harnessing) self-determination is of the essence in any attempt to improve health behavior, including those made in the perioperative setting.

Variability of Motivation

While a grasp of fundamental and universal tenets of motivation (such as we understand them) is important to the healthcare provider or caregiver invested in helping their patient, recognizing, respecting—and leveraging—differences between "what makes people tick" is arguably even more important. This section begins with a survey of pertinent interpersonal trait variance influencing the what, why, and how of people's goal pursuits. We examine this briefly from a biopsychosocial-spiritual perspective, no dimension of which exists in isolation from the others.

We then switch gears and examine dynamic intrapersonal factors that vary within the individual over both the short and long term. What we hope and purpose to do, as well as our fidelity to those intentions often waxes and wanes from morning to evening, in proximity to January 1, and in different stages of life. These short-term fluctuations and longer-term malleability are also influenced by inseparable biopsychosocial-spiritual factors, which are also fluid. Our knowledge base, belief system/worldview, priorities, self-efficacy, organizational abilities, capacity for delayed gratification, and so on, are mutable, with self-development and growth (or regression) being one of the defining features of humanity. Recognition of this multifactorial inconstancy is critical to efforts on the part of both patient and provider to improve health behavior.

Interpersonal Variability

Though every human being is unique at many levels, from a large scale, "wide-angle" perspective, somatic phenotypes have been used since the dawn of our existence to categorize people (e.g., by gender, race, body mass index, physical/athletic prowess and so forth). Psychosocial categories have been applied in every civilization as well throughout recorded history (e.g., sanguine, choleric, melancholic, phlegmatic), and so too have ethical/moral and religious categories. This systemization helps to make sense out of our heterogeneity and facilitate the analysis of associations between commonly acknowledged differences and outcome variables of interest. Similarly, while innumerable goals and motives exist among individuals at "high-resolution," lumping them together into big-picture groupings such as Maslow's tiers affords the opportunity to draw rough inferences from observation and experiment. In similar fashion, motivational trait (a quality relatively stable over time) categorization has been proposed, with various schema interdigitating with singular or combined biopsychosocial-spiritual axes [56, 57].

Biological

No one is an island, and biological behaviors and motivations are not independent of psychological and spiritual underpinnings; furthermore unless one lives alone on a deserted island there are confounding social influences and ramifications. Attempting to tease out strands for the sake of component categorization is artificial and frustrating at best, yet as with all such exercises, organization is essential for meaningful analysis, and thus we will start with the most basic/primal arena of physiology.

Perhaps the purest such "biological stratification" of motivation is that of age, and yet again, such arrangement is not without inherent connectivity to other dimensions of personhood. For example, goal-pursuit skills including tactical and strategic thought, concentration, resilience, and many more psychological factors generally follow a timeline of development. Nonetheless there are some frequently observed and generally consistent motivational differences between the arbitrary categories of young versus old, that seem to be best explained by phase of life and perspective, such as gain promotion versus loss prevention [58]. The young exist in a state of potential yet generally possess few resources and have achieved fewer goals; as such, the accumulation of material goods, a mate and family, a career, and so on, tends to dominate their pursuit. The old on the other hand more often tend to have accomplished many of these fairly ubiquitous objectives and focus on maintenance and avoiding attrition [59]. A piercing observation with direct relevance to the overall theme of health behavior (often evidently erroneously attributed [60] to the Dalai Lama) sums it up well: "Man . . . sacrifices his health in order to make money. Then he sacrifices money to recuperate his health."

Another difference that appears to correlate with age is extrinsic (or controlled, to use the language of SDT discussed previously) versus intrinsic (or autonomous in SDT parlance) motivation, with apparent shift toward the latter over time and with maturation [58, 59, 61].

Tailoring motivational enhancement to different age groups is thus theoretically sensible, with a more directive and growth/building focus presented to the young, in contrast to a more nuanced evocative and maintenance/loss-prevention approach to the elderly.

Psychological

This vast and perhaps best-studied arena in terms of motivation is not independent from physiologic needs and wants, nor certainly social and spiritual incentives. In other words as with any of the other dimensions, an isolated analysis is artificial, albeit useful to a degree in clarifying component effects.

Cognition is not separate from emotion in human experience and both are influenced by underlying personality traits. Again, an attempt to analyze "pure" cognitive determinants apart from these other psychological variables is essentially impossible in practice, nonetheless we briefly discuss the apparent association (or lack thereof) of trait cognitive function with health behavior and outcomes. Higher intelligence quotient (IQ) has been shown to predict increased health behavior performance and outcome measures in some studies [62, 63], while others have shown little to no effect [64] or subset effect, namely executive function [65–67]. From a more short-term/therapeutic perspective, individual cognitive (and emotional) process fluidity certainly contributes to motivational dynamic, and this is discussed in greater detail in the intrapersonal variability section later.

From a trait/dispositional standpoint, numerous multipolar schema exist, but within this discussion we only consider two personality theories that have been studied extensively in relation to health behavior (and apparent motivation) and outcomes, and that show reasonable if not good predictive value.

The first theory considered comes from the self-regulatory school of thought, and classifies people according to promotion versus prevention orientation [68, 69]. Promoters are characterized by an eager pursuit of "making good things happen," with a gain or happiness focus. Preventers are marked by a more cautious and vigilant guarding against adverse outcomes, as the term implies. Promoters tend to be explorers, whereas preventers are more likely to remain committed to a course of action or the status quo. Given their strong achievement focus, preventers are motivated and energized by success, and paralyzed by failure; conversely preventers do not seek high-yield (and high-risk) situations, but are more apt to be galvanized by failure into stronger efforts. Promoters are more vulnerable to depression, whereas preventers are more vulnerable to anxiety [69]. While a given individual almost always possesses and uses qualities and strategies of each system, an overall alignment toward one or the other is typical [68, 70]. Again, the orientation is not independent of social influence and in fact has been strongly linked to nurturance and advancement/accomplishment-focused upbringing in the case of promoters versus security and duty/responsibility-focused upbringing in the case of preventers [71, 72].

From a health behavior standpoint, promoters tend to more readily meet challenges of behavioral alteration (e.g., smoking cessation, weight loss) [73, 74] yet paradoxically have more difficulty tuning out and refusing pleasurable distractors or risky behaviors [75, 76]. Preventers on the other hand are more apt to pursue health maintenance behaviors (e.g., preventive medicine screenings, etc.) and to sustain change (including smoking cessation, dietary modification) once initiated [74, 75, 77].

The widely adopted five factor model of personality ("The Big Five") has perhaps been studied even more in relation to health behavior (and numerous other disciplines). The theory categorizes five overarching personality traits: openness (curiosity, preference for novelty), conscientiousness (goal-orientation, self-discipline, and perseverance), surgency (extraversion), agreeableness (sympathy and compassion, trust and cooperation), and neuroticism (emotional instability with a tendency to experience negative emotions more readily) [78, 79]. Conscientiousness has been shown in numerous investigations to correlate with higher levels of healthy behaviors and outcomes [64, 80, 81] and in experimental studies including a placebo intervention, conscientious adherents to placebo had outcomes comparable to the treatment group [82] suggesting potentially higher predictive value for the trait than a specific behavior. Conversely, neuroticism is associated with notably worse health behavior and outcomes [64, 83] and the more recent construct of the "Type D personality" (high negative affect proclivity combined with social inhibition), which correlates strongly with positive neuroticism/negative conscientiousness scores also showing significant and widespread health behavior deficits and adverse outcomes [84].

The infinite complexity and diversity of human psyche renders tailoring motivational enhancement accordingly a difficult prospect at best. While formal psychological analysis within a multidisciplinary team setting is certainly the gold standard and will provide exponentially better results, in many cases this will not be possible. It is thus incumbent on every clinician interested in cultivating improved health behavior among their patient population to recognize that at every step of contemplation, preparation, action, maintenance, and so forth, in addition to highly dynamic psychological incentives, facilitators, and obstacles (including their degree of self-efficacy, considered in the next section) there are also more entrenched basic personality and other cognitive issues that interface with both initiation and continuation of change. Aligning education/coaching with these varying phenotypes will only help facilitate the core psychological needs of autonomy and competence that are highly predictive of both initiation and maintenance of change [52].

Social
Human association provides a vast opportunity for motivational variability, as unlimited as the degree of affection versus enmity. From the standpoint of the individual, relationship to another may elicit competitive or collaborative goals, encouragement or discouragement, enhancement, distraction, or

reprioritization of goals. A considerable body of evidence as well as the common human experience confirms that socialization itself is a basic human goal and need in its own right [85, with deprivation predictive of morbidity and mortality [86, 87]. Self-determination theory, introduced briefly earlier, is arguably the most widely researched and validated motivational and behavioral paradigm in use today, with core constructs comprising or at least inseparable from social factors. The autonomous versus controlled behavior (and intrinsic vs. extrinsic motivation) dichotomy requires a relational or at least associative context, competence is judged by most by way of comparison and feedback, and finally relatedness is nothing but social.

Most social determinants of motivation at least in our fast-paced day appear to be dynamic ones involving peers, media, teachers, bosses, healthcare providers, and others. Furthermore, with the advent of the Internet and social media, we are inundated with unprecedented information availability (overload?) and transfer, with integrated network effect yielding the potential for cognitive and behavioral sway on a scale heretofore unseen [88, 89]. This section, however, is about more concrete and entrenched influences of family of origin, socioeconomic status, culture, and religion that pose significant and likely less malleable effects. All of these have been shown in numerous investigations to influence health behaviors in a profound manner [27, 81, 90–92]. From the standpoint of the sociocultural milieu, economic and other disparities frequently correlate with poor health-behavior modeling and lack of resources, and such an environment (where long-term health goals are generally subjugated to sometimes daily survival concerns) often results in profound "imprinting" that can be difficult to modify.

From the outset of our lives we learn from observing others [35, 93]. In early/ formative life the choice of those models (e.g., parents, siblings, teachers) is outside of our control. As within most axes of life, the imprint of early nurture (or lack thereof) is profound, and family health behaviors or interventions have a strong and sustained effect on the health behaviors of offspring [94–96]. The interrelated influence of culture has also been increasingly studied, with variance of "expectations, norms and sanctions" representing the majority of proposed mediating effects on health behaviors [97].

As we mature we increasingly seek out (or at least desire to) the company of those whose attributes we appreciate or whom we perceive benefit us. At any rate, comparison of oneself to a peer group, either self-selected or assigned (e.g., in the classroom) or to role models often serves as a powerful motivator for adopting behavioral change by way of imitation, with conscious attempts at maximizing a sense of social identity and congruence with group norms [27]. Accountability is a related but distinct social influence on behavior whereby expected interaction and evaluation is intended to improve effort and adherence to a goal or plan

[98]. Such arrangement may be highly formalized (and correspondingly often controlled) such as in a military or business setting, or informal (and generally more autonomous), such as a shared interest group.

A variety of social goals may motivate health behavior, and they certainly may metamorphose over the lifespan. The desire for self-esteem or external validation may drive one toward dieting and exercise, with aesthetics and interpersonal feedback, or achievements and trophies as the currency. As noted earlier, socialization is a motivation unto itself, and any number of activities whether beneficial or harmful may be adopted simply for the sake of friendship, belonging to a certain group, or love. With personal growth and development often comes a desire to improve one's health (including psychosocial health) for the sake of others' welfare and ensuring the ability to care for loved ones or interact with them in their activities.

Perhaps more often, however, the effect of social factors on health (or unhealthy) behaviors are unconscious or subconscious, and there is evidence [99, 100] supported by common experience that the relative contribution of cognitive and deliberate processes pales in comparison to that of habits or other impulsive/emotional drivers [101], which are much more likely to be elicited by social cues. Smoking, snacking, and so on, are often indulgences performed impulsively or compulsively under the influence of one's crowd, or even perfect strangers.

The impact of social factors on behavior is difficult to overstate, and it behooves clinicians to seek to understand and use these complex dynamics in motivational enhancement, both in terms of undergirding the therapeutic relationship with self-determination enhancement and accountability (which are not mutually exclusive), and in enlisting reinforcing alliances from the individual's network. It must also be remembered that for many, reshaping health behaviors requires reshaping one's place in culture and community, when that environment fosters and perpetuates disease-promoting behaviors.

Spiritual
Spiritual motivation (incorporating religious, moral, and ethical components for the purposes of this discussion) must be considered separately from psychosocial in that its primary object has to do with the Divine/transcendent; other entities including human beings and animals, and material goods are certainly relevant to and interconnected with spirituality but are secondary objects. A discussion of metaphysical/transcendent and religious factors (and related sociocultural influences) is beyond the scope of this book but merits consideration within any effort to apply a biopsychosocial framework to human behavior; history bears witness to the profound impact and even world-changing power of these issues on society, let alone the individual.

Moral and ethical influences on motivation have historically been the province of philosophers and religious leaders; nonetheless the underlying issues of right and wrong, virtuous versus dissolute behavior are intricately involved in the majority of peoples' choices and habits (in creed if not practice.)

Religiosity and spirituality appear in many studies to correlate with improved health metrics, reduced morbidity/mortality and longer lifespan [102–106], and this association is likely multifactorial with direct effects on physiology [107] and improved coping with disease [108, 109] but also, more germane to this discussion, via effects on adherence to health behavior [110–112].

Most organized religions are heavily focused on the exercise of the will in self-denial, the pursuit of personal virtue, and contribution to societal good. As such, we consider the phenomenon of willpower within this section. Willpower is a multidimensional construct clearly linked to psychological state but mutable in response to perturbations in other dimensions (e.g., diminished by physical duress; augmented by social reinforcements). The null hypothesis of no relationship between spiritual influences and willpower cannot be proven, and evidence from essentially every society throughout history supports the association.

Willpower is intricately linked with motivation in popular thought and frequently (and oversimplistically) considered to be a highly stable trait, and furthermore an "all-or-none" quality. In point of fact, willpower is a phenomenon with considerable process-specific (let alone goal-specific) interpersonal differences in expression. For example, as discussed in the psychology section, promoters might be described as excelling in moxie pertaining to new challenges and endeavors while more frequently lacking in persistence. Conversely, preventers tend to excel in grit and perseverance (more often associated with "willpower"). Nor is willpower a constant phenomenon within the individual even as pertains to a specific motivation, as we all know from personal experience; this is examined further in the next section.

A distinct but related phenomenon is the capacity to tolerate delayed gratification; this is also considered within this section, as it is a frequently defining component of many religions' practices and may be enhanced by certain religious or spiritual commitment [113, 114]. Delay discounting describes the reduced salience of reward that is temporally distant; correlating with impulsivity, this characteristic is associated with reduced health behaviors in virtually all arenas including poor diet, lack of exercise, nonadherence to medical treatment, substance use, risky sexual behaviors, and so forth [115–122].

Understanding an individual's spiritual and religious leanings and commitment is obviously an essential component of a biopsychosocial-spiritual approach, and particularly relevant in the arena of chronic disease or symptom management. While discussion of these matters has been generally avoided within medicine in the modern era for a number of reasons; we have found that use of the MI approach in discussing spirituality and religion, with open-ended questions, reflective listening, and respect for autonomy to be widely accepted by patients and frequently beneficial in enhancing motivation for healthy change.

Intrapersonal Variability

In this section, we change our perspective from a dimensional (biopsychosocial-spiritual) and interpersonal analysis to a situational and intrapersonal one. The axes are not at all exclusive; rather they display considerable overlap (e.g., biologic drive with incentive salience, psychosocial milieu with self-efficacy and regulation); nonetheless, for organizational purposes we have chosen to consider the following topics within this final section.

A given individual will experience inconstancy in goals and motivation from minute to day to year. In considering the dynamic nature of intrapersonal motivational variability it is worth stepping back and viewing the playing field, so to speak. Many factors and processes inherent to our existence and well-being are autonomic and outside of our control for practical purposes (e.g., genetics, the Krebs cycle, breathing.) Many others, however (e.g., eating, movement), are much more dependent on choice and the exercise of will, and subject to self-regulation. Motivation is of course more relevant to these activities that we can influence, and assumes a degree of control over process. It has to do with assigning significance and allocating resources toward a goal, or in more colloquial terms, intent and follow-through. Both of these are subject to fluctuation. Motivational variance in any context but certainly in terms of health behaviors may be affected by a number of different and interrelated factors including but not limited to:

- Incentive salience of the goal
- Perception of attainability of/proximity to the goal
- Resources/reserve

These factors are subject to both short- and long-term variability in their own right.

Incentive Salience and Related Factors

Most frequently discussed in the addiction field, the concept of incentive salience describes the desirability and attractiveness of a goal. It is that which captures and maintains attention, induces approach, and sustains effort. From the perspective of neurobiology, motivation is generally seen as the conditioned pursuit of reward or the avoidance of perceived harms, mediated by various structures such as the mesolimbic system and the neocortex. Biologically, the desirability of the goal is established by short-term neurotransmitter flux and longer-term synaptic plasticity; essentially by experiential learning.

Relative desirability/salience of the goal is of course affected by competing biologic or comfort drives. Again borrowing Maslow's construct, survival and love/belonging needs seem to exert dominance over esteem and self-actualization ones in terms of prioritization of pursuit, with deprivation of lower-tier needs accordingly exerting more dynamic influence on behavior. One's intention to exercise may be compromised by discomfort or pain, and study or task plans may be disrupted by a more acutely felt desire for socialization.

From a cognitive perspective, in the context of volitional behaviors (as opposed to autonomic processes) there must first be awareness of the goal in order for there to be desirability or pursuit. While awareness of some goals, whether positive (approach goals) or negative (avoidance goals) is stumbled into experientially, that of others (especially in a more developed society) is transmitted by an educational process. Education and the assimilation of new beliefs or values can alter motives, for example, alteration of diet or initiation of an exercise routine based on classes, or religious conversion, either positively (enhancement) or negatively (suppression). And yet unidimensional appeals to logic or abstract benefits seem to motivate the minority.

Emotions constitute one of the least understood or agreed on phenomena central to the human experience, and yet one that permeates nearly every aspect and minute of our lives. The relationship of emotion and motivation is vast (etymologically both share the Latin root "to move") and beyond the scope of this discussion; suffice it to say that direction of attention and expenditure of effort toward a goal (either approach or avoidance) have to do with how desirable the goal is, and that strength of attraction or repulsion is best measured in affective terms [123, 124]. As Caroll Izard, one of the preeminent research psychologists in the field of emotion, puts it, "Emotions . . . largely determine the contents and focus of consciousness throughout the life span. . . . Emotion feelings constitute the primary motivational component of mental operations and overt behavior" [125].

In terms of the variability of motivation, emotion plays a significant role both over the short term and the duration. From a moment-by-moment standpoint, emotions energize a more rapid (even impulsive) redirecting of perception, attention, and reaction [126–128.] While this undeniably profound impact on behavior may influence health behavior more frequently (e.g., anxiety leading to overeating or smoking) it is the interaction between emotion and cognitive learning [129, 130] leading to long-term, sustained change efforts that interest us. Educators at every level understand that strong emotional valence increases interest and persistence of learning effort, as well as memory and recall [131, 132]. Sustainability of change is much greater when reinforced by positive emotional reward, and especially when that reward is perceived early in the process of change [27, 133–135].

While we agree that increasing the emotional content of health education yields increased participatory dividends on the part of the learner, our experience in terms of trying to educate our chronic pain patient populace about the association between poor health maintenance and pain (arguably one of the most poignant stimuli we experience) has been frequently disappointing. Other emotionally laden incentives, for example, the well-being of loved ones, often seem similarly impotent in eliciting change. If these highly salient issues do not spur one to improve their health, to what then do we appeal? Understanding the complexities of self-determination factors as discussed previously, as well as self-efficacy, self-regulation of competing interests and resource management, ego depletion, and perhaps most importantly habit (the subject of next chapter) are crucial to effective motivational enhancement.

Self-Efficacy and Self-Regulation

Wanting to do something, or assent to the proposition that it is in one's best interest is not the same as believing one can, let alone committing to the course of action. Self-efficacy (SE), the confidence that the attainability of a goal lies within the power of the individual [136], is a major determinant affecting motivation often considered a trait-level "predictor variable." It is considered here, however, at the level of an intrapersonal factor, as it is dynamic within a given individual and may be augmented by success and encouragement, or diminished by failure and censure. Such waxing and waning may occur generally within the person's psyche over time, or more specifically within the context of the pursuit of a given objective. Self-efficacy furthermore is not a global characteristic but rather a "domain-specific" one with poor correlation between different objectives [137], for example, regulating diet versus smoking. Self-efficacy has also been shown to be more correlative of behavior initiation than maintenance [81, 137]. This is not to say that SE is not important in developing sustained behaviors; on the contrary, positive feedback and reinforcement of competence are generally essential to continued effort, and of course maintenance does not occur without initiation.

As represented graphically in Figure 3.3, SE is a key component of the health belief model (HBM), which is the most established framework for predicting an individual's likelihood of participating in a health behavior. The original HBM

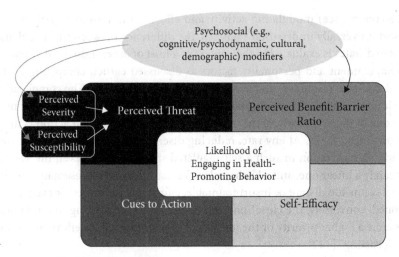

Figure 3.3. Health Belief Model

as conceived in the 1950s did not include the concept of SE among its predictor variables, but over the next few decades it became evident to the model's creators that SE has tremendous interaction not only with the magnitude of control in overcoming perceived barriers, but also with both perceived outcome benefit [138, 139]. The more likely a person believes themselves capable of influencing a desired outcome, the more likely they are to attempt and maintain effort, and as such, tailoring objectives to their confidence level is of the essence. Other tactics advisable in any situation but certainly in the perioperative period (which may predispose to a more passive mindset) include rehearsing desired behavior in situations where SE may be low, relaxation training to combat situational anxiety in the behavior change process, and encouragement/verbal reinforcement of efficacy [138].

Closely related to SE and strongly influenced by the construct [140] is the superfamily of theories labeled self-regulatory theory (SRT). Self-regulatory theory considers not only the attainability and proximity of a specific goal and how these factors influence motivation, but also how goal-directed behavior is influenced by obstacles and temptations to modify or abandon the behavior in question, and also by conflict between competing goals.

One of the underlying assumptions in most SRT is the idea of homeostasis as applied to effort. Borrowing from the engineering world, the complex phenomenon of human motivation has been compared to a cybernetic control system [141, 142]. The key concept here is that of a feedback loop, where outcomes are constantly being monitored and compared to a goal, with discrepancy (or congruence) modulating activity and effort; a thermostat is perhaps the most universally understood example. The difference between the actual and desired states is evaluated in the context of a host of other individual variables (temperament and personality factors as discussed earlier, competing goals, and available resources) and behavior is altered accordingly. The complexities of human motivation are not reducible to a formula, and health behavior may be one of the arenas where the incongruity between intent and action is most pronounced [140]. At any rate, reducing discrepancy is theoretically the underlying motivation in such a self-regulated state [143]; however, the system is rarely a linear one, and a U-shaped curve may be more representative. If the goal seems too distant or insurmountable, effort may be limited or even abandoned; conversely, the closer one gets to the target, competing interests may assume a higher priority or the individual may simply reduce effort and resort to "coasting" [142].

Resources and Ego Depletion

One of the more profound factors affecting motivation is resource levels. Humans do not possess unlimited willpower. Physical and emotional fatigue from a host of sources including illness state or increased stress can radically diminish the salience and pursuit of most goals, certainly one with apparently significant delay discounting (remote benefit) such as health maintenance. The pursuit of health—physical, psychological, relational/societal and spiritual—requires a degree of effort exceeding that of many simpler pursuits such as sitting down to watch a movie or eating a bowl of ice cream. A trade-off, or sacrifice is required that presumably incorporates several intertwined conscious and subconscious processes including exercise of willpower and tolerance of delayed gratification, self-regulation, and a host of social inputs.

"Ego depletion," a concept arising from observations of the attenuating effects of persistent self-control efforts in one arena (e.g., dieting) on another (e.g., concentration, emotional regulation, ethical behavior) [144, 145] posits essentially that the more things we try to restrict or manage, the quicker we wear ourselves out.

Conversely, rejuvenation/replenishment of glucose stores, sleep, emotional well-being, and so forth, frequently has salutary effects on our ability to persevere in our various aims. And in contrast to ego depletion, the practice (and habit formation) of self-control may in fact result in reduced resistance. This may be due to increasing reserve, "like a muscle" [146], or due to adoption of a new hedonic goal of self-esteem, and so forth, from repetitive success [147].

The Effect of Chronic Pain on Motivation

Chronic pain has the potential to exert deleterious effects on all four dimensions of a person's well-being (biological, psychological, social, and spiritual) and alter motivation accordingly. Again, few things get people's attention quite like pain does, and reprioritization of needs and goals, and resource depletion from the struggle to avoid or reduce painful stimuli often overwhelm any desire or effort to improve (biopsychosocial-spiritual) health.

The skillful clinician will try to appeal to cognitive and emotional bases to enlist initiation and facilitate maintenance of health behavior in the face of such opposition, tailoring both information transfer and prescription as well as motivational evocation according to where the patient is from a multidimensional standpoint. No matter where that may be, the ability to communicate understanding and express both insight and empathy facilitates rapport, and with that as noted earlier, increased effort and adherence.

References

1   Bauer UE, Briss PA, Goodman RA, Bowman BA. Prevention of chronic disease in the 21st century: elimination of the leading preventable causes of premature death and disability in the USA. Lancet. 2014;384:45–52.

2   Shi Y, Weingarten TN, Mantilla CB et al. Smoking and pain: pathophysiology and clinical implications. Anesthesiology. 2010;113:977–92.

3   Varrassi G, Fusco M, Skaper SD, et al. A pharmacological rationale to reduce the incidence of opioid induced tolerance and hyperalgesia: a review. Pain Ther. March 28, 2018. doi:10.1007/s40122-018-0094-9.

4   Arranz LI, Rafecas M, Alegre C. Effects of obesity on function and quality of life in chronic pain conditions. Curr Rheumatol Rep. 2014;16(1):390. doi:10.1007/s11926-013-0390-7.

5   Higgins DM, Buta E, Dorflinger L, et al. Prevalence and correlates of painful conditions and multimorbidity in national sample of overweight/obese Veterans. J Rehabil Res Dev. 2016;53:71–82.

6   Dean E, Söderlund A. What is the role of lifestyle behaviour change associated with non-communicable disease risk in managing musculoskeletal health conditions with special reference to chronic pain? BMC Musculoskel Disord. 2015;16:87. doi:10.1186/s12891-015-0545-y.

7   Finan PH, Goodin BR, Smith MT. The association of sleep and pain: An update and a path forward. J Pain. 2013; 14:1539–52.

8   Wertli MM, Burgstaller JM, Weiser S, Steurer J, Kofmehl R, Held U. Influence of catastrophizing on treatment outcome in patients with nonspecific low back pain: a systematic review. Spine (Phila Pa 1976). 2014;39:263–73.

9   Tønnesen H, Nielsen PR, Lauritzen JB, Møller AM. Smoking and alcohol intervention before surgery: evidence for best practice. Br J Anaesth. 2009;102:297–306.

10 Wilson JL, Poulin PA, Sikorski R, et al. Opioid use among same-day surgery patients: prevalence, management and outcomes. Pain Res Management. 2015;20:300–304.

11 Darnall BD. Pain psychology and pain catastrophizing in the perioperative setting: a review of impacts, interventions and unmet needs. Hand Clin. 2016;32:33–39.

12 Miller WR, Rollnick S. Motivational Interviewing: Helping People Change. 3rd ed. New York: Guilford Press; 2013.

13 Rollnick S, Miller WR, Butler CC. Motivational Interviewing in Health Care: Helping Patients Change Behavior (Applications of Motivational Interviewing). New York: Guilford Press; 2007.

14 Clifford D, Curtis L. Motivational Interviewing in Nutrition and Fitness. New York: Guilford Press; 2016.

15 Arkowitz H, Westra HA, Miller WR, Rollnick S. Motivational Interviewing in the Treatment of Psychological Problems. 1st ed. (Applications of Motivational Interviewing). New York: Guilford Press; 2007.

16 Prochaska JO, DiClemente CC. Stages and processes of self-change of smoking: toward an integrative model of change. J Consult Clin Psychol. 1983;51:390–5.

17 Prochaska JO, Norcross JC, DiClemente CC. Applying the stages of change. In Koocher GP, Norcross JC, Greene BA, eds., Psychologists' Desk Reference, 3rd ed. New York: Oxford University Press; 2013.

18 Lundahl B, Moleni T, Burke BL, et al. Motivational interviewing in medical care settings: a systematic review and meta-analysis of randomized controlled trials. Patient Educ Couns. 2013; 93:157–68.

19 Lindson-Hawley N, Thompson TP, Begh R. Motivational interviewing for smoking cessation. Cochrane Database Syst Rev. 2015;(3):CD006936. doi:10.1002/14651858.CD006936.pub3.

20 O'Halloran PD, Blackstock F, Shields N, et al. Motivational interviewing to increase physical activity in people with chronic health conditions: a systematic review and meta-analysis. Clin Rehabil. 2014;28:1159–71.

21 Armstrong MJ, Mottershead TA, Ronksley PE, Sigal RJ, Campbell TS, Hemmelgarn BR. Motivational interviewing to improve weight loss in overweight and/or obese patients: a systematic review and meta-analysis of randomized controlled trials. Obes Rev. 2011;12:709–23.

22 Alperstein D, Sharpe L. The efficacy of motivational interviewing in adults with chronic pain: a meta-analysis and systematic review. J Pain. 2016;17:393–403.

23 Rollnick S, Miller WR. What is motivational interviewing? Behav Cognit Psychother. 1995;23:325–34.

24 Horvath AO, Symonds BD. Relation between working alliance and outcome in psychotherapy: A meta-analysis. J Counseling Psychol. 1991; 38: 139–149.

25 Lambert MJ, Barley DE. Research summary on the therapeutic relationship and psychotherapy outcome. In Norcross J, ed., Psychotherapy Relationships That Work: Therapist Contributions and Responsiveness to Patients (pp. 17–32). New York: Oxford University Press; 1999.

26 Moyers TB, Miller WR, Hendrickson SML. How does motivational interviewing work? Therapist interpersonal skill predicts client involvement within motivational interviewing sessions. J Consult Clin Psychol. 2005;73:590–8.

27 Kwasnicka D, Dombrowski SU, White M, Sniehotta F. Theoretical explanations for maintenance of behaviour change: a systematic review of behaviour theories. Health Psychol Rev. 2016;10:277–96.

28 World Health Organization Regional Office for Europe. Health Promotion: a Discussion Document on the Concept and Principles: Summary Report of the Working Group on Concept and Principles of Health Promotion, Copenhagen, July 9–13, 1984. Copenhagen: WHO Regional Office for Europe; 1984.

29 US Department of Health and Human Services, Office of Disease Prevention and Health Promotion. Healthy People 2020. ODPHP Publication No. B0132. https://www.healthypeople.gov/sites/default/files/hp2020_brochure_with_LHI_508_FNL.pdf. Accessed May 26, 2018.

30 Schunk DH, Pintrich PR, Meece JL. Motivation in Education: Theory, Research and Application. 3rd ed. Upper Saddle River, NJ: Pearson Education; 2008.

31 Gollwitzer PM, Oettingen G. Goal pursuit. In Ryan RM, ed., The Oxford Handbook of Human Motivation. New York: Oxford University Press; 2012.

32 Hull C. Principles of Behavior: An Introduction to Behavior Theory. New York: Appleton-Century-Crofts; 1943.

33 White RW. Motivation reconsidered: the concept of competence. Psychol Rev. 1959;66:297–333.

34 Silvia PJ. Curiosity and motivation. In Ryan RM, ed., The Oxford Handbook of Human Motivation. New York: Oxford University Press; 2012.

35 Bandura A. Social Learning Theory. Englewood Cliffs, NJ: Prentice Hall; 1977.

36 Aristotle. Nichomachean Ethics. Translation with Introduction and Commentary by S Broadie and C Rowe. Oxford, UK: Oxford University Press; 2002.

37 Wahl J. Philosophies of Existence: An Introduction to the Basic Thought of Kierkegaard, Heidegger, Jaspers, Marcel, Sartre. Translated by FM Lory. London: Routledge; 1969.

38 Csikszentmihalyi M. Beyond Boredom and Anxiety. San Francisco: Jossey-Bass; 1975.

39 Frankl VE. Man's Search for Meaning. New York: Simon and Schuster; 1963.

40 Kesebir P, Pyszczynski T. The role of death in life: existential aspects of human motivation. In Ryan RM, ed., The Oxford Handbook of Human Motivation. New York: Oxford University Press; 2012.

41 Berridge KC, Robinson TE, Aldridge JW. Dissecting components of reward: "liking," "wanting," and learning. Curr Opin Pharmacol. 2009;9:65–73.

42 Berkman E, Lieberman M. The neuroscience of goal pursuit: Bridging gaps between theory and data. In Moskowitz G, Grant H, eds., The Psychology of Goals (pp. 98–126). New York: Guilford Press; 2009.

43 Powley TL. Hunger. In Berntson GG, Cacioppo TJ, eds., Handbook of Neuroscience for the Behavioral Sciences, Vol. 2. Hoboken, NJ: Wiley; 2009.

44 Hollerman JR, Schultz W. Dopamine neurons report an error in the temporal prediction of reward during learning. Nature Neurosci. 1998;1: 304–9.

45 Montague PR, Hyman SE, Cohen JD. Computational roles for dopamine in behavioural control. Nature. 2004;431:760–7.

46 Maslow AH. A theory of human motivation. Psychol Review. 1943;50:370–96.

47 Ryan RM, Deci EL. Self-Determination Theory: Basic Psychological Needs in Motivation, Development and Wellness. New York: Guilford Press; 2017.

48 Kasser VG, Ryan RM. The relation of psychological needs for autonomy and relatedness to vitality, well-being and mortality in a nursing home. J Applied Soc Psychol. 1999;29:935–54.

49 Chirkov V, Ryan RM, Kim Y, Kaplan U. Differentiating autonomy from individualism and independence: a self-determination theory perspective on internalization of cultural orientations and well-being. J Personality Soc Psychol. 2003;84:97–110.

50 Williams GC, McGregor H, Sharp D, et al. A self-determination multiple risk intervention trial to improve smokers' health. J Gen Intern Med. 2006;21:1288–94.

51 Fortier MS, Sweet SN, O'Sullivan TL, Williams GC. A self-determination process model of physical activity adoption in the context of a randomized controlled trial. Psychol Sport Exercise. 2007;8:741–57.

52 Ryan RM, Patrick H, Deci EL, Williams GC. Facilitating health behavior change and its maintenance: interventions based on self-determination theory. Eur Health Psychol. 2008;10:2–5.

53 Markland D, Ryan RM, Tobin VJ, Rollnick S. Motivational interviewing and self-determination theory. J Social Clin Psychol. 2005;24:811–31.

54 Vansteenkiste M, Sheldon KM. There's nothing more practical than a good theory: Integrating motivational interviewing and self-determination theory. Brit J Clin Psychol. 2006;45:63–82.

55 Patrick H, Williams GC. Self-determination theory: its application to health behavior and complementarity with motivational interviewing. Int J Behav Nutr Phys Act. 2012;9:18. doi: 10.1186/1479-5868-9-18.

56 Cattell RB, Radcliffe JA, Sweney AB. The nature and measurement of components of motivation. Genet Psychol Monograph. 1963;68: 49–211.

57 Mayer JD, Faber MA, Xu X. Seventy-five years of motivation measures (1930–2005): a descriptive analysis. Motiv Emot. 2007;31:83–103.

58 Freund AM, Hennecke M, Mustafic M. On gains and losses, means and ends: goal orientation and goal focus across adulthood. In Ryan RM, ed., The Oxford Handbook of Human Motivation. New York: Oxford University Press; 2012.

59 Heckhausen J, Schultz R. A life-span theory of control. Psychol Rev. 1995;103: 284–304.

60 Fox M. An Interview with God—I Stand Corrected. https://centerforglobal leadership.wordpress.com/2012/06/30/an-interview-with-god-i-stand-corrected/. Accessed June 6, 2018.

61 Crockett LJ. Agency in the life course: concepts and processes. Nebr Symp Motiv. 2002;48:1–29.

62 Batty GD, Deary IJ, Gottfredson LS. Premorbid (early life) IQ and later mortality risk: systematic review. Ann Epidemiol. 2007; 17:278–88.

63 Deary IJ, Gow AJ, Taylor MD, et al. The Lothian Birth Cohort 1936: a study to examine influences on cognitive ageing from age 11 to age 70 and beyond. BMC Geriatr. 2007;7:28. Review. PubMed PMID: 18053258; PubMed Central PMCID: PMC2222601.

64 Hall PA, Fong GT, Epp LJ. Cognitive and personality factors in the prediction of health behaviors: an examination of total, direct and indirect effects. J Behav Med. 2014;37:1057–68.

65 Duff K, Mold JW, Gidron Y. Cognitive functioning predicts survival in the elderly. J Clin Exp Neuropsychol. 2009;31:90–5.

66 Menon CV, Jahn DR, Mauer CB, O'Bryant SE. Executive functioning as a mediator of the relationship between premorbid verbal intelligence and health risk behaviors in a rural-dwelling cohort: a Project FRONTIER study. Arch Clin Neuropsychol. 2013;28:169–79.

67 Liang J, Matheson BE, Kaye WH, Boutelle KN. Neurocognitive correlates of obesity and obesity-related behaviors in children and adolescents. Int J Obes (Lond). 2014;38:494–506.

68 Higgins ET. Beyond pleasure and pain. Am Psychol. 1997;52:1280–300.

69 Scholer AA, Higgins ET. Too much of a good thing? trade-offs in promotion and prevention focus. In Ryan RM, ed., The Oxford Handbook of Human Motivation. New York: Oxford University Press; 2012.

70 Cunningham WA, Raye CL, Johnson MK. Neural correlates of evaluation associated with promotion and prevention regulatory focus. Cognit Affect Behav Neurosci. 2005;5:202–11.

71 Manian N, Strauman TJ, Denney N. Temperament, recalled parenting styles, and self-regulation: testing the developmental postulates of self-discrepancy theory. J Personality Social Psychol. 1998;75:1321–32.

72 Keller J. On the development of regulatory focus: the role of parenting styles. Eur J Social Psychol. 2008;38:354–64.

73 Foster GD, Wadden TA, Vogt RA, Brewer G. What is a reasonable weight loss? Patients' expectations and evaluations of obesity treatment outcomes. J Consult Clin Psychol. 1997;65:79–85.

74 Fuglestad PT, Rothman AJ, Jeffery RW. Getting there and hanging on: the effect of regulatory focus on performance in smoking and weight loss interventions. Health Psychol. 2008;27(3S):S260–70.

75 Freitas A, Liberman N, Higgins ET. Regulatory fit and resisting temptation during goal pursuit. J Experim Social Psychol. 2002;38:291–8.

76 Sengupta J, Zhou R. Understanding impulsive eater's choice behaviors: The motivational influences of regulatory focus. J Market Res. 2007;44:297–308.

77 Uskul AK, Keller J, Oyserman D. Regulatory fit and health behavior. Psychol Health. 2008;23:327–46.

78 Digman JM. Personality structure: emergence of the five-factor model. Annual Review Psychol. 1990;41:417–40.

79 Goldberg LR. The structure of phenotypic personality traits. Am Psychol. 1993;48: 26–34.

80 Bogg T, Roberts BW. Conscientiousness and health-related behaviors: a meta-analysis of the leading behavioral contributors to mortality. Psychol Bull. 2004;130: 887–919.

81 Leventhal H, Weinman J, Leventhal EA, Phillips LA. Health psychology: the search for pathways between behavior and health. Annu Rev Psychol. 2008;59:477–505.

82 Simpson SH, Eurich DT, Majumdar SR, et al. A meta-analysis of the association between adherence to drug therapy and mortality. BMJ. 2006;333(7557):15. Epub 2006 Jun 21.

83 Lahey BB. Public health significance of neuroticism. Am Psychol. 2009;64:241–56.

84 Mols F, Denollet J. Type D personality in the general population: a systematic review of health status, mechanisms of disease, and work-related problems. Health Qual Life Outcomes. 2010;8:9. doi: 10.1186/1477-7525-8-9. Review. PubMed PMID: 20096129; PubMed Central PMCID: PMC2822747.

85 Gable SL, Prok T. Avoiding the pitfalls and approaching the promises of close relationships. In Ryan RM, ed., The Oxford Handbook of Human Motivation. New York: Oxford University Press; 2012.

86 Berkman LF, Syme SL. Social networks, host-resistance, and mortality: a 9 year follow-up study of Alameda County residents. Am J Epidemiol. 1979;109:186–204.

87 House JS, Landis KR, Umberson D. Social relationships and health. Science. 1988;241:540–5.

88 Laranjo L, Arguel A, Neves AL, et al. The influence of social networking sites on health behavior change: a systematic review and meta-analysis. J Am Med Informatics Assoc. 2015;22:243–56.

89 Maher C, Ryan J, Kernot J, Podsiadly J, Keenhian S. Social media and applications to health behavior. Current Opin Psychol. 2016;9:50–5.

90 Barkley GS. Factors influencing health behaviors in the National Health and Nutritional Examination Survey, III (NHANES III). Soc Work Health Care. 2008;46:57–79.

91 Braveman P, Gottlieb L. The social determinants of health: it's time to consider the causes of the causes. Public Health Rep. 2014;129(Suppl 2):19–31.

92 Iwelunmor J, Newsome V, Airhihenbuwa CO. Framing the impact of culture on health: a systematic review of the PEN-3 cultural model and its application in public health research and interventions. Ethnic Health. 2014;19:20–46.

93 Bandura A. Social Foundations of Thought and Action: A Social Cognitive Theory. Englewood Cliffs, NJ: Prentice Hall; 1986.

94 McPherson KE, Kerr S, Morgan A, McGee E, Cheater FM, McLean J, Egan J. The association between family and community social capital and health risk behaviours in young people: an integrative review. BMC Public Health. 2013;13:971. doi: 10.1186/1471-2458-13-971

95 Larsen JK, Hermans RC, Sleddens EF, Engels RC, Fisher JO, Kremers SP. How parental dietary behavior and food parenting practices affect children's dietary behavior: INTERACTING sources of influence? Appetite. 2015;89:246–57.

96 Thomas RE, Baker PRA, Thomas BC. Family-based interventions in preventing children and adolescents from using tobacco: a systematic review and meta-analysis. Acad Pediatr. 2016;16:419–29.

97 Hruschka DJ. Culture as an explanation in population health. Ann Hum Biol. 2009;36:235–47.

98 Oussedik E, Foy CG, Masicampo EJ, Kammrath LK, Anderson RE, Feldman SR. Accountability: a missing construct in models of adherence behavior and in clinical practice. Patient Prefer Adherence. 2017;11:1285–94.

99 Hardeman W, Johnston M, Johnston DW, Bonetti D, Wareham NJ, Kinmonth AL. Application of the theory of planned behaviour in behaviour change interventions: a systematic review. Psychol Health. 2002;17:123–58.

100 Sheeran P, Gollwitzer PM, Bargh JA. Nonconscious processes and health. Health Psychol. 2013;32:460–73.

101 Strack F, Deutsch R. Reflective and impulsive determinants of social behavior. Personality and Social Psychology Review. 2004;8:220–47.

102 Chida Y, Steptoe A, Powell LH. Religiosity/spirituality and mortality: a systematic quantitative review. Psychother Psychosom. 2009;78:81–90.

103 Bonelli RM, Koenig HG. Mental disorders, religion and spirituality 1990 to 2010: a systematic evidence-based review. J Relig Health. 2013;52:657–73.

104 Unterrainer HF, Lewis AJ, Fink A. Religious/spiritual well-being, personality and mental health: a review of results and conceptual issues. J Relig Health. 2014;53:382–92.

105 Zimmer Z, Jagger C, Chiu CT, Ofstedal MB, Rojo F, Saito Y. Spirituality, religiosity, aging and health in global perspective: a review. SSM Popul Health. 2016;2:373–81.

106 Mishra SK, Togneri E, Tripathi B, Trikamji B. Spirituality and religiosity and its role in health and diseases. j Relig Health. 2017;56:1282–301.

107 Seeman TE, Dubin LF, Seeman M. Religiosity/spirituality and health: a critical review of the evidence for biological pathways. Am Psychol. 2003;58:53–63.

108 Büssing A, Ostermann T, Koenig HG. Relevance of religion and spirituality in German patients with chronic diseases. Int J Psychiatry Med. 2007;37:39–57.

109 Unantenne N, Warren N, Canaway R, Manderson L. The strength to cope: spirituality and faith in chronic disease. J Relig Health. 2013;52:1147–61.

110 Powell LH, Shahabi L, Thoresen CE. Religion and spirituality: linkages to physical health. Am Psychol. 2003;58:36–52.

111 Park CL, Edmondson D, Hale-Smith A, Blank TO. Religiousness/spirituality and health behaviors in younger adult cancer survivors: does faith promote a healthier lifestyle? J Behav Med. 2009;32:582–91.

112 Janssen-Niemeijer AJ, Visse M, Van Leeuwen R, Leget C, Cusveller BS. The role of spirituality in lifestyle changing among patients with chronic cardiovascular diseases: a literature review of qualitative studies. J Relig Health. 2017;56:1460–77.

113 Weatherly JN, Plumm KM. Delay discounting as a function of intrinsic/extrinsic religiousness, religious fundamentalism, and regular church attendance. J Gen Psychol. 2012;139:117–33.

114 Paglieri F, Borghi AM, Colzato LS, Hommel B, Scorolli C. Heaven can wait: how religion modulates temporal discounting. Psychol Res. 2013;77:738–47.

115 Reynolds B. A review of delay-discounting research with humans: relations to drug use and gambling. Behav Pharmacol. 2006;17:651–67.

116 Bradford WD. The association between individual time preferences and health maintenance habits. Med Decis Making. 2010;30:99–112.

117 Epstein LH, Salvy SJ, Carr KA, Dearing KK, Bickel WK. Food reinforcement, delay discounting and obesity. Physiol Behav. 2010;100:438–45.

118 Tate LM, Tsai PF, Landes RD, Rettiganti M, Lefler LL. Temporal discounting rates and their relation to exercise behavior in older adults. Physiol Behav. 2015;152(Pt A):295–9.

119 Dariotis JK, Johnson MW. Sexual discounting among high-risk youth ages 18–24: implications for sexual and substance use risk behaviors. Exp Clin Psychopharmacol. 2015;23:49–58.

120 Lebeau G, Consoli SM, Le Bouc R, et al. Delay discounting of gains and losses, glycemic control and therapeutic adherence in type 2 diabetes. Behav Processes. 2016;132:42–48.

121 Bruce JM, Bruce AS, Catley D, et al. Being kind to your future self: probability discounting of health decision-making. Ann Behav Med. 2016;50:297–309.

122   Jones J, Guest JL, Sullivan PS, M Sales J, M Jenness S, R Kramer M. The association between monetary and sexual delay discounting and risky sexual behavior in an online sample of men who have sex with men. AIDS Care. 2018;30:844–52.

123   Zajonc RB. Feeling and thinking: preferences need no inferences. Am Psychol. 1980;35:151–75.

124   LeDoux JE. The Emotional Brain. New York: Simon & Schuster; 1996.

125   Izard CE. Emotion theory and research: highlights, unanswered questions, and emerging issues. Annual Rev Psychol. 2009;60:1–25.

126   Epstein S. The self-concept revisited: or a theory of a theory. Am Psychol. 1973;28:404–16.

127   Epstein S. Integration of the cognitive and the psychodynamic unconscious. Amer Psychologist. 1994;49:709–24.

128   Metcalfe J, Mischel W. A hot/cool-system analysis of delay of gratification: dynamics of willpower. Psychol Review. 1999;106:3–19.

129   Antonacopoulou EP, Gabriel Y. Emotion, learning and organizational change: Towards an integration of psychoanalytic and other perspectives. J Organizational Change Management. 2001;14:435–51.

130   Linnenbrink EA. Emotion research in education: theoretical and methodological perspectives on the integration of affect, motivation, and cognition. Educ Psychol Rev. 2006;18:307–14.

131   Pekrun R. The impact of emotions on learning and achievement: towards a theory of cognitive/motivational mediators. Applied Psychol. 1992;41:359–76.

132   Dolan RJ. Emotion, cognition, and behavior. Science. 2002;298:1191–4.

133   Weinstein ND. The precaution adoption process. Health Psychol. 1988;7:355–86.

134   Rothman AJ. Toward a theory-based analysis of behavioral maintenance. Health Psychol. 2000;19:64–9.

135   Hall PA, Fong GT. Temporal self-regulation theory: a model for individual health behavior. Health Psychol Rev. 2007;1:6–52.

136   Bandura A. Self-efficacy: toward a unifying theory of behavioral change. Psychol Rev. 1977;84:191–215.

137   Baldwin AS, Rothman AJ, Hertel AW, et al. Specifying the determinants of the initiation and maintenance of behavior change: an examination of self-efficacy, satisfaction, and smoking cessation. Health Psychol. 2006;25:626–34.

138   Strecher VJ, DeVellis BM, Becker MH, Rosenstock IM. The role of self-efficacy in achieving health behavior change. Health Educ Behav. 1986;13:73–92

139   Rosenstock IM, Strecher VJ, Becker MH. Social learning theory and the health belief model. Health Educ Quart. 1988;15:175–183.

140   De Ridder DTD, De Wit JBF. Self-regulation in health behavior: concepts, theories, and central issues. In De Ridder DTD, De Wit JBF, eds., Self-Regulation in Health Behavior. West Sussex, UK: John Wiley and Sons; 2006.

141   Cybernetics: Or, Control and Communication in the Animal and the Machine. 2nd ed. Cambridge, MA: MIT Press; 1965.

142   Carver CS, Scheier MF. Cybernetic control processes and the self-regulation of behavior. In Ryan RM, ed., The Oxford Handbook of Human Motivation. New York: Oxford University Press; 2012.

143   Carver CS. Self-regulation of action and affect. In Baumeister RF and Vohs KD, eds., Handbook of Self-Regulation: Research, Theory, and Applications (pp. 13–39). New York: Guilford; 2004.

144 Baumeister RF. The self. In Gilbert D, Fiske ST, Lindzey G, eds., Handbook of Social Psychology, 4th ed. Boston: McGraw Hill; 1998.

145 Muraven M, Baumeister RF. Self-regulation and depletion of limited resources: does self-control resemble a muscle? Psychol Bull. 2000;126:247–59.

146 Gailliot MT, Mead NL, Baumeister RF. Self-regulation. In John OP, Robbins RW, and Pervin LA, eds., Handbook of Personality: Theory and Research (pp. 472–91). New York: Guilford Press; 2008.

147 Rothman AJ, Baldwin AS, Hertel AW. Self-regulation and behavior change. In Baumeister RF and Vohs KD, eds., Handbook of Self-Regulation: Research, Theory, and Applications (pp. 130–148). New York: Guilford; 2004.

4

The Pragmatism of Habit in Preoperative Optimization

Heath B. McAnally and Beth Darnall

Introduction/Abstract

The past two decades have seen considerable focus on enhancing individuals' motivation to improve their health; however, concomitant with a growing recognition of the inability of education and cognitive-focused interventions to enact consistent behavioral change, more recently there has been a proliferation of interest in harnessing the power of habit toward that end. In both the United States and the United Kingdom there is an increasing call for large-scale public health interventions incorporating behavioral strategies designed specifically to bolster healthy habit formation [1–4].

As discussed at length in the previous chapter, motivation (that which energizes and directs goal-oriented behavior) is complex, dynamic and flexible/adaptable, and unpredictable. Habit would therefore seem to represent the polar opposite: simple and reflexive, inflexible, and predictable. These two discrepant "governors" appear to direct two distinct behavioral regulatory systems [5, 6]; motivation has to do frequently with conscious reflection and deliberation, while habit appears essentially independent of cognition and emotion. While certainly a crude and imperfect metaphor, we think of motivation as the artistic community of the psyche, and habit as the engineering department of the brain. They serve distinct purposes, occasionally at odds in terms of form versus function, but may certainly operate in unison—especially under the direction of a skilled architect.

Perhaps a more utilitarian analogy is represented pictorially in Figure 4.1. We conceptualize motivation—essential for the initiation phase of change—as the booster rockets shown lifting the space shuttle off of the launch pad and through the earth's atmosphere.

Without motivation the ship would never get off the ground. Conversely, without the establishment of habit (pictured here as orbit) the journey will be a short-lived one.

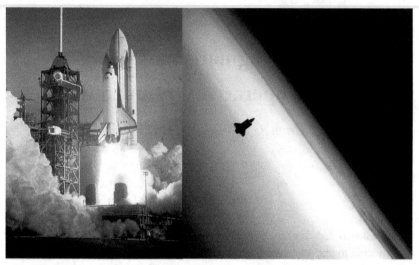

Images Courtesy of NASA - Great Images in NASA, Public Domain, and by NASA/Crew of Expedition 22 Public domain, via Wikimedia Commons

Figure 4.1. Motivation and Habit

In this chapter we explore the critical role of habit in directing behavior in general and, in particular, health behaviors. We examine what is currently known about the psychology and neurobiology of habit formation and maintenance. We then turn our attention to a brief overview of the application of these concepts to the perioperative optimization of patients with chronic pain, which constitutes the remaining subject of this book and the underlying effort of our program.

The Critical Role of Habit in Directing Behavior

The Importance of Habit in Daily Life

Certain human activities (e.g., deciding how to vote on a new proposed ballot measure) may require considerable effort in conscious concentration and decision-making, whereas others (e.g., an infant's crying in response to hunger or discomfort) are "instinctive" and require no evident cognition nor learning whatsoever. Somewhere in between these two extremes lies the vast majority of our day-to-day behavioral experience, which seems to fluctuate between states of consciousness and unconsciousness; even the same action (e.g., consuming food or lighting up a cigarette) may require deliberation in some circumstances and proceed automatically in others. As we have all experienced, with repetition of behavior and consistency of context, actions initially characterized by thoughtful (or impulsive) choice may become regimented and habitual. While estimates of the proportion of mindless/automatic behavior throughout our day may range as high as 95% [7], 40%–50% is more frequently quoted [8–10]. Regardless of the number, the literature supports the notion that we are all to some extent creatures of habit.

It is increasingly appreciated that habit formation and the development of automaticity serves a highly adaptive function yielding increased efficiency, and not infrequently even survival advantage [11–13]. Performance of a piano concerto, gymnastic routine, or crisis response protocol would be sketchy at best without automaticity, especially with the added context of stress. Beyond such specialized examples, we can all relate to the truism that daily mundane activities such as walking or driving everyday pathways, hygiene routines, and the innumerable minute-by-minute interactions with our environment would overwhelm our capacity for higher thought were they not relegated to our subconscious. Conversely habit formation can confer negative benefit, for example obsessive-compulsive disorder [12,13] and addiction [14,15].

The Tension and Cooperation Between Reflective and Reflexive Processes

Dual systems models (conscious vs. subconscious behavioral guidance) have become well accepted within modern psychology [5, 16–18]. Intention and habits jointly predict behavior [19], and the individual (and cooperative) roles of these distinct dual processes on both initiation and maintenance of new behaviors are well analyzed in Rothman et al's analysis of dietary change [20]. Their frequently cited 2×2 behavior change matrix summarizing these activities is depicted in simplified form in Figure 4.2.

A division of labor appears to parallel adaptation to routine. The cognitive-reflective system (with accompanying self-regulatory efforts) appears to exert greater traction and potency in early/initiation stages of change [21, 22], perhaps especially when the action is infrequent [19]. During this nascent phase, intentional behavior modification proceeds "slowly and effortfully" [23] in directing (or redirecting) actions provided satisfactory self-determination theory principles reinforce motivation. During long-term maintenance of behavior, mindful contribution appears to attenuate for the most part [24].

Conversely, within initiation phases, automatic or subconscious processes indeed also exert effects [20, 25]—if nothing else via inertia—but confer significantly more weight of impact on maintenance, when habits and their efficiency dominate [8, 24, 26, 27].

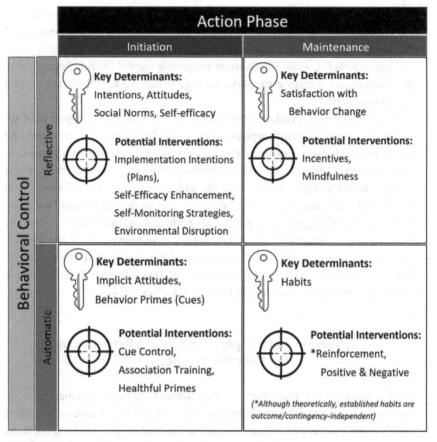

Figure 4.2. 2 × 2 Behavior Change Matrix
Adapted from Rothman et al [20].

Evidence of the Importance of Habit in Health Behavior

Evidence in support of the crucial role of habit in maintaining health behavioral change is both indirect (lack of efficacy of intention alone) and direct. Few systematic reviews/meta-analyses demonstrating effect sizes of habit formation on health behaviors exist, but those that are available at the time of this writing are presented at the end of this section.

Evidence for the Inefficacy of Good Intentions
In the 1990s and early part of this century it was widely assumed that intentions and plans mediated the majority of health-related and other behaviors [28, 29].

Recent investigations, however, have shown that at best, half of the variability of health behaviors is predicted by cognitive factors [30–32].

In a landmark review and meta-analysis, Webb and Sheeran [33] evaluated the effects of interventions designed to result in positive health behaviors (e.g., sunscreen use, self-examinations, diet and exercise improvements, smoking cessation, etc.) on outcomes of both intention and behavioral changes with a mean follow-up period of 15 weeks. Data from 47 studies ($n = 8,802$) meeting inclusion criteria—which among other things required evidence of positive change in intention—were pooled and analyzed. Within these studies a medium-to-large change in intention (Cohen's d statistic $= 0.66$) was found, however only a small-to-medium change in behavior ($d = 0.36$) resulted. The authors concluded, "intention has a significant impact on behavior, but the size of this effect is considerably smaller than correlational tests have suggested."

More recent analyses have shown similar or larger "intention–behaviour gap." Michie et al in 2009 [34] examined 122 experimental or quasi-experimental studies ($n = 44,747$) targeting physical activity and healthy eating interventions. Overall behavior change intervention effect sizes of 0.32 and 0.31 were shown, respectively, and it should be noted that (presumably as only 60% of the studies involved intention formation data gathering) effect sizes or comparisons involving intention change were not reported. Of interest, however, the authors did note that the incorporation of self-regulation techniques (prompt intention formation, prompt specific goal setting, and especially self-monitoring of behavior not otherwise specified) was associated with improved effectiveness. When self-monitoring and one other self-regulation technique were involved, the effect sizes rose to 0.38 and 0.54 for physical activity and healthy eating; 0.42 overall. As Rothman et al noted [20], "strong goal intentions are not sufficient to overcome self-regulatory problems that frequently undermine intention realization."

Rhodes and Dickau in 2012 [35] performed a meta-analysis of 11 studies ($n = 2,167$) focusing on interventions targeting physical activity. In this data pool, the effect of interventions on intention were somewhat weaker ($d = 0.45$), however the effect on behavior was notably weaker ($d = 0.15$). In a follow-up meta-analysis in 2013 [36], examining 10 studies ($n = 3,899$) only 54% of subjects forming change intention were able to successfully perform that intended behavior. The authors concluded, "this is strong evidence that intention is a necessary, but often insufficient construct to produce behavioural enactment." However, it should be noted that in this analysis, 6 of the 10 studies comprised college students, and the generalizability of these findings may thus be limited.

Along those lines, it has been demonstrated recently that behavioral models attempting to predict health behaviors based on cognitive control mechanisms (e.g., the theory of planned behavior [37]) show reasonable fit among younger, healthier, and more affluent groups in the short term, while losing predictive value over time, and also among less advantaged populaces [38, 39].

Finally it should be noted that intentions and habit may certainly correlate, and the studies cited thus far are unable to separate out the relative contributions of reflexive versus reflective behaviors in these contexts. In fact, as has been pointed out by leading investigators in the field [40], much of the variability in the predictive power of intention may well be related to the establishment (or lack) of habit.

Evidence for the Power of Habit

Numerous investigations [41–46] attest to the power of habit in routine health (or unhealthy) behaviors. Tremendous imprecision and heterogeneity of definition exists, however, within the literature, and determining the contribution of habit requires some means of (ideally objective, practically subjective) standardization of effect [40]. Accordingly, most current studies and reviews of the topic appear to be coalescing toward a definition that includes necessary components of contextual cueing, subconscious processing, frequency of performance, and some evidence of a learned association [23]. In human subjects, free of the tightly controlled experimental conditions that animals may be subjected to, subjective and self-report measures form the mainstay of independent variable collection. Currently the Self-Report Habit Index (SRHI [47]) constitutes the most commonly used measure of habit in health behaviors. This 12-item questionnaire solicits congruence of a given action with automaticity, frequency, and relevance to self-identity. It does not/cannot capture cue-behavior associations.

Gardner et al in 2011 [40] performed a systematic review and meta-analysis of reports linking SRHI data to indices of nutrition and physical activity and whether habit appears to moderate the intention-behavior relationship those studies. Twenty-two studies (n = 6,869), all of which reported an association between SRHI value and concordant or discordant behavior, or which explored the role of the SRHI in moderating an association between intention and outcome, were included. General conclusions were that habit as determined by SRHI confers moderate to strong effect (average weighted correlation between habit and behavior across all studies was estimated at $r+$ = 0.46). In eight of nine tests studies examining the question of interaction between habit and the intention-behavior relationship, a moderating effect (increasing habit strength was associated with decreasing effect of intention on behavior) was seen.

Rebar et al [48] carried out a systematic review of the effects of nonconscious regulatory processes in physical activity. Fifty-two very heterogeneous and brief studies (follow-up 2 weeks or less in most cases) measuring some aspect of habit (e.g., lack of awareness, degree of automaticity, cue consistency) as an independent variable were evaluated. Most used the SRHI or a derivative, and the authors reported median bivariate associations between automated processes and physical activity at $d = 0.67$. Subanalyses indicated that nonconscious regulatory processes maintained statistically significant effect after accounting for conscious regulation in the majority of studies, and were complementary and supportive of the intention-behavior association, as would be expected.

Prospective studies examining the influence of habit-based interventions on behavior modification are more scarce, although increasingly called for. In a systematic review and meta-analysis investigating the effects of various behavioral interventions to increase antihypertensive pharmacotherapeutic regimen adherence (156 studies, $n = 60,876$) one group reported, "Habit-based interventions were effective (habit $d = 0.477$; no habit $d = 0.181$) in improving diastolic outcomes ($p < .001$)" [49]. The authors conducted a similar analysis in a more focused population group of "subjects with adherence problems" [50]; 53 studies ($n = 8,243$) were examined. Again they reported that interventions using prompts or cues for taking medications had larger effect sizes than those that did not ($d = 0.497$ vs. 0.234, $p = 0.034$) and interventions in which participants' daily habits were linked to taking medications were also effective in increasing medication adherence compared to those that did not ($d = 0.574$ vs. 0.222, $p = 0.007$). Specific interventions for instilling habit, however, were not well characterized, and furthermore no means of assessing purported contributory habit components (e.g., frequency, automaticity, cue-responsiveness) were reported.

One well-designed series of prospective investigations from the United Kingdom involved a simple intervention consisting of a single flyer with dietary modifications and ways to make them habitual. The program, titled "Ten Top Tips" (10TT) encouraged low-fat options, low-calorie snacks, low-calorie drinks, five servings of fruit and vegetables a day, small portions and no second helpings, walking 10,000 steps a day, sitting for no more than 50 min of each hour, reading food labels, avoidance of performing other activities while eating, and eating at the same times each day. Specific planning/implementation intention and self-monitoring advice was also provided. In the initial pilot study [51], 104 participants were randomized to usual clinical care, or to one of two interventional arms each receiving the same 10TT program, but with one group being weighed weekly and the other monthly (controls were also weighed monthly.) At 8 weeks, participants receiving the 10TT intervention lost significantly more weight than those in the control condition (mean loss 2.0 kg vs. 0.4 kg), with no difference between the weekly and monthly weighing subgroups. To assess the development of habits, SRHI automaticity scores were followed from baseline through the completion of the 8-month study period and increased by an average of 9 points on the 42 point scale. Average automaticity change was significantly correlated with total weight loss (Spearman's $r = 0.424$, $p = 0.028$). The experimental group was followed for another 6 months and on average lost a total of 3.8 kg.

In a larger follow-up study [52], 537 participants were randomized to 10TT intervention or usual care. At the primary endpoint (3 months) the experimental group had lost significantly more weight (0.87 kg greater loss than control group, $p = 0.004$), however this difference was not seen at 24 months—the usual care group caught up to the 10TT group in terms of weight loss rather than the experimental group regaining weight. The experimental group registered a significantly greater degree of automaticity of target behaviors compared to the control group (adjusted difference = 8.45; 95% CI = 2.59, 14.32)

In an intriguing prospective trial of weight loss interventions in the United States [53], 59 participants were randomized to either a habit-based intervention (Transforming Your Life, TYL) or to a cognitive-based intervention (New Perspectives, NP.) The SRHI was used to grade both eating and physical activity habits in each group; no significant differences were reported. At the conclusion of the experimental period (3 months) the habit-based TYL group had lost 12 pounds more than the NP group, although the difference was not statistically significant ($p = 0.08$). However, at the 6-month follow-up visit the outcome difference was notably and significantly ($p = 0.05$) accentuated: the TYL group maintained an average weight loss of 4.8 pounds compared to an average weight gain of 4.7 pounds in the NP group.

In a prospective multiarm trial conducted in Australia [54], 75 participants were randomized to 3 months of the 10TT program (which focuses on forming new habits), or to an alternative habit-based program called "Do Something Different" (DSD, which focuses on breaking old nondiet and nonexercise habits) or to a control group. Both experimental groups achieved and maintained significantly more weight loss ($p < 0.001$) than the control group at the 6-month mark and continued to lose weight beyond that at 12-month follow-up. "Habits" were measured using a nondisclosed instrument and showed positive increase in both experimental groups at 6- and 12-month marks, both significantly greater than in the control group.

Summary of the Evidence

It appears, then, that both intentional/consciously controlled and habitual/subconscious generators power health behaviors. While the infinite complexity and variability of human beings' psyches likely obviates any universally applicable conclusions, recent work supports the resurgence of interest in the role of habit. Suffice it to say that it clearly serves as a significant determinant of human activity, and to ignore its role in health and disease at both population and individual levels is naive at best.

Habit Theory and Science

Current Habit Psychology

Definition and Components of Habit

Colloquial understanding of habit generally takes the form of "something I do regularly" or "something I do without thinking." Habit certainly includes the characteristic of repetition [27, 55] and automaticity [27, 47, 56], and while these phenomena may superficially identify habitual behavior, they are not specific nor sufficient to explain the construct. As a pain interventionalist, I (HM) can attest to the fact that I have performed certain procedures thousands of times and yet I still think through (often by necessity due to heterogeneous anatomy and other circumstances) the routine, to lesser or greater degree every single time. Spinal, corneal, and neonatal (e.g., Moro) reflexes are automatic but do not represent learned behavior.

Not captured in those components, but nonetheless representing a necessary component of habits—defined by leading researchers Wendy Wood and Dennis Runger as "implicit associations between contexts and responses that develop through repeated reward learning" [57]—is cue. As a learned response, habits by definition require a stimulus of some sort to respond to, and typically develop only in the context of a stable or at least consistent input pattern [58, 59]. In other words, a recurring antecedent must be present.

In many if not most cases, a recurring (at least initially) result providing enough reward to engender repetition of the behavior is also required. Essentially all of the work done in experimental habit psychology/biology in lower species involves initial enticement of the animal to adopt a certain behavioral pattern by providing reward (either positive or negative, e.g., escape from a painful stimulus.) The manipulation of both antecedent cue and resultant reward form the mainstay of such investigation. By general consensus, however, there comes a point when the reward or goal is no longer necessary ("goal-devaluation") to perpetuate the action sequence and in fact this switch from goal-oriented to goal-independent activity repetition is held by many researchers to mark the transition to habit [13, 60].

It is important to note that habit is defined by experts in the field not as behavior, but as a *process that determines behavior* [61]. In summation, habit reflects adaptation of behavior from an initial goal-directed/goal-sensitive pursuit with reward reinforcement to an automatic cue-directed and goal-insensitive process (Figure 4.3).

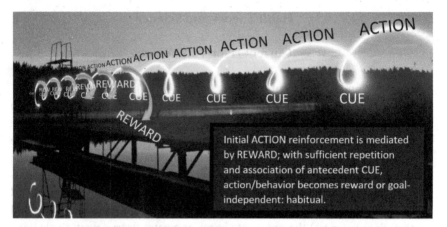

Initial ACTION reinforcement is mediated by REWARD; with sufficient repetition and association of antecedent CUE, action/behavior becomes reward or goal-independent: habitual.

Figure 4.3. Transition from Goal-Directed to Habitual Behavior
Modified from photo by Axel Antas-Bergkvist on Unsplash.

Natural History of Habit Formation

Debate persists as to the necessity of extrinsic reward in the process of habit formation—in other words many hold that the process of developing routine may hold sufficient intrinsic reward (e.g., personal satisfaction, perceived congruence with ideals or remote goals, increased efficiency, etc.) obviating the need for the proverbial "carrot." Furthermore, one is hard-pressed to conceptualize reward in the common sense for the establishment of many daily routines such as driving to work by one's normal route, or as William James pointed out over a century ago, always preferentially putting either right or left leg into one's trousers first.

Nonetheless, it is generally agreed on that some sort of outcome is inherent in the phenomenon of habit, as a process. It has also generally been accepted for over a century (and likely longer) that habit formation comprises instrumental learning [62]. And despite the evident inverse correlation between goal-directed behavior and habit as discussed in the next section, reward of some sort, whether extrinsic or intrinsic, incentive-salient (i.e., desirable, perceptibly pleasurable) or subconscious (e.g., increased efficiency of a necessary task), entrains repetition, which in time solidifies into routine. As alluded to previously, simple reward, however, is not sufficient to establish habit. An association between the action (or sequence of actions) and outcome, prompted by a consistent antecedent cue must be developed, and this process relies on multiple determinants both environmental and personal, which are discussed at greater length in the next section.

For the purposes of this section, which attempts to provide only a basic generalization of the process congruent with the current cognitive-behavioral dual-systems paradigm (i.e., not relying on animal model stimulus-response evidence) we consider some basic aspects of habit formation derived and culled from current models based on observational and experimental human data.

Leading health habit researchers Phillippa Lally and Benjamin Gardner have devised a four-stage model for the formation of habit [63, 64] in some ways superimposable on the transtheoretical model (TTM) discussed in the previous chapter, with the caveat that habit formation does not require conscious goal orientation or motivation to change and we are discussing two entirely distinct conceptual issues here.

The first stage is marked by reflection or deliberation as to whether to perform a new action (similar to the contemplative stage of the TTM). Once intention has solidified, the second stage commences, marked by implementation intention activities, that is, planning (similar to the planning stage of the TTM). The third and fourth overlapping stages (similar to the action and maintenance phases of the TTM) involve repetition of the behavior with the development of association between cue and action sequence wherein ultimately "regulation of behaviour is successfully transferred from conscious to non-conscious mental processes" [64]. The authors note that habit may be better conceptualized as a continuous rather than categorical outcome variable, that is, there exist varying degrees or strengths of habit that remain dynamic. Along those lines, it is possible for habit to be "undone" or at least overcome (competitively inhibited in biochemical terms) by other behavioral determinants—including other habits.

As early as the 1940s [65] evidence of an asymptotic curve (a distinct but perhaps overlapping phenomenon to the popular notion of a "learning curve") was seen in animal models, with large gains in automaticity measured at earlier intervals/with fewer cumulative repetitions, and subsequent "diminishing returns" or plateauing of the resultant strengthening of association. More recently, this asymptotic relationship has been demonstrated in human subjects, with recent prospective investigations [66, 67] corroborating these early findings.

The former study by Lally et al [66] has been widely cited recently in its finding that the median duration to establishment of 95% of the asymptote was 66 days in their sample of 96 primarily graduate-level students choosing a health behavior to practice. The range, however, was 18 to 254 days in this study (with the upper end extrapolated from existing data terminated at the 12-week mark). In the second study [67] the time to mean peak automaticity was 105 days for a task assigned to morning repetition and 154 days for an evening task among a sample of 42 students randomized to time-of-day grouping. The authors also measured cortisol levels (by salivary assay) and concluded that (physiologically) higher morning cortisol levels are associated with more rapid acquisition of habit.

Another recent study [68] showed significantly shorter duration (6 weeks) to development of evidence of exercise habit, provided at least four efforts per week occurred. The authors reported, "although affect was found to be the strongest predictor at baseline, consistency was the most important factor for predicting changes in habit."

These studies demonstrate that as would be expected from anecdotal experience, there is substantial variability in "aptitude" of or proclivity to habit formation, and these factors are discussed in the next section.

Factors That Strengthen or Weaken the Expression of Habit

At the outset of this section it should be noted that the literature by nature and necessary limitation will primarily reflect associations between independent variables of interest and novel habits whose covariance can be measured. Human beings come to the table, so to speak, with innumerable habits already in place which may or may not be desirable, and which may either enhance or impede formation of the new, studied habit. All that to say, while a certain personality trait (e.g., low self-control) may inhibit establishment of a desired habit such as regular exercise, it may conversely facilitate other habits such as dietary or other indiscretions and as such are likely to exhibit differing predictive value depending on the outcome behavior in question.

Personal Factors

Having said that, as discussed earlier and in greater detail within this section, the literature demonstrates that the development of automaticity may be facilitated or hampered by numerous factors. Personal factors, environmental/cue factors, task or routine factors and reward factors have all been shown to affect the expression of habit.

Similar to the interpersonal motivational variance factors reviewed in the previous chapter, it appears that some people are just more habit-prone also [69, 70]. There is ample popular notion (with scant research evidence [71, 72]) that people with stronger trait self-regulatory ability control are more apt to develop "good" or desirable habits. However, it has been argued (with ample face-validity) that this characteristic may in fact be selecting for increased ability to implement intentions and cultivate habits more congruent with expressed/desirable goals [64]. It also seems to correlate with greater ability to extinguish undesirable behavior patterns/habits. Conversely, individuals with less willpower or other self-regulatory strengths (as well as those with limitations in performance ability) may rely more on habits given the increased importance of efficiency [57] or again, may more readily establish habits incongruent with expressed/desirable goals.

Inflexible personality types have also been shown to predispose to more habit-dependence [73]. Habit propensity has been correlated in numerous investigations with various neurologic (e.g., Parkinson's disease [74] and psychiatric disorders as well, including obsessive-compulsive and related disorders [75–77] and substance abuse disorders [78, 79].

Cue Factors

While cues form the antecedent stimulus that the subject becomes (classically) conditioned to respond to, quite distinct from the reward (and operant conditioning mechanism) which in habit becomes progressively devalued, there seem to be certain characteristics of cues/environment that facilitate the development of habit to a greater or lesser degree.

In my (HM) clinical practice as a (very) part-time addictionologist, I have heard from numerous persons with an alcohol or heroin use disorder that some of the strongest factors leading to their addiction (and correspondingly often the strongest trigger for relapse or habit reinstatement) are unique environmental cues, for example driving by the usual liquor store or bar, or the sight of a spoon. Certain cues (such as overhearing other people discussing getting high) seem to be more universally potent, whereas others (spoons) trigger different heroin addicts to differing degrees reflecting the complexity of interpersonal variables. Alcoholics Anonymous lingo and literature is replete with references to "people, places, things" serving as relapse triggers (which generally served as initial culprits for the development of the habit) and the importance of discovering (and avoiding) one's individual cues is stressed.

In experimental habit formation, cues with a higher degree of convenience factor [80, 81] and consistency [82, 83] seem to be more readily associated with development of the new routine.

Other Environmental Factors

Stress appears to increase reliance on habitual response mechanisms [84], and this preference seems to be accentuated in chronically stressed individuals [85] and also those with memory challenges [86]. There is no evidence at present that stress facilitates new habit formation [57], however the literature has shown association between higher cortisol levels and more ready habit formation [67, 87].

The literature explicitly linking social influences to habit formation per se is remarkably scarce, at least in terms of investigation of automaticity development (e.g., SHRI-measured) and other metrics (strength, speed, and consistency of habit acquisition.) Nonetheless, despite the fact that formal psychological work in the field of social learning, modeling, and imitation has more frequently taken the course of cognitive theory [88], it has been essentially universally acknowledged across cultures and time periods that social determinants of habit formation are profound. Our "crowd" markedly influences both reflective and reflexive behavior. Human beings tend to imitate others, and, as with all behavior, this imitation may well begin as a conscious effort but progress to automaticity given adequate reward and repetition. A wealth of literature on innumerable topics spanning (but certainly not limited to) alcohol, tobacco, and other substance use [89, 90] and healthy and unhealthy dietary patterns [91, 92] supports the well-accepted belief that model behavior is a strong determinant of the development of habit in the imitator.

Behavior (Routine) Factors
More attention has been paid historically to behavior/task or routine factors than to other determinants of habit formation, and it is likely that this empiric focus correlates with actual importance. If habit is indeed a progressively goal/ outcome-devalued association (with salience variance as unique as the subject), and if cues can be as obscure and variable as they appear to be, from a pragmatic and application standpoint it makes sense to hone in on the action process.

Consistency of behavior/sequence is one of the key determinants of habit establishment as demonstrated by numerous animal experiments and more recently human investigations [66, 93–95]. To varying degrees, depending on a number of complex interactions, lapses in routine performance hinder habit formation [66, 94]. While not expressly shown in the literature, the adage that "practice makes perfect" likely holds applicability in habit formation in more ways than one, including the consideration that increased facility of/skill in the behavior should increase intrinsic reward from the process, reinforcing its performance.

Simplicity of the behavior has been shown to predict adoption and habituation [11, 93, 96]; the more complex the behavior the less likely automaticity is to occur, at least initially. Similarly, restricting options/multiplicity of behavioral responses supports the development of habit [58, 97] presumably through a concentration (as opposed to dilution) of association between a singular behavior/ routine and the cue.

Reward Factors
While perhaps not necessary for habit formation [64], reward certainly mediates habit formation in its initial stages at least; as noted elsewhere in this chapter the transition from goal/reward-directed behavior to automatic and goal-devalued behavior marks the boundary between cognitive and habitual behavior to many investigators. Conversely, continued reward salience or at least "deliberating that keeps rewards salient can hinder habit formation" [98].

Reward in the context of habit development may be extrinsic (post facto reinforcement, whether material or social) or intrinsic (derived from the action itself) and the two categories are not mutually exclusive: praise for a job well done may certainly coincide with self-satisfaction. It has been theorized that extrinsic rewards are more likely to predispose to goal-directed automatic action rather than goal-independent routine [58, 99] whereas conversely intrinsic reward is more likely to confer habit [64, 100].

Also of interest is the observation (reported as early as Skinner's operant conditioning experiments [101]) that intermittent reinforcement or reward confers automaticity or habit more reliably [99, 102]. Numerous explanations for this phenomenon have been proposed, including relative selection of intrinsic reward mediation; it is also conceivable that when extrinsic reward isn't "taken for granted" then more consistency of effort transpires in an attempt to secure the goal. A fascinating recently animal study [103] showed that random interval training resulted in habit formation (as opposed to continued goal-sensitive behavior in the control group subjected to "random ratio training") and that the former group showed alteration of dopamine receptors—consistent with reduction in dopaminergic activity seen in diminution of goal-sensitive behavior as discussed in the neurobiology section.

Habit Chunking and Keystone Habits
Of particular interest in health promotion (including preoperative optimization) is the fact that many habits (e.g., smoking and drinking, poor diet, and sedentary lifestyle) tend to cluster. Furthermore in many cases it appears that one habit (e.g., exercise, or diet journaling [104, 105]) may serve as a cue for another, and a hierarchy of sorts may exist such that one habit holds not only operational but even maintenance influence over others.

While not finding representation nor strong support in the scientific literature, the popular concept of a "Keystone habit" (a term coined by journalist and author Charles Duhigg [10]) has gained tremendous momentum over the past few years—a recent Internet search revealed over 1.4 million distinct unique record locators for the phrase. Such keystone activity of course need not necessarily be habitual or automated, although frequently repetition has solidified the behavioral pattern.

Reciprocal Relationship Between Habit and Outcome-Directed Behavior
The concept of a dual-process regulatory system [5,6] involving parallel and competing modes of reflective/cognitive and reflexive/automatic behavior has been discussed in this chapter and the previous one. The normal progression of intentional to habitual governance (with practical applications such as those suggested by Rothman's integrative 2×2 model) has also been previously discussed. What has not been explicitly covered so far is the observation (first expressed in the modern era by Triandis [26]) of an apparent inverse correlation

between the systems such that as habits form and grow, intention and goal-oriented deliberative contribution wanes to the point that the habitual action becomes outcome-insensitive [12, 57], that is, occurs with or without reward (and in many cases, e.g., addictive behaviors, despite negative consequences).

This phenomenon is so consistently observed in laboratory settings that in many experimental paradigms habit is not considered to be established so long as goal-directed pursuit still appears to be mediating behavior. This "outcome-devaluation" is observed not only in experimental animal models but also in human beings [105] and again is exemplified in the tragic case of addictive behaviors whereby compulsive drug use or gambling persists despite lack of reward and intention to the contrary.

The apparent disparate neurobiologic circuitry underlying these reciprocal pathways is discussed briefly in the next section.

Habit Neurobiology

Given the lack of current practical translational application, in this chapter we do not explore the neurobiology of habit in great detail. Nonetheless, an introduction to the neurocircuitry (such as we understand it) is presented for those interested.

Early work within the field focused on the basal ganglia and in particular the dorsal striatum. Methodology limited to lesioning studies (primarily in rodents) demonstrated that the dorsomedial striatum seems to be the major sub-cortical area associated with goal-directed pursuit [106, 107]. With entraining of behavior, neuronal activity typically switches to a dorsolateral striatal (DLS)-mediated pattern [107, 12] as habit-based behavior begins to manifest. Numerous lesioning studies and other investigative modalities (e.g., alteration of dopaminergic input) have corroborated the central role of the DLS in the establishment of habit: abolishment of this region and/or its function results in disruption of habits and restoration of "outcome-sensitive" and deliberative behavior [108, 109].

Within the DLS, after repetitive performance of a behavioral routine, neuronal activity has been shown to taper off in the middle of the sequence while maintaining or increasing activity toward the beginning and end [110]. This task-bracketing pattern has led to the hypothesis that the formation of habit/automated behavior involves "chunking" of a sequence of component actions into a single output engram [111].

More recent work has focused on the medial prefrontal cortex (mPFC) and its connections to the dorsal striatum (Figure 4.4). The dorsomedial area of the mPFC, often interchangeably labeled the prelimbic cortex (PL) is also

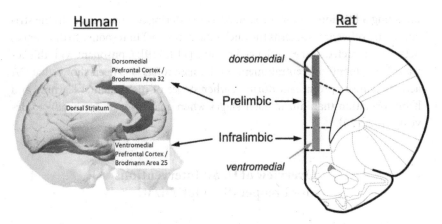

Figure 4.4. Habit Neurocircuitry

Adapted/modified from Gass and Chandler. The plasticity of extinction: contribution of the prefrontal cortex in treating addiction through inhibitory learning. Frontiers in Psychiatry. 2013;4. doi 10.3389/fpsyt.2013.00046 CC BY 3.0.

instrumental in directing goal-oriented and deliberative actions, and receives direct communication from the dorsomedial striatum [60]. Similarly, although the pathways remain incompletely elucidated (with proposed intervening circuitry involving the ventral striatum, substantia nigra, and/or amygdala [60]) the ventromedial area of the mPFC—also labeled the infralimbic cortex (IL) seems to be associated with the DLS, and together these two entities constitute the "habit highway" of the brain as we understand it at present. Lesioning experiments involving the IL demonstrate loss of previously established habits and inability to form new habits [112, 113].

The IL demonstrates "chunking" patterning of activity concurrent with the behavioral evidence of habit formation, similar to the DLS. In comparison to the DLS, however, its pattern appears later, only after "overtraining," and its consolidation appears more flexible and plastic [114].

The PL/deliberative and IL/automated systems appear to function in a sort of concurrent activation and tension [60, 115], lending support to dual-regulatory system models [5, 6]. Growing evidence indicates that the circuitry is highly complex and almost certainly involves areas of the brain not yet elucidated [114].

The catecholamine neurotransmitter dopamine (DA) is implicated in learning and plasticity throughout the central nervous system, however its activity in the DLS (with projection from the subtantia nigra and other basal ganglia neurons [116, 117] is particularly implicated in habit formation.

Once held to be the mediator of reward and in particular hedonic stimuli such as pleasurable activities and drugs of abuse, DA's role in habit acquisition including addiction is now recognized as registering learning traces in the striatum (and other areas such as the nucleus accumbens) in response to differences between predicted and experienced reward [118, 119]. Consonant with this reward "enjoyment" and entrainment mechanism it has also been shown that DA activity is more prominent during earlier stages of instrumental learning and habit formation than during later stages when goal-insensitivity begins to develop [102, 120].

Overview of Habit Interventions for Preoperative Optimization

The great thing, then, in all education, is to make our nervous system our ally instead of our enemy . . . we must make automatic and habitual, as early as possible, as many useful actions as we can, and guard against the growing into ways that are likely to be disadvantageous to us, as we should guard against the plague.
—William James [11]

Preoperative optimization of the chronic pain patient invariably requires behavioral change, and this must begin with motivation. The desire for elective surgery may in some cases supply sufficient (extrinsic) motivation to initiate change, however eliciting intrinsic motivation as discussed in the previous chapter yields greater dividends and is worth the minor investment on the time of the healthcare team.

Similarly, planning (the subject of chapter 11) is required to translate good intentions into action, but implementation still requires deliberation and commitment, which remain vulnerable to attenuation. Resource limitations and fatigability [7] can override conscious desires and plans.

Ultimately the effect sizes of purely cognitive and self-regulatory approaches to behavioral change interventions are typically small [33, 35, 121, 122, 123]. As such, to cite a recent systematic review examining 100 behavior theories, "The most sustainable mechanism for maintenance is to develop automaticity for the newly adopted behaviour" [22]. Sustained change in the chronic pain patient, however, also requires maladaptive habit elimination (e.g., pain catastrophizing, toxic substance use, toxic dietary habits, etc.)—not just advantageous habit instillation (e.g., adequate sleep, regular exercise, healthy and balanced nutrition, etc.). These topics constitute the remainder of the book. In the last few paragraphs of this chapter we outline basic principles for harnessing habit, catalyzing "fitness for surgery."

The Delicate Role of Reward

Habit formation almost universally begins with extrinsic and/or intrinsic re-ward reinforcement, as discussed previously. (Conversely, behavior that is met with negative or even neutral initial feedback is far less likely to engender rep-etition.) Identifying and clarifying the reward by education (e.g., "reduced pain and increased self-esteem") is relatively easy to do, but translating that into a tangible and believable outcome that builds self-efficacy and reinforces action requires some consistency of positive experience, which may be directly achiev-able in some cases, and in others may call for compromise of the provider's ideal means. For example, brief (and ideally intermittent) pharmacotherapy may be beneficial in the establishment of normal sleep architecture or exercise patterns. Conversely from the standpoint of negative reinforcement (i.e., the mitigation of an aversive stimulus in the language of operant conditioning) nicotine replace-ment or varenicline may be required for cigarette abstinence, and buprenorphine may play a role in preoperative opioid reduction or elimination. Without actual goal attainment it is difficult to sustain (or possibly even initiate) action. We view these means to an end much like "training wheels" on a child's first bicycle.

We are certainly not looking to create dependence on artificial reinforcement aids—to further the bicycle analogy, we hope that coordination, core strength, and so forth, obviate the need for the training wheels. However, a critical theo-retical point (and one that translates into practical application as well) that bears repeating is that the objective is not to achieve dependence on the reward either. While an initial desire to arrive at the destination, or satisfy the need for autonomy and achievement, and so forth, is useful to initiate practice (and to keep getting up off the ground after spills), the objective in this situation is for the child to develop the automatic, subconscious "motor memory" skills—the habit of riding a bicycle.

Extrinsic reward is often easier to identify and certainly to manipulate, but may carry a greater risk of continued conscious association and pursuit, with the behavior contingent on consistent (or even increasing) reward. Under the incen-tive of price reduction, consumers will adopt changes in purchase patterns but stop doing so when the cost increases. Habit formation is more likely to occur when reinforcement comprises a "low level of experienced instrumental contin-gency" [121] and when "rewards incentivize performance but are not highly sa-lient. . . . Motivated cognitions yield flexible orientations."

Finally, as discussed previously, intrinsic reward is more likely to confer habit [64, 99] as opposed to goal-directed automatic action from extrinsic re-ward reinforcement [58, 98]. Increasing task enjoyment, or at least associated positive affect [122, 124] and sense of fulfilment thus represents a more logical point of intervention, and calls for tailored, nuanced, and subtle (so as to not become a reward in itself) cultivation and encouragement on the part of the healthcare team.

Cues: Going Below the Surface

The association of cues with the (desirable or undesirable) behavior generally develops unconsciously or subconsciously, and in theory at least, the more unobtrusive the stimulus the better. Subconscious or unconscious automaticity is the goal and thus the least amount of intervention into the process may be the best strategy.

Nonetheless, in some cases just as with the "training wheel" reinforcement strategies discussed in the previous section, manipulation of the cueing process may at times be beneficial. Prompts, which comprise simple planned cues (e.g., bringing one's tennis shoes to work for a lunchtime walk, or putting one's vitamin bottle in front of the alarm clock to ensure noticing it) may be very beneficial in habit formation [3]. If, however, habit represents a consistent cue-driven activity, the potential for establishment of dependency on the prompt should engender careful consideration of practical and sustainable prompting. Along those lines, since repetition of behavior in a stable context may be the most important factor in habit development (see what follows), maximizing consistency in environment and conditions—which become natural cues—is of the essence.

Conversely, the breaking of undesirable habits is greatly facilitated by the identification of and avoidance of cues [10, 125]—a guiding principle of relapse prevention in substance abuse recovery [126, 127], and one that also holds relevance to less dramatic situations such as maladaptive dietary or activity patterns, or even shopping patterns [121]. The identification of cues is not surprisingly a generally difficult and labor-intensive task [128], given their subconscious association; in many cases the cues are not as straightforward as "people, places and things" (from Alcoholics Anonymous lingo) but may comprise internal stimuli such as negative emotions [127] for which there may be strong innate disincentive for identification. Strong psychological/counseling/spiritual support is ideal in such situations.

Establishing Routine: Practice Makes Perfect

Given the centrality of performance repetition in habit formation [66, 68, 93–94], concentrating efforts on this determinant makes sense.

Planning (discussed at greater length in chapter 11) is essential for at least initial adoption of a new and unfamiliar routine and overcoming the intention-behavior gap [20, 129]. Building frequency into the plan is of the essence; the more intermittent the behavior the less likely it is to become habitual [19].

Establishing the simplest suitable routine is more likely to result in repetition and habituation as discussed previously [8, 68, 95]. Given that there are likely multiple risk factors that need to be mitigated in the preoperative optimization of chronic pain patients, this consideration takes on added weight. Realistically in the context of the 2- to 3-month period we generally have to help facilitate readiness for surgery, few if any habits will be well formed by the time the operation is scheduled for many individuals, and many of the health behaviors we are working to instill will remain under conscious control, subject to motivational levels. Nonetheless, care should be taken to simplify focus and not attempt too many new behavioral patterns at once, especially in response to a given cueing process, as this may serve to both dilute habit formation [58, 96] and certainly confer motivational fatigue.

Ensuring stability of the environment is important when trying to form new habits [66, 130], presumably as repetition within the same context not only increases cue association but also likely increases (initial) consistent reward association as well. Conversely, when attempting to break undesirable habits, environmental alteration has been shown in numerous settings to disrupt the cue-action sequence [131]; this does not necessarily require tremendous upheaval, for example, moving one's residence; simply placing the cigarettes and lighter in the refrigerator under a bag of baby carrots has been a viable strategy for many of our patients.

References

1 Marteau TM, Hollands GJ, Fletcher PC. Changing human behavior to prevent disease: the importance of targeting automatic processes. Science. 2012;337:1492–5.

2 Gardner B, Lally P, Wardle J. Making health habitual: the psychology of "habit-formation" and general practice. Br J Gen Pract. 2012;62:664–6

3 Martin LR, Haskard-Zolnierek KB, DiMatteo MR. Improving health through the development and management of habits. In Martin LR, Haskard-Zolnierek KB, DiMatteo MR, eds., Health Behavior Change and Treatment Adherence: Evidence-Based Guidelines for Improving Healthcare. Oxford Scholarship Online, February 2010. doi: 10.1093/acprof:oso/9780195380408.001.0001

4 National Institutes of Health. Creating healthy habits make better choices easier. NIH News in Health. March 2018. https://newsinhealth.nih.gov/sites/nihNIH/files/2018/March/NIHNiHMar2018.pdf Accessed September 10, 2018.

5 Strack F, Deutsch R. Reflective and impulsive determinants of social behavior. Personality and Social Psychology Review. 2004;8:220–47.

6 Carver CS, Scheier MF. Cybernetic control processes and the self-regulation of behavior. In Ryan RM, ed., The Oxford Handbook of Human Motivation. New York: Oxford University Press; 2012.

7 Baumeister RF, Bratslavsky E, Muraven M, Tice DM. Ego depletion: is the active self a limited resource? J Personality Social Psychol. 1998;74:1252–65.

8 Wood W, Quinn JM, Kashy DA. Habits in everyday life: thought, emotion, and action. J Pers Soc Psychol. 2002;83:1281–97.

9 Verplanken B, Wood W. Interventions to Break and Create Consumer Habits. J Public Policy Marketing. 2006;25:90–103.

10 Duhigg C. The Power of Habit: Why We Do What We Do in Life and Business. New York: Random House; 2014.

11 James W. Habit. In The Principles of Psychology. London: Macmillan; 1890.

12 Graybiel AM. Habits, rituals, and the evaluative brain. Annu Rev Neurosci. 2008;31:359–87.

13 Smith KS, Graybiel AM. Habit formation. Dialogue Clin Neurosci. 2016;18:33–43.

14 Dunnington K. Addiction and virtue: beyond the models of disease and choice. Westmont, IL: Intervarsity Press; 2011.

15 Lewis M. The biology of desire: why addiction is not a disease. New York: Public Affairs; 2015.

16 Rothbart MK, Ahadi SA, Evans DE. Temperament and personality: origins and outcomes. J Personality Social Psychol. 2000;78:122–35.

17 Epstein S. Integration of the cognitive and the psychodynamic unconscious. Amer Psychologist. 1994;49:709–24.

18 Metcalfe J, Mischel W. A hot/cool-system analysis of delay of gratification: dynamics of willpower. Psychol Review. 1999;106:3–19.

19 Oullette JA, Wood W. Habit and intention in everyday life: the multiple processes by which past behavior predicts future behavior. Psychol Bulletin. 1998;124:54–74.

20 Rothman AJ, Sheeran P, Wood W. Reflective and automatic processes in the initiation and maintenance of dietary change. Ann Behav Med. 2009;38:S4–17.

21 Hunt SM, Martin CJ. Health-related behavioural change: a test of a new model. Psychology Health. 1988;2:209–30.

22 Kwasnicka D, Dombrowski SU, White M, Sniehotta F. Theoretical explanations for maintenance of behaviour change: a systematic review of behaviour theories. Health Psychol Rev. 2016;10:277–96.

23 Gardner B. A review and analysis of the use of "habit" in understanding, predicting and influencing health-related behaviour. Health Psychol Rev. 2015;9:277–95.

24 Lally P, Wardle J, Gardner B. Experiences of habit formation: a qualitative study. Psychol Health Med. 2011;16:484–9.

25 Wood W, Labrecque JS, Lin PY, Runger D. Habits in dual process models. In Sherman JW, Gawronski B, Trope Y, eds., Dual Process Theories of the Social Mind. New York: Guilford; 2014.

26 Triandis HC. Interpersonal Behavior. Monterey, CA: Brooks/Cole; 1977.

27 Verplanken B, Aarts H. Habit, attitude, and planned behaviour: is habit an empty construct or an interesting case of goal-directed automaticity? Eur Rev Soc Psychol. 1999;10:101–34.

28 Triandis HC. Values, attitudes, and interpersonal behavior. In Howe HE, Page M, eds., Nebraska Symposium of Motivation (Vol. 27, pp. 195–259). Lincoln: University of Nebraska Press; 1980.

29 Ajzen I. The theory of planned behavior. Organiz Behav Human Decision Process. 1991;50:179–211.

30 Sheeran P. Intention-behavior relations: a conceptual and empirical review. Eur Rev Social Psychol. 2002;12:1–36.

31 Rebar AL, Loftus AM, Hagger MS. Cognitive control and the non-conscious regulation of health behavior. Front Hum Neurosci. 2015;9:122. doi:10.3389/fnhum.2015.00122.

32 Sheeran P, Maki A, Montanaro E, et al. The impact of changing attitudes, norms, and self-efficacy on health-related intentions and behavior: a meta-analysis. Health Psychol. 2016;35:1178–88.

33 Webb TL, Sheeran P. Does changing behavioral intentions engender behavior change? A meta-analysis of the experimental evidence. Psychol Bull. 2006;132:249–68.

34 Michie S, Abraham C, Whittington C, McAteer J, Gupta S. Effective techniques in healthy eating and physical activity interventions: A meta-regression. Health Psychol. 2009;28:690–701.

35 Rhodes RE, Dickau L. Experimental evidence for the intention-behavior relationship in the physical activity domain: a meta-analysis. Health Psychol. 2012;31:724–7.

36 Rhodes RE, de Bruijn GJ. How big is the physical activity intention-behaviour gap? A meta-analysis using the action control framework. Br J Health Psychol. 2013;18:296–309.

37 Ajzen I. From intentions to actions: a theory of planned behavior. In Kuhl J, Beckmann J, eds., Action Control. SSSP Springer Series in Social Psychology. Berlin: Springer; 1985.

38 McEachan RRC, Conner M, Taylor N, Lawton RJ. Prospective prediction of health-related behaviors with the theory of planned behavior: a meta-analysis. Health Psychol Rev. 2011;5:97–144.

39 Sniehotta FF, Gellert P, Witham MD, Donnan PT, Crombie IK, McMurdo MET. Psychological theory in an interdisciplinary context: how do social cognitions predict physical activity in older adults alongside demographic, health-related, social, and environmental factors? Internat J Behavioral Nutrition Phys Activity. 2013;10(1):106. 10.1186/1479-5868-10-106.

40 Gardner B, de Bruijn GJ, Lally P. A systematic review and meta-analysis of applications of the Self-Report Habit Index to nutrition and physical activity behaviours. Ann Behav Med. 2011;42:174–87.

41 Towler G, Shepherd R. Modification of Fishbein and Ajzen's theory of reasoned action to predict chip consumption. Food Qual Prefer. 1991–2;3:37–45.

42 Verplanken B. Beyond frequency: habit as mental construct. Brit J Social Psychol. 2006;45:639–56.

43 De Bruijn GJ, Van den Putte B. Adolescent soft drink consumption, television viewing and habit strength. Investigating clustering effects in the Theory of Planned Behaviour. Appetite. 2009;53:66–75.

44 Hearst MO, Patnode CD, Sirard JR, Farbakhsh K, Lytle LA. Multilevel predictors of adolescent physical activity: a longitudinal analysis. Int J Behav Nutr Phys Act. 2012;9:8. doi: 10.1186/1479-5868-9-8.

45 van Bree RJ, van Stralen MM, Bolman C, Mudde AN, de Vries H, Lechner L. Habit as moderator of the intention-physical activity relationship in older adults: a longitudinal study. Psychol Health. 2013;28:514–32.

46 Cleo G, Isenring E, Thomas R, Glasziou P. Could habits hold the key to weight loss maintenance? A narrative review. J Hum Nutr Diet. 2017;30:655–64.

47 Verplanken B, Orbell S. Reflections on past behavior: a self report index of habit strength. J Appl Soc Psychol. 2003;33:1313–30.

48 Rebar AL, Dimmock JA, Jackson B, et al. A systematic review of the effects of non-conscious regulatory processes in physical activity. Health Psychol Rev. 2016;10:395–407.

49 Conn VS, Ruppar TM, Chase JAD. Blood pressure outcomes of medication adherence interventions: systematic review and meta-analysis. J Behav Med. 2016;39:1065–75.

50 Conn VS, Ruppar TM, Enriquez M, Cooper P. Medication adherence interventions that target subjects with adherence problems: systematic review and meta-analysis. Res Social Adm Pharm. 2016;12:218–46.

51 Lally P, Chipperfield A, Wardle J. Healthy habits: efficacy of simple advice on weight control based on a habit-formation model. Int J Obes (Lond). 2008;32:700–7.

52 Beeken RJ, Leurent B, Vickerstaff V, et al. A brief intervention for weight control based on habit-formation theory delivered through primary care: results from a randomised controlled trial. Int J Obes (Lond). 2017;41:246–54.

53 Carels RA, Burmeister JM, Koball AM, et al. A randomized trial comparing two approaches to weight loss: differences in weight loss maintenance. J Health Psychol. 2014;19:296–311.

54 Cleo G, Glasziou P, Beller E, Isenring E, Thomas R. Habit-based interventions for weight loss maintenance in adults with overweight and obesity: a randomized controlled trial. Int J Obes (Lond). April 23, 2018. doi: 10.1038/s41366-018-0067-4.

55 Aarts H, Verplanken B, Knippenberg A. Predicting behavior from actions in the past: repeated decision making or a matter of habit? J Applied Social Psychol. 1998;28:1355–74.

56 Aarts H, Dijksterhuis A. Habits as knowledge structures: automaticity in goal-directed behavior. J Pers Soc Psychol. 2000;78:53–63.

57 Wood W, Rünger D. Psychology of habit. Annu Rev Psychol. 2016;67:289–314.

58 Wood W, Neal DT. A new look at habits and the habit-goal interface. Psychol Rev. 2007;114:843–63.

59 Neal DT, Wood W, Labrecque JS, Lally P. How do habits guide behavior? Perceived and actual triggers of habits in daily life. J Exper Social Psychol. 2012;48: 492–8.

60 Dolan RJ, Dayan P. Goals and habits in the brain. Neuron. 2013;80:312–25.

61 Rebar AL, Gardner B, Verplanken B. Habit in exercise behavior. In Tenenbaum G, Eklund RC, eds., Handbook of Sport Psychology (Vol. 4). Hoboken, NJ: Wiley; 2018.

62 Thorndike EL. Animal intelligence: an experimental study of the associative processes in animals. Psychol Monogr Gen Appl. 1898;2:1–109.

63 Lally P, Gardner B. Promoting habit formation. Health Psychol Rev. 2013;7(Suppl 1), S137–58.

64 Gardner B, Lally P. Modelling habit formation and its determinants. In Verplanken B, ed., The Psychology of Habit. Springer Nature: Cham Switzerland, 2018.

65 Hull C. Principles of Behavior: An Introduction to Behavior Theory. New York: Appleton-Century-Crofts; 1943.

66 Lally P, van Jaarsveld CHM, Potts HWW, Wardle J. How are habits formed: modelling habit formation in the real world. Eur J Social Psychol. 2010;40:998–1009.

67 Fournier M, d'Arripe-Longueville F, Rovere C, et al. Effects of circadian cortisol on the development of a health habit. Health Psychol. 2017;36:1059–64.

68 Kaushal N, Rhodes RE. Exercise habit formation in new gym members: a longitudinal study. J Behavioural Med. 2015;38:652–63.

69 Gardner B, Lally P. Does intrinsic motivation strengthen physical activity habit? modeling relationships between self-determination, past behaviour and habit strength. J Behavioral Med. 2013;36:488–97.

70 Radel R, Pelletier L, Pjevac D, Cheval B. The links between self-determined motivations and behavioral automaticity in a variety of real-life behaviours. Motiv Emotion. 2017;41:443–54.

71 Tangney JP, Baumeister RF, Boone AL. High self-control predicts good adjustment, less pathology, better grades, and interpersonal success. J Personality. 2004;72:271–324.

72 Galla BM, Duckworth AL. More than resisting temptation: beneficial habits mediate the relationship between self-control and positive life outcomes. J Personality Social Psychol. 2015;109:508–25.

73 Linnebank FE, Kindt M, de Wit S. Investigating the balance between goal-directed and habitual control in experimental and real-life settings. Learn Behav. 2018;46:306–19.

74 de Wit S, Barker RA, Dickinson AD, Cools R. Habitual versus goal-directed action control in Parkinson disease. J Cogn Neurosci. 2011;23:1218–29.

75 Gillan CM, Papmeyer M, Morein-Zamir S, et al. Disruption in the balance between goal-directed behavior and habit learning in obsessive-compulsive disorder. Am J Psychiatry. 2011;168:718–26.

76 Gillan CM, Morein-Zamir S, Kaser M, et al. Counterfactual processing of economic action-outcome alternatives in obsessive compulsive disorder: further evidence of impaired goal-directed behavior. Biological Psychiatry. 2014;75:639–46.

77 Robbins TW, Gillan CM, Smith DG, de Wit S, Ersche KD. Neurocognitive endophenotypes of impulsivity and compulsivity: towards dimensional psychiatry. Trends Cogn Science. 2012;16:81–91.

78 Sjoerds Z, de Wit S, van den Brink W, et al. Behavioral and neuroimaging evidence for overreliance on habit learning in alcohol dependent patients. Trans Psychiatry. 2013;3(12):e337. https:// doi.org/10.1038/tp.2013.107.

79 Ersche KD, Gillan CM, Jones PS, et al. Carrots and sticks fail to change behavior in cocaine addiction. Science. 2016;352:1468–1471.

80 McDaniel MA, Einstein GO. Strategic and automatic processes in prospective memory retrieval: A multiprocess framework. Applied Cogn Psychol. 2000;14:S127–44.

81 Schüz B, Sniehotta FF, Wiedemann A, Seemann R. Adherence to a daily flossing regimen in university students: effects of planning when, where, how and what to do in the face of barriers. J Clin Periodontol. 2006;33:612–9.

82 Judah G, Gardner B, Aunger R. Forming a flossing habit: an exploratory study of the psychological determinants of habit formation. Br J Health Psychol. 2013;18:338–53.

83 Pimm R, Vandelanotte C, Rhodes RE, Short C, Duncan MJ, Rebar AL. Cue consistency associated with physical activity automaticity and behavior. Behav Med. 2016;42:248–53.

84 Schwabe L, Wolf OT. Stress and multiple memory systems: from "thinking" to "doing." Trends Cogn Sci. 2013;17:60–8.

85 Radenbach C, Reiter AMF, Engert V, et al. The interaction of acute and chronic stress impairs model-based behavioral control. Psychoneuroendocrinol. 2015;53:268–80.

86 Otto AR, Raio CM, Chiang A. Working-memory capacity protects model-based learning from stress. PNAS. 2013;52:20941–6.

87 Quirarte GL, Ledesma de la Teja IS, Casillas M, Serafín N, Prado-Alcalá RA, Roozendaal B. Corticosterone infused into the dorsal striatum selectively enhances memory consolidation of cued water-maze training. Learning Memory. 2009;16:586–9.

88 Bandura A. Toward a psychology of human agency: pathways and reflections. Perspect Psychol Sci. 2018;13:130–6.

89 Kandel DB, Andrews K. Processes of adolescent socialization by parents and peers. Int J Addict. 1987;22:319–42.

90 Seo DC, Huang Y. Systematic review of social network analysis in adolescent cigarette smoking behavior. J Sch Health. 2012;82:21–7.

91 McGowan L, Cooke LJ, Gardner B, Beeken RJ, Croker H, Wardle J. Healthy feeding habits: efficacy results from a cluster-randomized, controlled exploratory trial of a novel, habit-based intervention with parents. Am J Clin Nutr. 2013;98:769–77.

92 Stein A, Woolley H, Cooper S, Winterbottom J, Fairburn CG, Cortina-Borja M. Eating habits and attitudes among 10-year-old children of mothers with eating disorders: longitudinal study. Br J Psychiatry. 2006;189:324–9.

93 Armitage CJ. Can the theory of planned behavior predict the maintenance of physical activity? Health Psychol. 2005;24:235–45.

94 Staples AD, Bates JE, Petersen IT. Chapter IX. Bedtime routines in toddlerhood: prevalence, consistency, and associations with nighttime sleep. Monographs Society Res Child Develop. 2015;80:141–59.

95 Verplanken B. Beyond frequency: habit as a mental construct. Brit J Social Psychol. 2006;45:639–56.

96 Mc Culloch KC, Fujita K, Aarts H, Bargh JA. Inhibition in goal systems: a retrieval-induced forgetting account. J Exp Soc Psychol. 2008;44:857–65.

97 Wood W. Habit in personality and social psychology. Personal Social Psychol Rev. 2017;21:389–403.

98 Dickinson A. Actions and habits: the development of behavioural autonomy. Philosoph Transact Royal Society London. Series B. Biol Sciences. 1985;308:67–78.

99 Wiedemann AU, Gardner B, Knoll N, Burkert S. Intrinsic rewards, fruit and vegetable consumption, and habit strength: a three-wave study testing the Associative-Cybernetic Model. Applied Psychol Health Well-Being. 2014;6:119–34.

100 Skinner BF. A case history in scientific method. Am Psychologist. 1956;11:221–33.

101 Balleine BW, Dickinson A. Goal-directed instrumental action: contingency and incentive learning and their cortical substrates. Neuropharmacol. 1998;37:407–19.

102 He Y, Li Y, Chen M, et al. Habit formation after random interval training is associated with increased adenosine A_{2A} receptor and dopamine D_2 receptor heterodimers in the striatum. Frontier Mol Neurosci. 2016;9:151. doi:10.3389/fnmol.2016.00151.

103 Blair SN, Jacobs DR Jr, Powell KE. Relationships between exercise or physical activity and other health behaviors. Public Health Rep. 1985;100:172–80.

104 Hollis JF, Gullion CM, Stevens VJ, et al. Weight loss during the intensive intervention phase of the weight-loss maintenance trial. Am J Prev Med. 2008;35:118–26.

105 de Wit S, Dickinson A. Associative theories of goal-directed behaviour: a case for animal-human translational models. Psychol Research, 2009;73:463–76.

106 Yin HH, Ostlund SB, Knowlton BJ, Balleine BW. The role of the dorsomedial striatum in instrumental conditioning. Eur J Neurosci. 2005;22:513–23.

107 Thorn CA, Atallah H, Howe M, Graybiel AM. Differential dynamics of activity changes in dorsolateral and dorsomedial striatal loops during learning. Neuron 2010;66:781–795.

108 Yin HH, Knowlton BJ, Balleine BW. Lesions of dorsolateral striatum preserve outcome expectancy but disrupt habit formation in instrumental learning. Eur J Neurosci. 2004;19:181–9.

109 Lingawi NW, Balleine BW. Amygdala central nucleus interacts with dorsolateral striatum to regulate the acquisition of habits. J Neurosci. 2012;32:1073–81.

110 Jog MS, Kubota Y, Connolly CI, Hillegaart V, Graybiel AM. Building neural representations of habits. Science. 1999;286:1745–9.

111 Graybiel AM. The basal ganglia and chunking of action repertoires. Neurobiol Learn Mem 1998;70:119–36.

112 Coutureau E, Killcross S. Inactivation of the infralimbic prefrontal cortex reinstates goal-directed responding in overtrained rats. Behav Brain Res. 2003;146:167–74.

113 Killcross S, Coutureau E. Coordination of actions and habits in the medial prefrontal cortex of rats. Cereb Cortex 2003;13:400–8.

114 Smith KS, Graybiel AM. Investigating habits: strategies, technologies and models. Front Behav Neurosci. 2014;8:39. Published online February 12, 2014. doi: 10.3389/fnbeh.2014.00039.

115 Wassum KM, Cely IC, Maidment NT, Balleine BW. Disruption of endogenous opioid activity during instrumental learning enhances habit acquisition. Neuroscience 2009;163:770–80.

116 Faure A, Haberland U, Condé F, El Massioui N. Lesion to the nigrostriatal dopamine system disrupts stimulus-response habit formation. J Neurosci. 2005;25:2771–80.

117 Shan Q, Christie MJ, Balleine BW. Plasticity in striatopallidal projection neurons mediates the acquisition of habitual actions. Eur J Neurosci. 2015;42:2097–104.

118 Hollerman JR, Schultz W. Dopamine neurons report an error in the temporal prediction of reward during learning. Nature Neurosci. 1998;1:304–9.

119 Montague PR, Hyman SE, Cohen JD. Computational roles for dopamine in behavioural control. Nature. 2004; 431:760–7.

120 Choi WY, Balsam PD, Horvitz JC. Extended habit training reduces dopamine mediation of appetitive response expression. J Neurosci. 2005; 25: 6729–33.

121 Wood W, Neal DT. The habitual consumer. J Consumer Psychol. 2009;19:579–92.

122 Custers R, Aarts H. Positive affect as implicit motivator: on the nonconscious operation of behavioral goals. J Pers Soc Psychol. 2005;89:129–42.

123 Hardeman W, Johnston M, Johnston DW, Bonetti D, Wareham NJ, Kinmonth AL. Application of the theory of planned behaviour in behaviour change interventions: a systematic review. Pscyhol Health. 2002;17:123–58.

124 de Bruijn GJ, Keer M, Conner M, Rhodes RE. Using implicit associations towards fruit consumption to understand fruit consumption behaviour and habit strength relationships. J Health Psychol. 2012;17:479–89.

125 Sun X, Prochaska JO, Velicer WF, Laforge RG. Transtheoretical principles and processes for quitting smoking: a 24-month comparison of a representative sample of quitters, relapsers, and non-quitters. Addict Behav. 2007;32:2707–26.

126 Marlatt GA. Determinants of relapse and skill-training interventions. In Marlatt GA, Gordon JR, eds., Relapse Prevention: Maintenance Strategies in the Treatment of Addictive Behaviors. New York: Guilford Press; 1985.

127   Gorski TT, Miller M. Staying Sober: A Guide for Relapse Prevention. Independence, MO: Herald House/Independence Press; 1986.

128   Quinn JM, Pascoe A, Wood W, Neal DT. Can't control yourself? Monitor those bad habits. Pers Soc Psychol Bull. 2010;36:499–511.

129   Gollwitzer PM, Sheeran P. Implementation intentions and goal achievement: a meta-analysis of effects and processes. Adv Exp Soc Psychol. 2006;38:69–119.

130   Danner UN, Aarts H, de Vries NK. Habit formation and multiple means to goal attainment: repeated retrieval of target means causes inhibited access to competitors. Pers Soc Psychol Bull. 2007;33:1367–79.

131   Rothman AJ, Gollwitzer PM, Grant AM, Neal DT, Sheeran P, Wood W. Hale and hearty policies: how psychological science can create and maintain healthy habits. Perspect Psychol Sci. 2015;10:701–5.

5

Pain Catastrophizing and Anxiety

Beth Darnall

Psychology and Perioperative Optimization

The optimization of perioperative patients involves targeting the modifiable individual factors that influence pain, function, and surgical outcomes. First, we should recognize that pain is a useful signal to alert a person to potential physical harm. Accordingly, pre- and post-surgical medical problems and underlying disease processes that may be driving the post-surgical pain experience should be assessed and either addressed and treated or ruled out. For ongoing chronic pain, in which pain is serving no useful purpose, and in perioperative timeframe, there are often many opportunities for behavioral intervention to reduce post-surgical suffering and enhance recovery. Indeed, psychological factors—including pain anxiety and pain catastrophizing—are among the most influential factors on surgical outcomes yet rarely are targeted in the perioperative timeframe. To date, research has largely focused on the *characterization* of behavioral risk factors that associate with or predict poor surgical outcomes, whereas fewer perioperative studies and programs have focused on perioperative *interventions*. As such, interventions that effectively address the highest-yield targets may meaningfully improve perioperative care and favorably alter the long-term trajectory of health after surgery. This chapter aims to elucidate key research to date for pain anxiety and pain catastrophizing and underscore their importance as therapeutic targets in the perioperative timeline; it also reviews data on their malleability and responsivity to intervention, and highlights promising relevant clinical programs.

Pain Catastrophizing Definition and Measurement

Pain catastrophizing is defined as *a maladaptive pattern of negative cognitive and emotional response to actual or anticipated pain* [1]. Often catastrophizing can lead to a focus on a "worst case scenario" such as, "What happens if my pain gets worse?" or "What if something is seriously wrong with me?" Catastrophizing is typically measured with one of three self-report questionnaires: the Pain Catastrophizing Scale (PCS), the Coping Skills Questionnaire

(CSQ)—Catastrophizing Subscale, and the newly created Pain Appraisal Scale (PAS).

Pain Catastrophizing Scale

The PCS is the most commonly used measure of pain catastrophizing. It includes 13 items, and respondents are directed to consider times in their lives where they have experienced pain (e.g., illness, injury, dental procedure, or surgery) and to consider how they tended to respond to pain. It is important to note that the PCS is not specific to chronic pain, nor does it assume that respondents have current pain. While most psychological measures direct respondents to consider a specific timeframe of reference for each scale items (e.g., the past week or past month) the PCS provides no specific chronological referent and for this reason it has been considered to assess pain catastrophizing as a "trait." However, "trait variable" suggests the construct maintains relative stability over time, and in fact studies that include repeated administration of the PCS show a fair degree of variance over time [2].

The PCS presents respondents with various statements and one is directed to rate the *frequency* with which their experience matches the content of the statement [1]. Examples: "I anxiously want the pain to go away," and "There's nothing I can do to reduce the intensity of the pain." (0 = not at all; 1 = to a slight degree; 2 = to a moderate degree; 3 = to a great degree; 4 = all the time). The 13 items of the PCS are distributed across three subscales: magnification of pain, feelings of helplessness about pain, and rumination. Scores for all individual items are summed to arrive at a total PSC score, ranging from 0 to 52. The total PCS score is clinically useful because it has moderate and strong associations with clinical outcomes. Results from research spanning decades has demonstrated that higher PCS scores predict an array of negative outcomes such as persistence of pain healthy populations [3], greater pain intensity in evoked pain studies in healthy volunteers [4], and a host of poor outcomes in patients with chronic pain and nonsurgical acute pain [5–8] as well as in surgical patients with and without preexisting chronic pain [9, 10].

It is notable that while there is shared variance between pain catastrophizing and depression, there is considerable unique variance and thus is a distinct construct [11].

While scoring the PCS is straightforward, interpretation and clear cut-off scores are less simple. Often, a clinical cut-score of 30 is used as an artificial threshold and index for treatment needs. However, pain catastrophizing is not binary and its effects should be considered within the context of each individual. The literature suggests that scores of 30 or higher are strongly associated with persistent *work-related disability* [12], and we argue that this is a poor index for treatment needs for patients with chronic pain wherein the goal is to restore function and prevent deterioration and major disability whenever possible. For context and framing, many outpatient chronic pain studies report mean PCS scores ranging from the low- to mid-20s; these are noted to frequently be pain-treatment-seeking populations. The PCS scale, scoring manual, and compilation of background science may be accessed here: http://sullivan-painresearch.mcgill.ca/pdf/pcs/PCSManual_English.pdf.

In surgical research, psychological measures are administered prior and proximal to one's surgery date and then examined in models of predictors for postsurgical outcomes, such as pain intensity, duration of pain, indices of function/recovery, and amount and duration opioid use. Results for perioperative research have shown that presurgical PCS scores of 14–15 associate with poor postsurgical outcomes [13], a strikingly lower threshold than is frequently described in the chronic pain literature. These findings suggest application of a low threshold for treatment in perioperative patients; this dovetails nicely with a conceptual shift from "treating an entrenched problem or 'psychopathology' " to simply focusing on optimizing the surgical outcomes for every single patient.

Pain is dynamically processed in the central nervous system with individual and psychological factors being foundational to the presence, strength, and direction of descending pain modulation. For instance, overfocus and attention to pain, and maladaptive beliefs about pain (e.g., "hurt equals harm"), oppose descending pain modulation and serve to amplify pain intensity and distress about pain. Catastrophizing stands as an important and measurable index of poor descending pain modulation. A low catastrophizing score suggests that in the context of pain, an individual generally refrains from pain rumination and worrying about the negative consequences, and they are able to adaptively regulate pain-related cognition and emotion. Adaptive self-regulation skills provide a degree of control over one's experience of pain. Use of adaptive self-regulatory pain management skills cultivates self-efficacy to self-manage aspects of one's pain experience, opposes feelings of helplessness about pain, and ultimately extinguishes patterns of pain catastrophizing. As such, it is useful to consider higher catastrophizing scores as indicative of a pain self-regulation skills *deficit*, whereas low catastrophizing scores point to adaptive self-regulation of pain. Pain self-regulation skills are learned, and lead to improved ability to reduce suffering and enhance personal control over pain-related distress. Few or no studies suggest a link between low PCS scores ≤10 and negative outcomes across care settings. For this reason, as a clinician, I (BD) encourage all patients to adopt a goal of reducing ideally to ≤10 for a total PCS score.

Perioperative patients with chronic pain have established, quantifiable patterns of responses to their preexisting chronic pain. As such, the presurgical optimization of the patient living with chronic pain can dually address acute pain after surgery and preexisting chronic pain, toward a goal of enhanced recovery after surgery.

Additional Pain Catastrophizing Measures

Coping Skills Questionnaire (CSQ) Catastrophizing Subscale. The CSQ Catastrophizing Scale [14] comprises six items across two subscales (helplessness and pessimism about pain).

Pain Appraisal Scale (PAS). Recent research employing cognitive interviewing techniques demonstrates that many patients abhor the term "pain catastrophizing" due it having a pejorative connotation that seems to imply that pain is either "psychological," "in one's head," "the patient's fault," or "exaggerated" [15]. To address these common concerns and barriers to patient engagement, the researchers consulted with patient advisors and adopted more neutral terminology to title their new catastrophizing scale the University of Washington Pain Appraisal Scale (UW-PAS). To further address patient concerns about the stigmatizing effect of negative pain appraisal, the authors clearly state in the clinician manual that "a high score on the UW-PAS does not diminish the importance of patient's report of chronic pain." Rather, a high score represents an opportunity to help patients reduce suffering. The UW-PAS exists in several versions, including 2-item, 6-item, 8-item, and 24-item banks. The authors suggest that a score >55 is greater than for most patients with chronic pain, and they supply crosswalk information to the PCS. The authors suggest that a score of 52 on the UW-PAS is equivalent to a score of 20 on the PCS, and a score of 57 on the UW-PAS is equivalent to a score of 30 on the PCS. The UW-PAS measures and scoring manual may be accessed here: https://uwcorr.washington.edu/wp-content/uploads/2018/12/uw-pas-userguide.pdf.

Anxiety and Fear

Anxiety is associated with greater pain intensity and poorer outcomes in patients with chronic pain, and it has established association with greater pain after surgery [16–18]. Depending on the scale used, anxiety may be measured as a trait or state variable, or specific to the context of pain (pain-related anxiety, fear of pain, or fear of movement). Pain catastrophizing is highly correlated with all measures of anxiety, general and pain-specific anxiety [19–23], and this is perhaps unsurprising when reflecting on the fact that an item for negative expectation or anticipatory pain is included in the measure: "I become afraid that the pain will get worse." Anticipation of pain dovetails closely with hypervigilance and exaggerated threat appraisal of pain, two components of anxiety and pain-specific anxiety, respectively. Furthermore, one prominent measure of pain-related anxiety, the Pain Anxiety Symptom Scale (PASS) [24], actually contains a catastrophizing subscale [1, 22], and as such there is little surprise in the strong correlations found between catastrophizing measures and the PASS.

Like catastrophizing, pain-related anxiety and fear of pain enhance the threat value of pain, and therefore pain itself. Prospective studies have shown that both fear of pain [3] and kinesiophobia (fear of movement) predict future back pain in population studies [25]. Pain-related anxiety and fear of pain may shape avoidance behavior, deconditioning, and disability [26–28]. The fear avoidance model posits that activity avoidance may contribute to physical changes (e.g., muscle tension, disuse, and atrophy) that may promote greater pain upon movement—and therefore confirm the patient's underlying fear-related bias [26, 27]. Researchers examining the impact of kinesiophobia after spine surgery found that early postoperative fear of movement (6 weeks) predicted pain intensity, pain interference, disability, and physical health at 6-month follow-up [29].

Cognitive-behavioral therapy for chronic pain and graded exposure therapy may effectively address these psychobehavioral factors, as can physical therapy with a therapist skilled in treating chronic pain [30–32]. Treatment typically involves gradual exposure to therapeutic movement and exercises. The goals are to help patients: (1) slowly begin appropriate movement; (2) gain strength and endurance; (3) challenge and extinguish maladaptive pain beliefs and fear of movement and/or pain and catastrophizing; (4) reduce avoidance behaviors; (5) understand that movement is vital to recovery of function; (5) increase self-efficacy for activity; (6) reduce pain-related interference and disability; (7) actively engage in a daily pain self-management plan.

The clinical purpose of anxiety measurement is to identify therapeutic targets and ideally deliver targeted interventions. Given the shared variance between pain catastrophizing and pain anxiety, and attention to survey burden for patients, and general superior predictive value for catastrophizing compared to anxiety, we recommend that pain catastrophizing be prioritized over general or pain-specific indices of anxiety in presurgical screenings and for outcomes research. For programs and studies that allow for deeper phenotyping, the following are useful and more specific self-report measures of pain-related anxiety.

- **Pain Anxiety Symptom Scale** (PASS-20) [33]—a validated 20-item measure of pain-related anxiety that includes subscales for fear/catastrophizing, cognitive anxiety, escape/avoidance, and physiological anxiety. The PASS-20 may be accessed here:
  https://www.exchangecme.com/resourcePDF/chronicpain/resource5.pdf.
- **Tampa Scale of Kinesiophobia** (TSK)—a validated 17-item measure that assesses fear of movement or (re)injury. Kinesiophobia is defined as

an "irrational, and debilitating fear of physical movement and activity resulting from a feeling of vulnerability to painful injury or re-injury."

The TSK may be accessed here: https://www.novopsych.com/tsk-2.html.
Additionally, a validated 11-item [34] version retains the psychometric properties of the 17-item scale with reduced response burden.

- Fear of Pain Questionnaire-9 [35]—a psychometrically sound and efficient measure fear and anxiety associated with pain: https://onlinelibrary.wiley.com/doi/full/10.1002/ejp.1074

Pain Catastrophizing, Anxiety, and Surgical Outcomes

Greater levels of pain catastrophizing have been shown to influence pain perception [11, 36–38], chronic pain treatment outcomes [39, 40], acute postsurgical pain [18, 41–46], length of hospital stay after total joint arthroplasty [47], and surgical recovery (either indexed by pain resolution and/or functional measures) [10, 18, 46, 48, 49]. One interesting meta-analysis aggregated 53 studies containing a total of 10,749 patients to examine pooled effects for presurgical psychological variables on acute postsurgical pain [44]. The presurgical psychological variables of interest included pain catastrophizing, anxiety (state and trait), optimism, expectation of pain, neuroticism, negative affect, and depression [44]. The authors noted that while every aforementioned psychological variable significantly associated with acute postsurgical pain, pain catastrophizing was noted to have the strongest association (OR = 5.00; 95% confidence interval 3.03–8.24; $p < 0.001$).

Results for research on the influence of presurgical pain catastrophizing scores on postsurgical opioid consumption are both mixed and sparse. Positive association between pain catastrophizing and in-hospital opioid use after surgery has been reported [45], while other studies have reported no association [18, 47], though a notable limitation in the data are differing cut-points for analytic models. While some studies suggest PCS scores of 14 confer risk for poorer outcomes after surgery, some studies have applied a cut-point of 30, an index for work-related disability due to chronic pain versus being empirically informed in perioperative studies.

In terms of prolonged use of opioids after surgery, researchers of one noteworthy study used logistic regression modeling (not including pain intensity) to examine predictors for prolonged postoperative opioid use after musculoskeletal surgery. The authors reported that in models that controlled for injury severity, fracture site, and treating surgeon, the single best predictor of reported opioid use 2 months after surgery was pain catastrophizing (odds ratio, 1.12 [95% confidence interval, 1.07–1.18]), which explained 23% of the variance ($p < 0.001$) [13].

Among the most important outcomes after surgery is recovery and resolution of pain. Roughly 10% of patients will experience chronic postsurgical pain, though this figure is known to vary up to fivefold largely based on the type of surgery and study methods. Chronic postsurgical pain is defined as de novo pain acquired after a surgical procedure and experienced for at least 2 months; it must not be a continuation of preexisting pain and has no other identifiable cause outside of the surgical event. Various investigations have characterized the importance of preexisting psychosocial factors on the development of chronic postsurgical pain and associated treatment needs.

One particular meta-analytic study examined whether preoperative anxiety (general or pain-specific) and pain catastrophizing predicted chronic postsurgical pain [10]. Theunissen and colleagues first examined 29 relevant studies (excluding dental surgeries) that included preoperative assessment of the psychological variables of interest and a measure of pain at 3 months after surgery. They reported that of these 29 studies, 16 evidenced a statistically significant association between presurgical anxiety or pain catastrophizing and the development of postsurgical chronic pain (55%) while 13 studies (45%) did not; interestingly, general anxiety was a better predictor of postsurgical chronic pain than pain-specific anxiety. Fifteen studies containing a total of 5,046 patients using similar analytic methods and assessment timepoints were included in their meta-analysis examining whether anxiety or pain catastrophizing was associated with chronic postsurgical pain. Pooled odds ratio (OR) analyses revealed total OR of 2.1 (95% CI, 1.49–2.95) for the maximum effect scenario and 1.55 (95% CI, 1.10–2.20) for the minimum effect scenario [10(p825)]. Furthermore, the ORs suggested relative superiority of pain catastrophizing as a predictor.

Finally, the Archer et al study [29] showing that postsurgical kinesiophobia (6 weeks) is predictive of disability at 6 months after spine surgery underscores the need to assess and address such factors to cultivate engagement in rehabilitative behavior and restoration of function after surgery.

Mechanisms of Pain Catastrophizing and Anxiety

Pain catastrophizing and anxiety exert their influence through multiple mechanisms, and here we touch on just two: behavioral and neurological mechanisms.

Pain catastrophizing and pain-related fear exert lasting impacts by shaping behavioral pathways, most notably illustrated by the fear-avoidance model of chronic pain (see Figure 5.1).

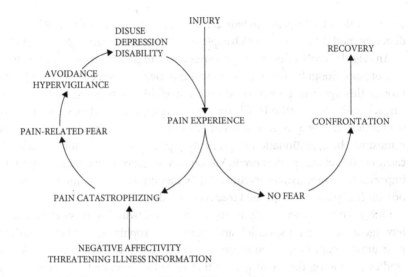

Figure 5.1. The Fear-Avoidance Model of Chronic Pain

From "Fear avoidance and its consequences in musculoskeletal pain: A state of the art", by J.W. Vlaeyen and S.J. Linton, 2000, Pain, 85, p. 329. Used with permission from IASP.

In the fear-avoidance model of chronic pain, these pain-related psychological constructs promote hypervigilance for pain and avoidance of rehabilitative behaviors (due to fear of greater pain or physical damage), thereby leading to reduced function, deconditioning, depression, and disability. Feelings of helplessness about pain may operate similarly to discourage engagement in active rehabilitation and cultivate passive strategies. As such, patients may have terrific physical therapy and medical treatments, but the underlying psychological factors can undermine patient engagement and response to their care [39]. As such, patients need access to multidisciplinary care, and data suggest that scalable psychological treatments should be applied first to ensure best response to medical care, including surgery.

While the fear-avoidance model was conceptualized within the context of chronic pain, it may be similarly applied to postsurgical acute pain. For instance, greater presurgical pain-related anxiety and pain catastrophizing have been associated with poorer postsurgical function across a variety of surgical types including total knee arthroplasty [46] and hand fracture surgery [50, and in musculoskeletal trauma surgery patients [13]. Conceptually, when considering perioperative patients, it may be useful to replace "injury" in Figure 5.1 with the term "surgery." It is vitally important to assess and address pain catastrophizing and pain-related fear to promote active engagement in rehabilitative strategies that facilitate recovery from surgery and enhance long-term function and wellness.

In terms of neurological mechanisms, functional magnetic resonance imaging studies conducted in healthy volunteers during evoked pain experiments show that pain catastrophizing increases blood flow in the regions of the brain associated with attention and the affective dimensions of pain [51]. The researchers reported that "during experiments that involved more intense pain, the prefrontal cortical regions implicated in the top-down modulation of pain were negatively correlated with catastrophizing." In other words, pain catastrophizing is an index of poor descending pain modulation and diminished ability to disengage from and suppress pain [52]. Instead, as one gives greater attention and negative focus to pain through catastrophizing, the result is amplified distress, increased pain processing in the brain [36, 51], and greater reports for in vivo pain intensity [51] as well as greater pain over time [22].

Other neuroimaging research conducted on patients with chronic pain has shown that catastrophizing—which should be considered a neurological pattern of pain facilitation—shapes brain functioning and alters the physical structure of the brain [52–54]—as well as the functioning of the brain even in resting states [54]—such that the individual is primed to experience greater pain. As one example, researchers compared functional and structural brain scans between healthy individuals and patients with chronic pain [54]. The authors noted that patterns of pain catastrophizing in individuals with chronic pain were associated with functional connectivity patterns that were akin to what is seen in people who have an anxiety disorder, despite anxiety disorder having been a criterion of exclusion. It is thought that the collective findings demonstrating altered structure and function of the brain provide a neurological basis for catastrophizing's role in the progression of pain to the chronic state [51].

Treating Pain Catastrophizing

While an exhaustive review of psychological treatment for pain is beyond the scope of this chapter, the interested reader may wish to review an in-depth clinical overview of this topic [55]. Pain catastrophizing and anxiety are both effectively treated with cognitive-behavioral therapy for chronic pain (pain-CBT) [56] delivered in individual or group settings, with the latter most often used in treatment research studies. Decades of research have demonstrated that, to date, pain-CBT enjoys the largest evidence base, and for this reason it is recommended by multiple national clinical guidelines and organizations [57, 58]. Pain-CBT is manualized and skills-based and includes several key components that help patients both increase engagement in self-management of pain and symptoms and increase function.

When delivered in group format, pain-CBT most commonly involves attending eight 2-hour group sessions. During pain-CBT participants are given pain education (which serves to challenge many underlying maladaptive pain beliefs, such as "pain = harm"). Often pain education underscores the importance of activity goal setting and gradually increasing movement as a critical component of pain management and restoring function, and as a pathway to reducing pain interference, goal attainment, and quality of life. Additional topics covered over the course of pain-CBT include goal-setting skills; problem-solving skills; relaxation skills; understanding mood and pain; sleep and pain; understanding how thoughts, emotions, and pain relate; identifying and challenging negative thoughts about pain; and creating action plans. Participants complete homework each week, and are encouraged to use their skills daily to begin to entrain new patterns of thought and behavior. Indeed, cognition and emotion regulation skills, coupled with behavioral action and movement plans, serve as the foundations of evidence-based pain-CBT.

Treatment outcomes research for pain-CBT has shown that it leads to improved cognitive, emotional, and physiological regulation. Moreover, pre-post treatment neuroimaging research has shown that after pain-CBT participants have significant volumetric increases in gray matter in the regions of the brain associated with pain control [52]. These adaptive structural brain changes were found to be mediated by reductions in pain catastrophizing and associated with reduced pain intensity. While replication of this study is needed, these findings suggest that pain-CBT favorably alters the function and structure of the brain, thereby reshaping the central nervous system toward relief. These pain-CBT neuroimaging findings also underscore pain catastrophizing as the primary therapeutic target for adaptive rewiring of the central nervous system.

Shaping the central nervous system toward pain relief requires regular use of pain-CBT skills in order to recondition some automatic and unhelpful responses to pain. Humans are hardwired to perceive pain as a threat and to mount protective responses. It is understandable that most people living with chronic pain would have a degree of catastrophizing tendencies, and those with highly protective nervous systems will naturally have greater vigilance and protective responses to pain. However, these hard-wired protective responses are counterproductive for long-term pain relief, restoration of function, and surgical recovery, and should be included in programs that aim to enhance recovery after surgery. Doing so requires new systems of care delivery and programming to transcend many of the barriers to mental healthcare that are experienced by outpatients with chronic pain [59]. Such barriers to effective psychological treatment for pain contribute to the overmedicalization of patients with chronic pain

[60] and to untreated mental health needs among those who become surgical candidates.

Brief and Scalable Behavioral Pain Treatment

My (BD) clinical work and research has focused on developing and investigating brief, accessible, scalable psychological treatments to meet the needs of patients with chronic pain and postsurgical pain. As one example, I created a single-session pain class that focally treats pain catastrophizing and enhances descending modulation of pain through application of acquired skills. The single-session class is called "Empowered Relief" (formerly called "From Catastrophizing to Recovery") [21]. The single-session in-person pain class is 2 hours in duration, and may be delivered en masse, and class size is limited by the size of your room (the largest class I taught had 85 attendees). The class is didactic and involves delivery of a manualized protocol and PowerPoint slide presentation. Patients are encouraged to bring a friend or family member with them to the class. Participants may ask questions for clarification, but due to the tight time constraints and volume of information that must be presented, participant interaction is relatively minimal. Benefits of this class format include rapid delivery, treatment is complete immediately after the session, and due to the classroom format and friends/family member attendance, there is reduced stigma attached to receiving "psychological treatment." I have observed much greater receptivity to class attendance because most barriers are eliminated with the unique design and format.

The "Empowered Relief" class includes pain education, and focal content on pain catastrophizing (what it is, how to know if you are catastrophizing, and how to stop it). Participants complete a Personalized Plan for Relief, an action plan for addressing catastrophizing in the moment as soon as it is identified. Participants also use relaxation daily to begin to encode the basics of cognitive, emotional, and physiological regulation and how to apply these skills when in pain or under duress. Importantly, "Empowered Relief" is not meant to replace longer-course pain-CBT—a modality that is proven to work well; rather, it provides effective, targeted behavioral medicine and focal pain treatment that ascribes minimal burden and therefore broadens access to pain care.

Early research on 57 mixed etiology patients with chronic pain who attended "Empowered Relief" had meaningful and large effect reductions in pain catastrophizing at 2- and 4-week follow-up (Cohen's d = 1.15), and results suggested that reductions strengthened over time [21]. This study served to challenge common perception that pain catastrophizing required longer-course treatment, and it opened the door to study the single-session pain class further.

We are now conducting an NIH-funded three-arm randomized controlled trial of "Empowered Relief" compared to 8-week pain-CBT and a health education control group [61]. Our main outcome is pain catastrophizing at 3 months, and we will be assessing its effects on pain intensity, pain interference, and function. [Note: "Empowered Relief" is owned and copyrighted by Stanford University. Only certified instructors may deliver the Empowered Relief program, and certification is available for all healthcare clinicians through Stanford University. Information on the certification workshops is found at: https://empoweredrelief.com/]

Brief and Scalable Interventions for Surgical Patients

For surgical candidates, it is generally infeasible for patients to access pain-CBT in the perioperative timeframe due to treatment intensity requirements and duration of care as well as patient travel and cost burdens and availability of skilled therapists. Indeed, the perioperative setting presents a unique set of challenges and limitations for physicians, patients, and mental health therapists alike, and such complexities underscore the need for brief and accessible treatments to address the psychological factors that influence pain after surgery and treatment needs.

To fill this gap and address the unmet needs of perioperative patients, I adapted "Empowered Relief" to the perioperative setting, digitized it, and named the online program "My Surgical Success" (MSS) The first iteration of the MSS website included a 90-minute skills-based video, a personalized plan for pain management, and a downloadable relaxation audio file. We conducted a randomized controlled clinical trial at Stanford University and Stanford Hospital comparing MSS to a digital health education (HE) control intervention in women scheduled for breast cancer surgery [62]. We assessed opioid use daily after surgery, and larger surveys occurred at 2, 4, 8, and 12 weeks after surgery. We randomized 127 women to one of the two treatment groups and found that attrition was greater in the MSS group due to its greater time burden; the HE control group did not require a 90-minute education video. Our analytic sample included 68 patients ($N = 36$ MSS, $N = 32$ HE control) who completed treatment and initiated opioid use after surgery.

Our primary study outcome was feasibility and acceptability of MSS (80% threshold for acceptability items). Secondary outcomes included time (in days) to opioid cessation after surgery for patients who initiated opioid use, and pain catastrophizing. Despite greater attrition for MSS, feasibility was demonstrated for the 56% of patients who engaged with the online treatment, and 80% thresholds for acceptability were met. "My Surgical Success" was associated with 86% increased odds of opioid cessation within the 12-week study period relative to HE controls (hazard ratio 1.86 (95% CI: 1.12–3.10), $p = 0.016$). There were no significant differences in psychological variables between the groups, and interesting, due to a floor effect for pain catastrophizing we were unable to meaningfully assess treatment impacts on catastrophizing. Importantly, MSS was associated with significantly briefer opioid exposure after surgery (5 day difference) relative to controls. These promising results signal that perioperative digital behavioral pain medicine may be a low-cost, accessible adjunct that could promote opioid cessation after surgery.

Based on these first results, we addressed the attrition rate by creating briefer and modularized videos; MSS now contains three 15-minute videos (45 minutes of total treatment time) for a 50% reduction in treatment burden. We are currently conducting a phase II randomized controlled trial of the updated version of MSS compared to digital HE in orthopedic trauma surgery patients at Stanford Hospital. The benefits of digital behavioral treatment include on-demand access to a virtually no-cost treatment that patients may engage with in the comfort of their own home, or in the hospital when recovering from their surgery. We are currently conducting a large, pragmatic study at Stanford whereby nurses offer all neurosurgery and orthopedic surgery patients a Stanford "Recovery Toolkit" that includes print education, a relaxation audiofile, and access to an iPad to view MSS. We are assessing patient engagement and patient satisfaction with the behavioral pain management program, and we are examining impacts on inpatient opioid use relative to a usual care cohort.

Enhancing Patient Engagement

One of the best ways to enhance patient engagement in behavioral medicine and/or self-management of pain is for all healthcare professionals to prioritize adaptive patient behaviors as paramount to their outcomes. Avoid the mistake of deferring topics related to behavioral pain management to behaviorists; in fact, the entire care team plays an important role in orienting patients to the importance of pain self-management. All members of the care team—surgeon, primary care physician, pain physician, nurse, physical therapist, occupational therapist, social workers—should endeavor to be educated about simple techniques and resources they can use to better engage patients in learning what they can do to begin to self-regulate cognition, emotion, and pain.

Behavioral/psychological optimization stands to benefit patients in a multitude of ways. Improved surgical outcomes are the main goal, of course. However, adaptive behavioral changes may become enduring patterns that yield improved management of preexisting (and often overlapping) chronic pain conditions. A surgical date offers a tangible, medical event that may motivate patients in ways that daily management of chronic pain does not. Further, in the surgical arena patients tend to receive focused medical, family, and social attention that far outweighs one's daily life experience—and this attention may support lasting behavioral changes. While many patients may be reticent to engage in *psychological treatment for pain* due to stigma, perceived lack of need, or other reasons, we argue that integration of psychological principles and cost-effective treatment options in the perioperative pathway as standard care may enhance patient engagement. At once patients are both normalized for engaging with the treatments and assured that they are being offered cutting-edge, personalized perioperative pain treatment that addresses their needs as a whole person. Language matters, as alluded to earlier, so rather than discussing with patients the need for psychological treatment for pain, we may simply promote the concept of integrated pain treatment for improved surgical outcomes and lifelong wellness. Accordingly, normalization and validation of patient distress about their pain is the first step to helping them engage with the information and skills that will lead to better self-regulation and long-term outcomes.

The pathway to normalizing patient distress about their pain begins with the definition of pain. The International Association for the Study of Pain defines pain as being "a noxious sensory and emotional experience" [63], thereby underscoring psychology as being integral to pain *proper*, versus being a separate, albeit related, experience or response. As such, it is useful to consider pain as a psychosensory experience, and to help patients understand this point.

Addressing the Stigma of Pain Catastrophizing

While this chapter has used pain catastrophizing as the clinical and scientific term, I avoid using the term with patients because it is difficult to pronounce and carries a pejorative connotation for some patients. Clinically, I have found using simpler terms such as "negative pain mindset" instead of pain catastrophizing, or used the term "recovery mindset" to describe adaptive cognitive, emotional, and behavioral patterns that are at the other end of the continuum. This relatively neutral language may increase patient receptivity, particularly when it is paired with a plain-language description of what it means.

Clinical Resources That Enhance Self-Regulation and Enhance a Recovery Mindset

Catastrophizing, negative pain appraisal, and anxiety are vitally important therapeutic targets in the perioperative context. Overcoming stigma related to these

Table 5.1. Clinical Toolkit for Enhancing Self-Regulation in the Perioperative Context

Table 5.1 provides a clinical toolkit to accomplish three main goals:
- Goal 1: Help patients understand why self-regulation of psychological dimensions of pain is important to their pain care and surgical outcomes.
- Goal 2: Extinguish pain catastrophizing/negative pain mindset
- Goal 3: Enhance self-regulation and descending modulation

Enhancing Self-Regulation in the Perioperative Context*

Goal 1: Help patients understand why self-regulation of psychological dimensions of pain is important to their pain care and surgical outcomes.

Clinician Communication with Patients	Patient Actions
• Using lay language, educate patients about the role of psychology in the experience of pain. • Establish psychological treatment and enhanced descending modulation of pain as *primary* pain treatment and important to surgical outcomes. • Provide education on how behavioral medicine and self-management skills can "boost" the effect of medical treatments for pain. • Provide education on how and why thought patterns influence pain after surgery, and surgical outcomes. • To assure comprehension, use simple lay language to explain complex concepts. Ask patients to explain their understanding of the concepts you describe to facilitate learning through verbal recall and allow you to positively reinforce their accurate comprehension, correct any misunderstandings, and identify and address any concerns they raise. Clinician Resource: *Psychological Treatment for Patients with Chronic Pain* ©2018 by Beth Darnall. American Psychological Association Press.	• Acquire a fundamental understanding of the importance of brain–body interactions on pain and recovery. • Understand that there are many simple, evidence-based skills that can be learned and that, when used over time, shape brain and body toward relief. • Create goals for daily use of skills after surgery to enhance comfort, cultivate self-regulation, and potentially reduce need for opioids.

(*continued*)

Table 5.1. Continued

Goal 2: Extinguish Pain Catastrophizing/Negative Pain Mindset

Clinician Communication with Patients	Patient Actions
• **Assess** pain-related cognition with the Pain Catastrophizing Scale or UW-Pain Appraisal Scale. • **Review** the patient's findings with them (e.g., "Your score tells me that we can help you learn to reduce your distress around pain, and can help you be more comfortable as you recover from surgery.") • **Validate** their distress—it is real and understandable—and help them understand that distress is a pain amplifier. • Using patient-friendly language, such as "negative pain mindset" or "pain appraisal" in lieu of the term "pain catastrophizing" may enhance receptivity to the concepts and the treatment plan. • **Use imagery and narrative:** "Nobody wants more pain, but having a negative pain mindset is like picking up the can of gasoline and pouring it on a fire. You can learn to put the can of gasoline down, and by doing so it changes your pain in the moment, and steers your nervous away from pain in the future." • **Remoralize** patients: "Research shows that applying some easy-to-use skills will help you shift these patterns toward pain relief and wellness." • **Prescribe patients a skills-based toolkit such as the following:** *The Opioid-Free Pain Relief Kit* ©2016 by Beth Darnall *The Pain Survival Guide* ©2006 by Dennis Turk and Fritz Winter Both are simple workbooks with accompanying relaxation audiofiles. These are good resources before or after surgery.	• Understand that negative thought patterns amplify pain processing and oppose relief. • Understand one's thought patterns around pain (e.g., receive score on PCS or UW-PAS with interpretation). • Receive reassurance that while it is not "all in your head," there is much you can do to impact brain-pain experience. • Become remoralized to reduce a negative pain mindset. "While some degree of pain may be inevitable, I can learn to put the can of gasoline down so that I am focusing on comforting myself instead of unwittingly feeding my own distress." • Obtain a skills-based book as homework and acquire and use simple behavioral tools to cultivate a pain relief mindset.

Table 5.1. Continued

Goal 3: Enhance self-regulation and descending modulation

Clinician Communication with Patients	Patient Actions

• **Prioritize self-management in the medical visit.** At every follow-up, *begin the visit* by asking patients about what they are learning, and assess their level of engagement with the skills. You are training patients to understand that what they do on a daily basis matters more than what you do to them.
• **Remind patients that results take time.** Brain studies show changes occur over the course of 2–3 months.
• **Provide encouragement.** If patients remain skeptical, review the evidence and content of previous conversations as needed.
• **Reinforce engagement.** Acknowledge challenges, and identify at least one positive behavior to celebrate with patients at each clinical visit.
• **Refer patients who are stuck or need a higher level of care.** Refer to a health or pain psychologist whenever possible, and to a general psychologist if pain specialists are not available. Lack of engagement may indicate depression, or the need for professional support and structure.
• **Encourage** *skills use and behavior change*—changes in pain come later; focusing on pain changes undermines the goal of shifting focus away from pain.
• **End every visit by asking patients to set one small, achievable goal.** Example: "I will use my audiofile twice a week." Smaller is better; the goal is to help patients feel successful. Begin the next visit by asking how they are doing with their small step.
• **Referral to a skilled physical therapist** may effectively reduce kinesiophobia and fear of pain with graded activity.
	• Through engagement in the homework and working with a therapist (when possible), acquire the ability to identify negative thoughts and reactions (physical, emotional) and apply adaptive strategies to interrupt negative pain mindset:
	  ✓ Cognitive reframing
	  ✓ Positive self-talk
	  ✓ Relaxation response
	  ✓ Mindfulness observing
	  ✓ Distraction
	  ✓ Self-soothing actions
	• Practice the relaxation response as a self-treatment tool to reduce distress. Skills strengthen over time, and positive effects build over the course of weeks.
	Both books listed here are written for patients, include relaxation resources, and are workbook style:
	The Opioid-Free Pain Relief Kit ©2016 by Beth Darnall
	The Pain Survival Guide ©2006 by Dennis Turk and Fritz Winter

---

*Adapted from Table 5.1 (pp. 22–23) of Darnall BD, Colloca L. Optimizing placebo and minimizing nocebo to reduce pain, catastrophizing, and opioid use: a review of the science and an evidence-informed clinical toolkit. Int Rev Neurobiol. 2018;139:129–57. PMID: 30146045 topics is an important aspect of patient engagement, and providers play a key role in this regard. Validation and normalization of the patient experience are paramount for all healthcare clinicians, while ensuring patients are given a roadmap to engage in self-treatment, self-soothing behaviors, and techniques that reduce distress and pain. While often relegated to the realm of "psychological treatment" or to mental health therapists, the clinical toolkit (Table 5.1) offers actionable steps for every healthcare clinician to begin engaging with patients and integrating principles of the biopsychosocial model into everyday pain care, and particularly in the perioperative context. And in fact, improvement in patient outcomes depends on it. It is through the integration of these principles—across multiple professional disciplines—that patients are able to fully encode how and why self-regulation is *primary* pain care, and thus their motivation to engage may be enhanced.

References

1 Sullivan MJ, Bishop SR, Pivik J. The pain catastrophizing scale: development and validation. Psychol Assess. 1995;7:524–32.

2 Wade JB, Riddle DL, Thacker LR. Is pain catastrophizing a stable trait or dynamic state in patients scheduled for knee arthroplasty? Clin J Pain. 2012;28(2):122–8.

3 Linton SJ. Do psychological factors increase the risk for back pain in the general population in both a cross-sectional and prospective analysis? Eur J Pain. 2005;9(4): 355–61.

4 Weissman-Fogel I, Sprecher E, Pud D. Effects of catastrophizing on pain perception and pain modulation. Exp Brain Res. 2008;186(1):79–85.

5 Wertli MM, et al. The influence of catastrophizing on treatment outcome in patients with non-specific low back pain: a systematic review. Spine (Phila Pa 1976). 2013.

6 Spinhoven P, et al. Catastrophizing and internal pain control as mediators of outcome in the multidisciplinary treatment of chronic low back pain. Eur J Pain. 2004;8(3):211–19.

7 Severeijns R, et al. Pain catastrophizing predicts pain intensity, disability, and psychological distress independent of the level of physical impairment. Clin J Pain. 2001;17(2):165–72.

8 Burton AK, et al. Psychosocial predictors of outcome in acute and subchronic low back trouble. Spine. 1995;20(6):722–8.

9 Khan RS, et al. Catastrophizing: a predictive factor for postoperative pain. Am J Surg. 2011;201(1):122–31.

10 Theunissen M, et al. Preoperative anxiety and catastrophizing: a systematic review and meta-analysis of the association with chronic postsurgical pain. Clin J Pain. 2012;28(9):819–41.

11 Geisser ME, et al. Catastrophizing, depression and the sensory, affective and evaluative aspects of chronic pain. Pain. 1994;59(1):79–83.

12 Sullivan M. The Pain Catastrophizing Scale User Manual. 2009. http://sullivan-painresearch.mcgill.ca/pdf/pcs/PCSManual_English.pdf.

13 Helmerhorst GT, et al. Risk factors for continued opioid use one to two months after surgery for musculoskeletal trauma. J Bone Joint Surg Am. 2014;96(6):495–9.

14 Rosenstiel AK, Keefe FJ. The use of coping strategies in chronic low back pain patients: relationship to patient characteristics and current adjustment. Pain. 1983;17(1):33–44.

15 Amtmann D, Jensen MP, Turk D, Bamer AM, Liljenquist KS. Pain Appraisal Scale (PAS) User Guide. 2018. http://uwcorr.washington.edu/sites/uwcorr/files/files/ UWPAS_UserGuide__v1_0.pdf.

16 Sommer M, et al. Predictors of acute postoperative pain after elective surgery. Clin J Pain. 2010;26(2):87–94.

17 Ip HY, et al. Predictors of postoperative pain and analgesic consumption: a qualitative systematic review. Anesthesiology. 2009;111(3):657–77.

18 Dunn LK, et al. Influence of catastrophizing, anxiety, and depression on in-hospital opioid consumption, pain, and quality of recovery after adult spine surgery. J Neurosurg Spine. 2018;28(1):119–26.

19 Darnall BD, et al. Development and validation of a daily pain catastrophizing scale. J Pain. 2017.

20 Sturgeon JA, et al. Physical and psychological correlates of fatigue and physical function: a Collaborative Health Outcomes Information Registry (CHOIR) study. J Pain. 2015;16(3):291–8 e1.

21 Darnall, BD, Sturgeon JA, Kao MC, Hah JM, Mackey SC. From Catastrophizing to Recovery: a pilot study of a single-session treatment for pain catastrophizing. J Pain Res. 2014;14(7):219–26.

22 Quartana PJ, Campbel CM, Edwards RR. Pain catastrophizing: a critical review. Expert Rev Neurother. 2009;9(5):745–58.

23 Suffeda A, et al. Influence of depression, catastrophizing, anxiety, and resilience on postoperative pain at the first day after otolaryngological surgery: A prospective single center cohort observational study. Medicine (Baltimore). 2016;95(28):e4256.

24 McCracken LM, Zayfert C, Gross R.T. The Pain Anxiety Symptoms Scale: development and validation of a scale to measure fear of pain. Pain. 1992;50(1):67–73.

25 Picavet HS, Vlaeyen JW, Schouten JS. Pain catastrophizing and kinesiophobia: predictors of chronic low back pain. Am J Epidemiol. 2002;156(11):1028–34.

26 Vlaeyen JW, Crombez G, Linton SJ. The fear-avoidance model of pain. Pain. 2016;157(8):1588–9.

27 Vlaeyen JW, Crombez G. Fear of movement/(re)injury, avoidance and pain disability in chronic low back pain patients. Man Ther. 1999;4(4):187–95.

28 Gheldof EL, et al. Pain-related fear predicts disability, but not pain severity: a path analytic approach of the fear-avoidance model. Eur J Pain. 2010;14(8):870 e1–9.

29 Archer KR, et al. Early postoperative fear of movement predicts pain, disability, and physical health six months after spinal surgery for degenerative conditions. Spine J. 2014;14(5):759–67.

30 Woods MP, Asmundson GJ. Evaluating the efficacy of graded in vivo exposure for the treatment of fear in patients with chronic back pain: a randomized controlled clinical trial. Pain. 2008;136(3):271–80.

31 George SZ, et al. Comparison of graded exercise and graded exposure clinical outcomes for patients with chronic low back pain. J Orthop Sports Phys Ther. 2010;40(11):694–704.

32 George SZ, et al. The effect of a fear-avoidance-based physical therapy intervention for patients with acute low back pain: results of a randomized clinical trial. Spine (Phila Pa 1976). 2003;28(23):2551–60.

33 Coons MJ, Hadjistavropoulos HD, Asmundson GJ. Factor structure and psychometric properties of the Pain Anxiety Symptoms Scale-20 in a community physiotherapy clinic sample. Eur J Pain. 2004;8(6):511–16.

34 Woby SR, et al. Psychometric properties of the TSK-11: a shortened version of the Tampa Scale for Kinesiophobia. Pain. 2005;117(1-2):137–44.

35 McNeil DW, et al. Fear of Pain Questionnaire-9: brief assessment of pain-related fear and anxiety. Eur J Pain. 2018;22(1):39–48.

36 Gracely RH, et al. Pain catastrophizing and neural responses to pain among persons with fibromyalgia. Brain. 2004;127(Pt 4):835–43.

37 Geisser ME, et al. Perception of noxious and innocuous heat stimulation among healthy women and women with fibromyalgia: association with mood, somatic focus, and catastrophizing. Pain. 2003;102(3):243–50.

38 Wade JB, et al. Role of pain catastrophizing during pain processing in a cohort of patients with chronic and severe arthritic knee pain. Pain. 2011;152(2):314–19.

39 Burns JW, et al. Do changes in cognitive factors influence outcome following multidisciplinary treatment for chronic pain? A cross-lagged panel analysis. J Consult Clin Psychol. 2003;71(1):81–91.

40 Burns JW, et al. Cognitive factors influence outcome following multidisciplinary chronic pain treatment: a replication and extension of a cross-lagged panel analysis. Behav Res Ther. 2003;41(10):1163–82.

41 Burns JW, Moric M. Psychosocial factors appear to predict postoperative pain: Interesting, but how can such information be used to reduce risk? Techniques in Regional Anesthesia and Pain Management. 2011;15:90–99.

42 Pinto PR, et al. Risk factors for persistent postsurgical pain in women undergoing hysterectomy due to benign causes: a prospective predictive study. J Pain. 2012;13(11):1045–57.

43 Pavlin DJ, et al. Catastrophizing: a risk factor for postsurgical pain. Clin J Pain. 2005;21(1):83–90.

44 Sobol-Kwapinska M, et al. Psychological correlates of acute postsurgical pain: A systematic review and meta-analysis. Eur J Pain. 2016;20(10):1573–86.

45 Papaioannou M, et al. The role of catastrophizing in the prediction of postoperative pain. Pain Med. 2009;10(8):1452–9.

46 Riddle DL, et al. Preoperative pain catastrophizing predicts pain outcome after knee arthroplasty. Clin Orthop Relat Res. 2010;468(3):798–806.

47 Wright D, et al. Pain catastrophizing as a predictor for postoperative pain and opiate consumption in total joint arthroplasty patients. Arch Orthop Trauma Surg. 2017;137(12):1623–29.

48 Bierke S, Petersen W. Influence of anxiety and pain catastrophizing on the course of pain within the first year after uncomplicated total knee replacement: a prospective study. Arch Orthop Trauma Surg. 2017;137(12):1735–42.

49 Sorel JC, et al. The influence of preoperative psychological distress on pain and function after total knee arthroplasty. Bone Joint J. 2019;101–B(1):7–14.

50 Roh YH, et al. Effect of anxiety and catastrophic pain ideation on early recovery after surgery for distal radius fractures. J Hand Surg Am. 2014;39(11):2258–64 e2.

51 Seminowicz DA, Davis KD. Cortical responses to pain in healthy individuals depends on pain catastrophizing. Pain. 2006;120(3):297–306.

52 Seminowicz DA, et al. Cognitive-behavioral therapy increases prefrontal cortex gray matter in patients with chronic pain. J Pain. 2013;14(12):1573–84.

53 Hubbard CS, et al. Altered brain structure and function correlate with disease severity and pain catastrophizing in migraine patients. eNeuro. 2014;1(1):e20 14.

54 Jiang Y, et al. Perturbed connectivity of the amygdala and its subregions with the central executive and default mode networks in chronic pain. Pain. 2016;157(9):1970–8.

55 Darnall BD. Psychological Treatment for Patients with Chronic Pain. Clinical Health Psychology Series. American Psychological Association; 2018.

56 Ehde DM, Dillworth TM, Turner JA. Cognitive-behavioral therapy for individuals with chronic pain: efficacy, innovations, and directions for research. Am Psychol. 2014;69(2):153–66.

57 IOM Committee on Advancing Pain Research, C.a.E. Relieving Pain in America: A Blueprint for Transforming Prevention, Care, Education, and Research. Institute of Medicine; 2011.

58 NIH Interagency Pain Research Coordinating Committee. http://iprcc.nih.gov/ National_Pain_Strategy/NPS_Main.htm. Accessed November 10, 2015.

59 Darnall BD, et al. Pain psychology: a global needs assessment and national call to action. Pain Med. 2016;17(2):250–63.

60 Darnall BD, Carr DB, Schatman ME. Pain psychology and the biopsychosocial model of pain treatment: ethical imperatives and social responsibility. Pain Med. 2017;18(8):1413–15.

61 Darnal BD, et al. Comparative efficacy and mechanisms of a single-session pain psychology class in chronic low back pain: study protocol for a randomized controlled trial. Trials. 2018;19(1):165.

62 Darnall BD, Ziadni MS, Krishnamurthy P, Mackey IG, Heathcote L, Taub CJ, Flood P, Wheeler A. "My Surgical Success": Impact of a digital behavioral pain medicine intervention on time to opioid cessation after breast cancer surgery. Pain Med. 2019 May 13. pii: pnz094. doi:10.1093/pm/pnz094. PMID: 31087093.

63 IASP. Part III: Pain terms, a current list with definitions and notes on usage. In Bogduk HMaN, ed., Classification of Chronic Pain (2nd ed., pp. 209–14). Seattle: IASP Press; 1994.

6

Sleep Optimization

Lyn Freeman

Introduction: Body, Mind, Emotion, Behavior

Few things are as critical for medical and psychological recovery as deep, restorative sleep. When things are going well, restorative sleep is experienced much like a rhythmic dance. We move in and out of wave patterns that occur in longer and longer time periods as the night progresses. Each wave state provides specific benefits to the body. For example, without attaining theta sleep, we cannot dream, and dreaming is a requirement for healing our emotions. Without attaining adequate deep delta sleep, we cannot heal our bodies and fight infection effectively [1].

If we do not experience the rhythms that constitute restorative sleep, we will be unable to perform mental tasks well the next day. Even more important, our motivation will be stunted, and behavioral change will become almost impossible. Without the motivation to implement behavioral change, patients will be unable to take responsibility for their health in ways that will support best medical and surgical outcomes.

Sleep Deprivation, Pain, and Behavior Change

The quality of our sleep is easily compromised by the very medical and psychological conditions that we seek to alleviate. The most common statement that I hear from pain patients who are sleep deprived is "don't ask me to do even one more thing." These patients are exhausted, unable to focus or concentrate, drained of motivation, and mesmerized by the suffering they want to escape. That is why addressing sleep is always the very first thing that I evaluate and address in patients that I treat. Improve sleep even a little, and everything else in treatment will move forward more easily.

Sleep deprivation is arguably the single most compromising event that prevents pain patients from changing behavior. So, how do you get the sleep deprived patient to take action to improve their sleep, and by design, become more capable of healthy change? You must approach the patient with the evidence of "what works," but on his or her own terms, in a language that he or she can understand and cognitively retain, and in a psychological manner that will inspire hope and increase motivation.

In this chapter, I will endeavor to accomplish the following: (1) review the scope of the problem; (2) clarify the frame of reference of the author; (3) explain how we function as living rhythm machines; (4) define circadian rhythms, chronobiology, and clock genes; (5) describe the challenges of improving sleep hygiene in a patient population; and (6) identify the methods of change that we use clinically, including motivational interviewing (MI).

The Scope of the Problem

There is no shortage of research to demonstrate that sleep dysregulation is common, with insomnia being reported by more than 30% of adults. Ten percent of those persons suffer from chronic insomnia [2, 3]. Obstructive sleep apnea is reported in up to 21% of women, and 31% of men, varying somewhat by study [4, 5].

Sleep deprivation contributes to short- and long-term health problems. Sleeping too much or too little impacts health and well-being in negative ways. Premature all-cause mortality is also increased on both ends of this sleep dynamic [6]. More specifically, too much or too little sleep are both correlated with coronary heart disease, stroke, hypertension, obesity, and diabetes [7, 8].

Quality of sleep also has significant effects on short-term and long-term surgical recovery. Poor sleep quality increases the risk of postoperative delirium, results in more cardiovascular events, increases patient pain, and produces poorer surgical outcomes including functional limitations and extended hospital stays. Unfortunately, opioid analgesia for pain management worsens postoperative sleep, decreasing REM sleep and increasing the apnea-hypopnea index [9].

It has been demonstrated that sleep promotion strategies as simple as use of ear plugs and eye masks can reduce likelihood of postsurgical delirium. Melatonin, a readily available over-the-counter medication, has been found to reduce postsurgical patient anxiety, decrease pain scores, and improve sleep [9].

These findings suggest that a strategic approach to sleep promotion may result in better surgical outcomes and an improved quality of life for surgical patients. Engaging with presurgical patients in the development of a sleep protocol to improve sleep before surgery and during the recovery period may improve surgical outcomes and overall quality of life.

The Author's Frame of Reference and Lens

It is important to understand the frame of reference of this writer, and the experiential "lens" that is used to view and interpret what is presented in what follows. The "lens" of experience was originally shaped by the creation, delivery, and publication of NIH-funded clinical research with sleep deprived, anxious, depressed, and chronically fatigued surgical and chronic pain patients with a current or previous diagnosis of cancer [10–12]. The "lens" was further honed by writing academic textbooks and medical manuals on mind/body and neuroplastic brain approaches to improve medical and psychological outcomes. In the textbooks, leaders in mind/body medicine were consulted and extensively interviewed as part of the writing process, and their expertise added to my "view" on these topics [13–15].

The "lens" was further polished by a decade of treating patients both in and outside of hospital settings. More "shaping" occurred as psychology interns and residents were trained and supervised to intervene at the hospital bedside of chronic pain patients in postoperative units at Alaska Regional Hospital. This particular "lens" adaptation required me to teach others how to refine what worked, or did not work, in real-life situations, such as chaotic hospital wards, while still individualizing treatment in a systematic and scientifically valid way. Finally, this author faced the challenges of caregiver after multiple surgical interventions and long-term chronic pain in her immediate family members.

Always at the forefront of this 30+ years of work, research and experience was the question: How can we impact the brain perceptually, and shift patient behavior in ways that produce better medical outcomes, less emotional suffering, and improved quality of life? It is within this frame of reference and "voice" that this chapter is presented.

Chronobiology, Rhythms, and Gene Clocks: What Dysregulates Them

We are all, quite literally, living rhythm machines, and our health depends on supporting our natural circadian (24-hour) and ultradian (90- to 120-minute) rhythms. There are also biological and chemical rhythms that are timed in minutes, seconds, or microseconds. For example, nerve cells exhibit rhythmic behavior with a period of a few tenths of a second. Smooth muscles of the stomach and intestines have a slightly longer contractual rhythm of 3–10 cycles per minute. There are daily, weekly, seasonal, and annual rhythms, and the combined studies of all these rhythms is called chronobiology [16].

Humans as Rhythm Machines

This 24-hour cycle regulates a wide range of behavioral, physiological and metabolic subrhythms that constitute the many biological "rhythms of life" [16]. In addition to the synchronization of our rhythms by daylight or dark, we also possess intracellular mechanisms via a set of clock genes that are organized in a system of feedback loops. These rhythms are intertwined and synergistic, meaning that humans both can and do impact their functioning based on how we live, what we do, and how we think and feel.

Synchronizing Our Two Clocks

We have two internal clocks that support the circadian rhythms of the body. There is the *neurological clock* that is controlled by light and our environment, which affect the rhythm of our body temperature, and changes throughout the day. This neurological clock is called the hypothalamic suprachiasmatic nuclei (SCN) and is synchronized by exposure to light and dark. This "reset" each day is accomplished by a photoreceptive system in the ganglion cells of the inner retina. We now know that the effect of light on sleep and wakefulness depends on light intensity as well as circadian time [17, 18].

There is also a *chemical clock*, where certain chemicals decay throughout the day and are replenished at night. This clock contributes to our sleep/wake behaviors as well as numerous other rhythmic systems in the body. The two clocks (neurological and chemical) are not perfectly aligned in time, and you need to synchronize them every day by exposure to light and dark in the correct "doses."

Regulating Our Rhythms

Our understanding of circadian cycles has changed with time. It was originally believed that the SCN controlled the "clocks" in our bodies. However, more recent discoveries of tissue- and organ-specific ultradian and circadian cycles have changed our understanding of how our rhythms become dysregulated. We now understand that the SCN coordinates rather than controls these rhythms; it helps to sustain them. This may well explain why bright light, at the correct times and doses, can alleviate some symptoms of mental health disorders including depression, schizophrenia, and even dementia [19]. Light (or the absence of it at specified times) can be used as a strong synchronizing agent, finessing our bodies back into a healthier rhythm, much like a conductor leading the orchestra so that all instruments play in harmony.

In modern society, the 24-hour circadian cycle is easily impacted by cultural interferences (light, noise, social interactions) and by stress. These issues must each be addressed in any effective sleep protocol so that our neurological and chemical clocks are not disrupted from their healthy cycles.

Although there are many clock-chemicals involved in maintaining circadian rhythms, the two clock hormones that we focus on most in this chapter are cortisol and melatonin [19].

Cortisol and Circadian Rhythms, and What Modifies Them

A review of cortisol rhythm and its effects on medical and psychological outcomes was a main focus of my earliest exploratory cancer research [12]. The protocols that evolved from that research sought to significantly improve patient circadian cycles as a means to improve health outcomes, mood state, and quality of life [10, 11]. This was accomplished by eliciting perceptual changes and empowering patients to modify their behaviors in ways that reinforced harmony with the circadian cycle. Aside from the pre-bedtime sleep rituals, attention was also given to the amount and timing of exercise to produce optimal sleep, as well as to food choices, timed to support energy in the day and melatonin rise at night. Stress reduction and mood enhancement strategies were also critical pieces of a circadian management approach, as stress interferes with sleep and the melatonin rise, and mood affects daytime energy, pain perception, and motivation to change. Many factors including those mentioned previously contribute to the proper maintenance of the circadian clock, and these factors are referred to as Zeitgebers, meaning "time keepers."

Zeitgebers

Zeitgebers are those things that help us reset the circadian and ultradian clocks and synchronize various bodily rhythms throughout each day. We can synchronize our clocks by exposing ourselves to daylight and dark in the optimal doses; by using Ericksonian-based imagery, metaphor and story as part of "change talk" to encourage the brain to reinforce healthy rhythms; and we can eat and exercise in a circadian supportive manner. We can also impact our emotional responses in ways that support daytime focus and energy, and nighttime relaxation in preparation for sleep. Positive emotional responses can be encouraging by simple practices, such as gratitude lists, and easy strategies such as a 30-second exercise, referred to as ANTS (Automatic Negative Thought Stomping). Both are quite powerful for shifting perception in a positive direction, with little effort required.

Further, both can be "automated" into patient life as part of their sleep plan to reduce ruminations and stress before bedtime.

Imagery, Story, and Metaphor for Stress Reduction

Ericksonian-based imagery has been extensively used in research to influence the subconscious mind in ways that reinforce the circadian "rhythms of life." The pre- to post-test daily cortisol rhythm of breast cancer patients in the Freeman study suggested that patients succeeded in modifying their cortisol rhythms by modifying their behaviors, thoughts, images, and emotions [12]. In that study, they also used their imagination, engaging all their senses and the emotions, to "see," their cortisol rhythm improving. For good or bad, the circadian sleep rhythm is readily modified by our behaviors and perceptions.

On the perceptual and emotional side, issues of rumination, anxiety, and depression can be addressed with imagery-based metaphor and story, stress reduction, and other psychological strategies [10–12]. It should not be a surprise that depression and anxiety are the two mental health conditions most often correlated with disrupted sleep patterns [20]. It is also generally understood that the correlation between quality of sleep and mental health is a two-way street. Sleep deprivation exacerbates existing mental health challenges, and anxiety and/or depression contribute to sleep dysfunction [21, 22].

Behavioral Change as Zeitgeber: Sleep Assessment and Environment

Of particular interest for this chapter are the societal issues that contribute to an ever-increasing rise in sleep disturbances. For example, the constant exposure to artificial light in the home and at work includes, but is not limited to, television sets, cell phones, computers, and work and home lighting systems. This ever-increasing exposure to artificial light, especially in the form of blue light, continues to drive our cortisol rhythm and degrade the natural melatonin rise of evening, modifying the quality and quantity of sleep [23–25]. We can make behavioral choices to modify the quality and quantity of light we are exposed to. We can control the timing of that exposure in ways that support healthy sleep rhythms. In the VALERAS program, patients are encouraged to avoid blue light for an hour before bedtime and are provided with information on how to purchase clinically tested blue-light-blocking glasses for use before bedtime, if they cannot break the TV/computer habits.

Sleep Assessment: Quantity and Quality as Zeitgeber

What constitutes restorative sleep varies in quantity from person to person. This issue must be addressed to assure that the optimal amount of sleep is sought as part of a sleep protocol. Is the patient naturally a "short-sleeper," requiring 6 hours or less sleep for full recuperation? Or is the patient a "long-sleeper," requiring more than 8 hours for full recuperation? This can also vary depending on health events such as surgery. This points to the importance of offering an individualized and systematic sleep strategy to address the problem of sleep deprivation.

From the behavioral side, presleep rituals, regular bedtimes, and bedrooms that block light and distraction can significantly improve the quality of sleep. These factors can be modified via behavioral change. Assessing the bedroom and the existing sleep habits is critical as a first step. Then, after environmental changes are made, a sleep ritual becomes part of the protocol.

Food and Exercise as Zeitgeber

Our cortisol rhythms and our sleep are also impacted by the types of food we eat and when we eat those foods. From the circadian perspective, it is important to feed the adrenergic chemical system in the morning for focus and alertness and to provide food for relaxation, repair, and sleep at the evening meal [1]. Both what is eaten and when it is eaten can have powerful effects on our cortisol rhythm and melatonin rise. This is described in greater detail in the nutrition chapter.

Challenges of Improving Sleep: Overcoming Patient Resistance

The information presented so far suggests that a sleep protocol needs to include education on specific Zeitgebers to manage the cortisol/melatonin clock hormones. Then, behavioral and perceptual change work, using metaphor, imagery-based story, stress reduction strategies, and a sleep ritual can be incorporated into an individualized protocol. Finally, food and exercise can be selected and timed to support the cortisol/melatonin cycle. These are important methods for improving cortisol rhythmicity, circadian function, and quality of sleep.

These approaches are actively incorporated in our clinical approach. However, for these approaches to translate into better sleep outcomes, the patient must apply and apply what is offered. The patient must do the work.

This raises the question: How do we overcome resistance in a presurgical patient population that is already challenged mentally, emotionally, and physically? The answer to this difficult question is in two parts: First, the mental health provider must speak in the language of the subconscious mind to help the patient overcome resistance. Second, the behavioral changes and perceptions that evolve must be "discovered" by the patient, rather than imposed by the provider. These two factors go a long way to mitigating patient resistance.

Speaking the Subconscious Language to Overcome Resistance

Use of metaphors and story, such as the metaphor of humans as "living rhythm machines," reference to the "rhythms of life," and imagery and story of the patient as "conductor of the rhythmic orchestra" is purposeful. Story and metaphor are more easily retained in memory and allow patients to recall information when cognitively challenged, as most sleep deprived patients are. It also inspires the patient to improve their sleep behaviors [11].

Metaphor and story were repeatedly used by Milton Erickson to speak directly to the unconscious mind; these approaches are powerful ways to move past resistance and elicit behavioral change [26]. Ernest Rossi and others have also written extensively on these approaches as psychological methods for modifying gene expression and biological rhythms [27].

Of additional interest for this chapter is the benefit of hypnotic imagery strategies as pain relief. Even in terminal cancer patients, Erickson demonstrated that pain can be partially suppressed via the method of storytelling, enriched with metaphor [26]. In this way, no hypnotic induction is necessary. Further, studies have been completed or are now underway to more precisely determine how hypnotic imagery, metaphor and story can be utilized to "reset" circadian rhythms in health benefitting ways [19].

Full hypnotic inductions are not used in the VALERAS program. However, the language of the subconscious mind, in the form of story and metaphor, is used extensively, as taught by Erickson. Story and metaphor are based on accurate scientific findings related to circadian rhythm, sleep, and mood enhancement, and are selected based on identified patient patterns of resistance.

Metaphor, story, and imagery engage patients more fully than "facts," reduce resistance, and allow the patient to hold much more information in memory. In fact, Erickson taught that story and metaphor could often produce deep communication with the subconscious mind without the need for a formal induction. We also address emotional and perceptual issues, such as ruminations, anxiety, and depression, that corrode the natural circadian rhythms of life. The key method of reducing these impactful emotions is to reframe these emotions and change perception of events via metaphor and story.

Motivational Interviewing: Helping Patients "Discover" Their Own Solutions

As stated earlier, the behavioral changes and perceptions that evolve from the sleep protocol, and all other VALERAS protocol components, must be "discovered" by the patient, rather than imposed by the provider. To do this, the therapeutic approach of MI is ideal for medical environments and for medical as well as psychological conditions. Additionally, metaphor and story (the language of the subconscious mind) are easily woven into the fabric of the summary statements of the motivational interview, blending both approaches to reduce patient resistance. We cover each in order. We begin by posing these questions: What is MI, and how do you use it in a sleep protocol?

Defining and Implementing A Motivational Interviewing Approach

Motivational interviewing has been defined as a collaborative conversation style for strengthening the patient's own motivation and commitment to change [28]. Within the context of medical environments, it has been described as "a skillful clinical style for eliciting from patients their own good motivations for making behavior changes in the interest of their health" [29]. This second definition is most applicable to our purposes here.

In this section, I describe how MI will be implemented for the sleep session. The form for MI remains the same for all VALERAS sessions, but the metaphors and stories presenting the scientific evidence would, of course, change, based on the topic at hand (e.g., nutrition, exercise, stress). As the need to preserve healthy circadian rhythms is pervasive across all sessions and chapters, the overarching theme of the "rhythms of life" will be the storyline and thread that is woven throughout the tapestry of the program. It is of interest to note that even our emotions have daily, event-related, and seasonal cycles. Simply understanding this gives patients a new perspective in relation to what they feel, and how they can take action to experience more pleasant emotions.

It is argued that a patient will not be persuaded to change behavior by what the physician or mental health professional will say, but only by what the patient discovers within themselves. This is experienced as what the patient is able to state out loud, in his or her own words. Solutions and the motivation to change must come from the patient's own internal realizations and be verbally expressed to move the motivational needle in the direction for change.

Motivate, Educate, Giftwrap, and Create the Plan

To move human consciousness in a direction that will result in change, you must *motivate* the patient via the MI interview; *educate* them by providing scientific information specific to their current problematic behaviors and perceptions (these emerge from the interview), and *"giftwrap"* this information in the language of the subconscious mind as metaphor and story, when possible. Finally, the provider and the patient must jointly *create* an individualized behavioral plan that is based on what the patient has "discovered" and verbalized from the session, and what they are willing to commit to.

Laying the Emotional Foundation: Core Values

To succeed in motivating the patient, it is important to take the first step of identifying and reinforcing the patient's "core values" in relation to how they want to live their life. The mental health professional "posture" must be that the patient already possesses and brings the strengths they need, but that they may not yet recognize it. Using the MI approach, the therapist and patient work together to draw out those strengths. Taking at least a few minutes to explore core values also serves to align the patient and provider as coequal partners, moving toward improved outcomes.

Basic "core values" can be explored quickly with any one of the following questions: "If you were to write out your goals or purpose in life, what would you write?" or "If your best friends were to tell me what matters most to you in life, what would they tell me?" My favorite "core values" question is "What are the basic principles that guide your life?" These principles can then be drawn on again and again in motivating the patient to change. Exploring core values as the first patient/professional interaction also sets a foundation that allows patient and provider to view the presenting medical condition from a broader perceptual level than ongoing pain and suffering alone. Core values questions are following by reflective listening. Reflective listening is an active exercise that is used throughout and across the MI process.

Digging Deeper: Reflective Listening

Reflective listening is described as the professional's "best guess" as to the deeper meaning of what the patient has just said. In relation to a surgical population, a reflective listening conversation may go something like this:

THERAPIST: How are you feeling about your upcoming surgery? (Open-Ended Question)

PATIENT: My last surgery went very badly, and I am fortunate to still be here.

THERAPIST: You easily could have died and are worried about surviving this next surgery.

PATIENT: They told me later that they thought I had a 10% chance of surviving my last surgery, but I beat the odds.

THERAPIST: You had luck on your side and hope to have luck again with this upcoming surgery.

PATIENT: Yes, because I have a lot to live for.

THERAPIST: Your family is really important to you and you want to live for their sake as well as your own.

PATIENT: Yes, I want to be here to watch my children grow up and to make sure they are cared for.

THERAPIST: And you are willing to do what you can to make sure you will be here for them.

PATIENT: Yes. I would do anything to protect my family.

THERAPIST: And you are here today because you want to learn what you need to do to get better so you can take care of them.

Reflection is more than simply repeating what the patient said in summary form. It is continuing the paragraph. In essence, you are adding what you believe will be the next sentence. This reflection is always done with statements, not questions, and the voice "drops" at the end of each sentence. As you listen deeply for the underlying meaning, and move the conversation forward, the patient will add to your statements, or clarify them for you if you have not understood them correctly. This leads to better understanding and an attuned form of listening.

The Overall Process: OARS

Once you have explored the patient's core values, and have actively engaged in reflective listening, it is time to dig deeper into the MI method. The backbone of the MI method is the OARS approach. O involves open-ended questioning. A means "affirming" what the patient has said in response to questions. R directs the therapist to "reflect" back verbally the deeper understanding of what the patient is saying. S means that at the end of the session, the mental health professional will summarize what the patient has said. The summary is what pulls everything together and affirms what the patient has shared in the interview (desires, abilities, reasons for change, and the strength of his or her needs). It is in the summary that you will use analogy, metaphor, and story to gain "buy-in" and to help the patient retain all key points in memory.

Post-Summary: Offering Advice and Implementing a Plan

After the summary, a next step can be, with patient permission, to provide information and evidence-based advice for changing behavior and moving toward implementing a plan. This will be advice or clarification that adds to the ideas already identified and "discovered" by the patient, via the MI process. Metaphor and story can again be used where appropriate to reinforce the evidence-based recommendations for change. Evidence-based information for offering advice is systematically organized as graphic power points, readily available to the mental health professional for display based on the advice that is to be given. What information is displayed will be based on a presession questionnaire, and on what is shared and learned in the interview itself.

Now that the overview of MI has been provided, let's dig deeper into how to select the open-ended questions, in the specific order intended to induce the most effective change talk.

Selecting Open-Ended Questions
DARN—Eliciting Change Talk
Systematic methods for selecting the open-ended questions are represented in the MI model by the acronym **DARN**. **DARN** is a way to identify questions that will generate and elicit ideas from the patient to mobilize change.

D stands for **Desire**. What does the patient want, wish, or hope for? For example, I may ask the patient what he or she hopes our work together will accomplish in relation to their sleep, or what they want from the preoperative optimization program to help with sleep quality.

A stands for **Ability** and may include questions like "What ideas do you have for how you could improve the quality of your sleep?" "How confident are you that you could change your sleep patterns, if you made up your mind to do that?" How the patient responds is key to understanding what they perceive their ability to succeed or follow-thru with change to be. "I can" or "I am able" type of patient statements suggest they think they are ready for and capable of doing what is under discussion. "I could" or "I would" statements do not represent as strong a recognition of ability. "I will get a new alarm clock tonight" is stronger and more promising change talk than "I could see if I might find a clock."

R refers to **Reasons** why the patient may genuinely want to change, such as to improve sleep as a way to gain more energy, improve health or mood state, or reduce pain. If I am unsure whether the patient has their own reasons for change, but may only be in session because others have told him or her to do so, I might ask the patient questions like this: "What is the down side of not getting restorative sleep?" Another way to elicit change talk is to ask, "Finish this sentence for me: I can't continue to be sleep deprived because . . . ." In patients who are somewhat but not strongly resistant to change, you might ask, "Why would you want to get better sleep?" As mentioned before, it is important that the patient verbalize the reasons that they need to change, and that it comes from them, not the provider.

N stands for patient identification of **Needs** and is successfully elicited when patients make statements with words like "I need to," "I want to," "I must," or "something has to change."

Need statements do not identify why change is important (that is a reason), nor whether they have the ability to change (the skill or motivation), or even the desire to do so. Need statements tell you how urgently the patient thinks change and action are required. For example, a patient may say, "I won't survive if I go on this way" which suggests that they know the urgency for acting is immediate. This still does not identify clearly their reasoning, desire, or ability to change. That said, recognizing that there is a timely need for change is still critical as one of the key components leading to change.

CAT—Mobilizing Change, Developing a Plan

At this point in the interview, the provider has (1) identified what the patient hopes for; (2) assessed the patient's abilities to change; (3) clarified the reasons for change; and (4), if all goes well, strengthened the motivation and need for change in the here and now. Next steps involve mobilizing the change talk into a developed plan. You begin by eliciting the patient's ideas for a change plan, by asking open-ended questions. You could ask "So, what do you think you are going to do about improving your sleep?" Or, more indirectly, "I wonder what you might decide to do now?"

Developing a Plan

For example, in a recent session on sleep with an Alaskan patient, the discussion in relation to those questions went something like this. (Note: Anchorage, Alaska, has as much as 20 hours of daylight in the summer). This was in response to the question "What do you think you should do about your sleep problems?"

PATIENT: Well, I could put up blackout curtains to keep the bright light from keeping me awake all night.
FREEMAN: Good idea. (Affirming) Is there anything else?
PATIENT: I could begin the stress reduction ritual we discussed, including turning off all computers and blue light devices, and listen to nature sounds for the hour before bedtime.
FREEMAN: Yes, those are good calming strategies. (Affirming) Have you decided on other strategies?
PATIENT? I could turn the temperature down and sleep in a cooler room.
FREEMAN: Yes, that would help you sleep more deeply. Any other thoughts?
PATIENT: No, I think that is about all that I can think of at the moment that would make a difference.

Advice and Education, with Permission

At this point, the patient has presented their ideas of what they want to do. You may, at this point, with permission, offer advice and additional education on how to improve their plan.

FREEMAN: I think you have some excellent ideas of things to do to help with your sleep. May I offer an additional suggestion, based on the research?

PATIENT: Yes, that would be appreciated.

FREEMAN: Well, you mentioned turning down the temperature as a way to make you sleep deeper, and that certainly does support deep sleep. But you also mentioned that you have a Jacuzzi in your bathroom that you use from time to time. Did you know that raising your body temperature in a Jacuzzi, sauna, or hot shower just before bedtime, and then sleeping in the cool room makes people sleep even better? Is that something you might want to do just before bedtime?

PATIENT: That is a great idea. It is really convenient for me to do that, and that would relax me even more. I can do that for 10 or 15 minutes just before bedtime.

FREEMAN: Yes, and it makes for a big drop in temperature, which is one of the reasons for sleeping in a cool room in the first place. Raising your temperature slightly before bed will lead to even deeper sleep, since it will be able to drop even more in the cool room.

CAT: Commitment, Activation, and Taking First Steps

If your patient has suggested they are ready to change, and based on the summary, what changes they are willing to take, you want to solidify and strengthen that commitment for change, based on the summary of what they have told you they can and will do. Again, what matters is what your patient tells you they will do, not what the provider tells them they should do. For C, you ask for a **Commitment** in a very straightforward manner. "Are you going to do that?" or "Is that what you intend to do?" are very important questions to ask. It is best to pose questions like this in relation to each change goal they are committing to make.

A stands for **Action** or **Activating**. "Are you willing to give it a try this week?" "How ready are you to do that?" These are the questions that move the patient from commitment to action.

T stands for **Taking Steps** to begin and implement the sleep changes. Examples of these questions might be: "What would be your first step?" "How will you go about doing that?" "When will you do it?" Again, these questions are posed for each part of the plan, until all steps are clearly outlined.

Following Through with a Plan

There are certain steps that can be taken to strengthen the likelihood of patient compliance. Those steps include, during the session, having the patient (1) write down the goal and subgoals agreed on in the session, (2) spell out options and steps for meeting each goal, (3) troubleshoot any issues that may interfere with implementation, and (4) summarize the overall plan. In the preoperative optimization program, the mental health professional documents the goals, subgoals, options, and steps agreed on and sends this written document to the patient as a "behavioral prescription."

Behavioral Prescriptions

It is important to assure follow-through on the behavioral prescriptions that the patient agrees to and that will be revisited in the next session. In this way, problems can be addressed and the protocol fine-tuned to produce best outcomes. The work from the previous session is always reviewed during the first 5 minutes of the follow-up session, before beginning with the next behavioral change topic. For example, after the sleep protocol, progress would be reviewed in the first 5 minutes of the next session before beginning with the nutritional protocol. Similarly, the nutritional protocol progress would be reviewed before beginning the next session on mood enhancement, and so forth.

The Challenges and Evidence for Potential Success

As with most research, the challenge is translating these findings into behavioral change in patients who are often living complicated, financially challenged, physically and emotionally painful lives. It is a great deal to ask that they make significant life changes and discipline themselves in new ways, in the face of what is often a strong sense of despair. I have learned that it is difficult, but not impossible, to move the behaviors of a challenged patient in the right direction. I learned this in the process of two decades of clinical research and patient care, and my experiences are also supported by other clinical research.

A 2015 meta-analysis of nonpharmacological treatment of insomnia in chronic pain patients suggested that the use of sleep protocols can benefit this population. The "interventions" assessed in the meta-analysis consisted of combinations of some or all of the following: education, stimulus control, relaxation training, sleep hygiene education, stress management, sleep restriction, and cognitive-behavioral therapy (CBT). There is also the issue of time and distance constraints faced by the patient and the provider. This meta-analysis found that face-to-face interventions achieved better outcomes than those delivered by phone or over the Internet, although the authors acknowledged that the small sample size might explain these nonsignificant effects in that subgroup [30]. In opposition to this last finding, the Freeman research has found that face-to-face telemedicine approaches can be as effective as in-office visits. In fact, the VALERAS program uses telemedicine to allow for immediate therapist support after being seen by the pain specialist.

Time Limitations

The time allotted for behavioral support in most such optimization efforts will be short, due to cost and time constraints. In our VALERAS program, there is only one session dedicated primarily to sleep, one for nutrition, and three other sessions canvassing stress reduction, exercise, and other components of the protocol.

Because time will be precious, it will be necessary to gather fact-based patient information in advance of sessions, so that all time can be process oriented. This is best accomplished with a patient presession questionnaire.

Patient Questionnaire

In a sleep protocol, there are certain key questions that need to be asked to identify basic causes of sleep disruption. For example, can the patient sleep, but just not when they want to? One patient reported that they could sleep deeply between six in the morning and two in the afternoon. Another patient reported falling asleep around 7 p.m. and being able to sleep until 1 a.m. but then being unable to complete a night of rest. Both patients needed to sleep between 10 p.m. and 6 a.m. to have energy for their work day but were unsuccessful in doing so. Often, with those patients, it was identified that due to blue light exposure, or lateness of the hour of eating or exercising, they were slowly resetting their neurological clocks to later and later hours. In other cases, their internal clocks were being reset because of staying up later each consecutive night of a weekend. As it takes a day per hour to reset the circadian clock, they were not able to get themselves back into a normal sleep rhythm during the next week. In some patients, their entire circadian rhythms were "flipped" in that they wanted to sleep all day but were wide awake all night. This is a common occurrence that I see in cancer patients who have had chemotherapy.

These types of detailed questions can readily identify whether environmental factors or emotional distress should be targeted during the time in session. The details in the previous paragraph point to disrupted sleep due to environment factors (light, late sleep hours, eating or exercise timing issues). However, having trouble getting to sleep, or getting back to sleep can also be related to anxiety. Sleeping in too long, or all day, is often an indicator of depression. As time is limited, and not all factors can be addressed, it is important to "choose your battles" in how you focus the majority of time in a session.

Summary

In this chapter, we (1) reviewed the scope of the problem of sleep deprivation; (2) clarified the frame of reference and personal experience of the author; (3) defined circadian rhythms, chronobiology, and clock genes; (4) explained how humans function as living rhythm machines; (5) described the challenges of improving sleep hygiene in a presurgical patient population and (6) identified the methods of change used in VALERAS for our preoperative optimization program. This included explanations of the therapeutic style of MI, along with patient/therapist session examples.

The VALERAS program was designed to provide a patient intervention that will result in behavioral change and improved surgical outcomes. The intervention is based on sound scientific evidence and created within a psychological framework to reinforce the greatest likelihood of patient motivation and compliance. This intervention represents the best of medical and psychological skillsets, synergistically applied to address a very complex and challenging medical problem and patient population. It is our hope that this information will inform and assist other medical and psychological providers in their practices in ways that benefit their patients.

References

1 Baker SM, Baar K. The Circadian Prescription. New York: Berkeley Publishing Group; 2000.
2 Ferrie JE, Kumari M, Salo P, Singh-Manoux A, Kivimaki M. Sleep epidemiology—a rapidly growing field. Int J Epidemiol. 2011;December:1431–7.
3 Brown DW. Insomnia: prevalence and daytime consequences. In MD Teofilo Lee-Chiong (Ed.), Sleep: A Comprehensive Handbook (pp. 93–98). New Jersey: John Wiley and Sons; 2006.
4 Li C, Ford, Earl S, Zhao G, Croft JB, Balluz LA, Mokdad AH. Prevalence of self-reported clinically diagnosed sleep apnea according to obesity status in men and

women: National Health and Nutrition Examination Survey 2005–2006. Prev Med (Baltim). 2010;51(1):18–23.

5 Young T, Palta M, Dempsey J, Skatrud J, Weber S, Badr S. The occurrence of sleep-disordered breathing among middle-aged adults. N Engl J Med. 1993;17(328):1230–5.

6 Galliccio L, Kalesan B. Sleep duration and mortality: a systematic review and meta-analysis. J Sleep Res. 2009;18(2):148–58.

7 Cappuccio FP, Daniel C. Sleep duration predicts cardiovascular outcomes: a systematic review and meta-analysis of prospective studies. Eur Heart J. 2011;32(12):1484–92.

8 Buxton OM, Marcelli E. Short and long sleep are positively associated with obesity, diabetes, hypertension, and cardiovascular disease among adults in the United States. Soc Sci Med. 2010;71(5):1027–36.

9 Su X, Wang D-X. Improve postoperative sleep: what can we do? Curr Opin Anaesthesiol. 2018;31(1):83–8.

10 Freeman LW, White R, Ratcliff CG, et al. A randomized trial comparing live and telemedicine delivery of an imagery-based behavioral intervention for breast cancer survivors: Reducing symptoms and barriers to care. Psychooncology. 2015;24(8):910–18.

11 Freeman LW, Cohen L, Stewart M, Link J, Palmer JL, Welton D. Imagery intervention for recovering breast cancer patients: Clinical trial of safety and efficacy. J Soc Integr Oncol. 2008;6(2):67–75.

12 Freeman LW, Cohen L, Stewart M, et al. The experience of imagery as a post-treatment intervention in patients with breast cancer: program, process, and patient recommendations. Oncol Nurs Forum. 2008;35(6):E116–21.

13 Freeman LW. Best Practices in Complementary and Alternative Medicine: An Evidence-Based Approach with CEs/SMEs. 2nd ed. Gaithersberg, MD: Aspen; 2003.

14 Freeman LW, Dirks L. Mind-body imagery practice among Alaska breast cancer patients: a case study. Alaska Med. 2006;48(3):74–83.

15 Morgan R, Freeman L. The healing of our people: substance abuse and historical trauma. Subst Use Misuse. 2009;44(1):84–98.

16 Refinetti R. Circadian Phsyiology. 2nd ed. Boca Raton: CRC Press; 2006.

17 Peirson S, Foster R. Melanopsin: another way of signaling light. Neuron. 2006;49(3):331–9.

18 Dijk D-J, Archer SN. Light, sleep, and circadian rhythms: together again. PLOS Biol. 2009;7(6):1–4.

19 Leglise A-A. Progress in Circadian Rhythm Research. New York: Nova Science; 2008.

20 Staner L. Comorbidity of insomnia and depression. Sleep Med Rev. 2010;14(1):35–46.

21 Jansson_Frojmark M, Lindblom K. A bidirectional relationship between anxiety and depression, and insomnia: a prospective study in the general population. J Psychosom Res. 2008;64(4):443–9.

22 Neckelmann D, Mykletun A, Dahl AA. Chronic insomnia as a risk factor for developing anxiety and depression. Sleep Res Soc. 2007;30(7):873–80.

23 Kronholm E, Partonen T, Laatikained T, et al. Trends in self-reported sleep duration and insomnia-related symptoms in Finland from 1972 to 2005: a comparative review and re-analysis of Finnish population samples. J Sleep Res. 2008;1(17):54–62.

24 Knutson KL, Van Cauter E, Rathouz PJ, DeLeire T, Lauderdale DS. Trends in the prevalence of short sleepers in the USA. Sleep Res Soc. 2010;1(33):37–45.

25 Ravan AR, Bengtsson C, Lissner L, Lapidus L, Bjorkelund C. Thirty-six-year secular trends in sleep duration and sleep satisfaction, and associations with mental stress and

socioeconomic factors—results of the population study of women in Gothenburg, Sweden. J Sleep Res. 2010;19(3):496–503.

26 Erickson MH. Hypnosis in painful terminal illness. Am J Clin Hypn. 1959;1(3):117–21.

27 Rossi EL. The Psychobiology of Gene Expression: Neuroscience and Neurogenesis in the Healing Arts. 1st ed. New York: Norton; 2012.

28 Miller WR, Rollick S. Motivational Interviewing: Helping People Change. 3rd ed. New York: Guilford Press; 2013.

29 Rollnick S, Miller WR, Butler CC. Motivational Interviewing in Health Care: Helping Patients Change Behavior. New York: Guilford Press; 2008.

30 Tang NK, Lereya TS, Boulton H, Miller MA, Wolke D, Cappuccio FP. Nonpharmacological treatments of insomnia for long-term painful conditions: A systematic review and meta-analysis of patient-reported outcomes in randomized controlled trials. Sleep Res Soc. 2015;38(11):1751–64.

7

Preoperative Physical Conditioning

Heath B. McAnally

Introduction

Physical fitness is increasingly recognized as a crucial and unfortunately diminishing component and contributor to overall biopsychosocial-spiritual well-being. Morbidity and mortality are closely linked to physical inactivity (PI), as are many chronic pain states; furthermore, there are complex and confounding relationships between PI and obesity, sleep disorders, depression, and anxiety, which all mediate chronic pain and other morbidity and mortality in their own right. Physical inactivity is also associated with worsened postoperative outcomes, and a growing body of evidence supports both rationale and effectiveness of improving physical fitness levels prior to surgery for optimal patient and overall system/economic outcomes. Recent evidence indicates that as little as 4 weeks of mild to moderate but regular physical activity can improve surgical outcomes.

As with many if not all lifestyle issues, PI is at its root a biopsychosocial-spiritual issue, and adequate understanding and accommodation of underlying motivational deficits, obstacles and competing factors, and habit factors are essential to supporting patients in improving their fitness for surgery.

Fitness, Health and Pain

Background/General Concepts of Physical Fitness

Physical fitness (PF), defined as "The ability to carry out daily tasks with vigor and alertness, without undue fatigue, and with ample energy to enjoy leisure-time pursuits and respond to emergencies" [1], is positively correlated with numerous health indices as discussed in greater detail in this chapter. Unfortunately, as the developed world becomes increasingly industrialized and automated, PF levels are steadily decreasing with diminishing physical activity requirements.

Physical fitness has multiple components including cardiorespiratory fitness (CRF), musculoskeletal fitness, flexibility, balance, and speed [1]. Of all these components, CRF has received by far the most attention in terms of clinical and epidemiologic research and constitutes the majority of the focus of this chapter as well. Objectively, CRF is best described in terms of maximum rate of oxygen consumption (VO_2 max), however this value is not readily measurable outside of advanced physiologic laboratories, and as such it is generally estimated in clinical studies by the maximum peak work rate achieved on a treadmill or a cycle ergometer. In the literature and in much clinical practice, a surrogate exercise tolerance measure known as metabolic equivalent of task (MET) is frequently used to judge PF. One MET is defined as the amount of energy expended while sitting at rest (generally corresponding to a VO_2 of 3.5 mL O_2/kg/min); activities are typically categorized by multiples of MET (which vary from individual to individual.) In general:

- 1.5–3 METs (light intensity) is typically achieved with walking or light household chores
- 3–6 METs (moderate intensity) examples include walking briskly (2.5 to 4 mph), playing doubles tennis, or raking the yard.
- >6 METs (vigorous intensity) examples include running, carrying heavy groceries or other loads upstairs, shoveling snow, or participating in a strenuous fitness class.

While it is increasingly recognized and communicated by health authorities that "some is better than none," current recommendations for adults include 150–300 minutes of moderate intensity, or 75–150 minutes of vigorous intensity aerobic exercise per week. In addition, muscle-strengthening activities involving all major muscle groups, of moderate or greater intensity are recommended on at least two days per week [1].

Physical Fitness and Biopsychosocial Health
Correlation Between Physical Fitness and Overall Health
An enormous array of literature over the past few decades overwhelmingly supports the benefits of regular exercise for cardiovascular, metabolic and endocrine, immunologic/anti-oncologic, musculoskeletal, and psychiatric functions, among others [2, 3]. Conversely, a low level of physical activity/CRF displays some of the greatest health risk in the developed world, thought to be a potentially stronger predictor of mortality than established risk factors such as smoking, hypertension, and diabetes [4]. The relationship between PI and increased all-cause mortality is independent of age and also independent of weight status [3]. A maximal exercise tolerance of < 5 METs is associated with particularly high mortality risk [4] and it has been estimated that physical inactivity (PI) is responsible for

9% of premature mortality globally, or greater than 5 million deaths per year [5] from causes such as cardiovascular disease, diabetes, and cancer. Besides CRF deficit, other forms of suboptimal conditioning such as decreased musculoskeletal fitness, balance, and flexibility also confer health risks (e.g., osteoporosis, increased likelihood of minor traumatic injuries, etc.).

Regular exercise is also highly important in maintaining other contributors to overall wellness such as sleep architecture, cognitive function and psychological health, and many others [6–11], and conversely, PI correlates with deficits in all of these arenas.

Deconditioning/Physical Inactivity and Chronic Pain

Physical inactivity is a strong independent predictor of postoperative morbidity and mortality, as discussed in greater detail later. The purpose of this section is to establish the association between PI and chronic pain, which we have previously shown predicts multiple poor operative outcomes. Sedentary lifestyle correlates strongly with an increased incidence of many painful states including chronic low back pain, fibromyalgia, rheumatoid arthritis and other autoimmune conditions, and migraine [12–16]. The association between PI and chronic pain is complex, multifactorial, and biopsychosocial in nature, and varies in pathophysiology between different states of disease/conditions.

Inactivity, Obesity, and Inflammation

One fairly obvious constellation of mechanisms whereby PI exerts pronociceptive effects is via the mediation of obesity. Besides the long-held attribution of increased mechanical load on the musculoskeletal system, along with altered force vectors [17], recent evidence is revealing a host of other complex direct and downstream systemic pro-inflammatory effects of obesity. In the obese state adipocytes (and in particular visceral ones) increase secretion of a vast and surprising array of pro-inflammatory cytokines including tumor necrosis factor, interleukin-6, plasminogen activator inhibitor-1, and leptin [18]; conversely they decrease secretion of protective adipokines such as adiponectin, and in concert this altered milieu results in phenotypic switch of the immune system to a pro-inflammatory and thus pronociceptive state (Figure 7.1).

Obesity (and associated poor diet) also alters the normal gut flora ("microbiome") in a reciprocal fashion [19, 20], and this alteration also confers a systemic inflammatory state thought currently to be mediated predominantly by increased lipopolysaccharide burden with resultant Toll-like receptor-4 activation and cytokine cascade. A downward spiral of oxidative stress and further chronic inflammation ensues [21, 22]. Skeletal muscle also undergoes immune cell infiltration and inflammatory myocyte changes [23]. Obesity is also strongly

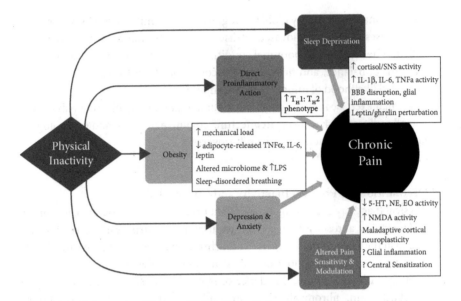

Figure 7.1. Relationship Between Physical Inactivity and Chronic Pain

5-HT = serotonin; BBB = blood-brain barrier; EO = endogenous opioid; LPS = lipopolysaccharide; NE = norepinephrine; NMDA = n-methyl-d-aspartate; IL = interleukin; SNS = sympathetic nervous system; TH = helper T-cell; TNF = tumor necrosis factor.

correlated with obstructive sleep apnea and other sleep disturbance states, which increase inflammation in their own right [24].

Besides these obesity-mediated effects, PI is independently associated with systemic inflammation [25, 26] with complex and still poorly understood pathophysiology [14].

Inactivity, Maladaptive Neural Plasticity, Altered Pain Perception, and Modulation

Maladaptive neural plasticity within the central nervous system is increasingly recognized as a major contributor to many chronic pain states [27], and, while far from well-characterized, convergent evidence supports a likely link between PI and such maladaptive neural plasticity [9, 28–33]. Intertwined with such neural plastic changes both structurally and functionally, there is reverse evidence of decreased pain perception and improved pain tolerance and modulation with exercise [32, 34, 35].

Inactivity, Adverse Psychological Effects, and Pain

Depression and anxiety are both increasingly linked to chronic pain in a reciprocal relationship, and both are also strongly associated with PI [10, 36].

Physical Activity and Pain Reduction

Conversely, a large and growing body of evidence reveals significant improvements in pain burden (as well as, and likely interdigitating with, improvements in depression, anxiety, insomnia, etc.) with regular exercise [37, 38].

Mechanisms for this hypoalgesic effect of physical activity are undoubtedly as complex as the mechanisms introduced previously underlying the relationship between PI and chronic pain. Many of these beneficial effects may be simply "mirror-image" phenomena of reversed pathology, for example, decreased inflammation [14, 39], improved pain sensitivity and modulation capacity [32, 34, 35], and improved affective state [10, 11]. Consistently increased physical activity invariably results in weight loss as well, and interesting and encouraging results have been replicated across varying conditions showing significant improvements on the order of ≥30% decrease in subjective pain ratings with a 10% reduction in weight [40–42].

However, there are other distinct mechanisms of physical activity–induced pain benefit that as of yet do not show convincing evidence of correlative pathophysiologic deficit states associated with PI. For example, activation/upregulation of the endogenous opioid system has been shown in several studies [35, 43] in response to regular exercise; corresponding evidence of endogenous opioid system dysfunction is lacking. Similarly, a strong role for the endogenous cannabinoids system has been proposed [44], again without corresponding evidence of dysregulation associated with PI.

Epidemiology of Physical Inactivity/Deconditioning

Prevalence of Physical Inactivity

The prevalence of PI has reached distressing proportions in the Western world; fewer than half of Americans meet minimum recommendations for aerobic activity, and fewer than one-quarter meet recommendations for joint aerobic and muscle-strengthening activities [3] (Figure 7.2). These figures do not vary significantly by gender nor by ethnicity, however there are statistically significant trends toward inactivity with increasing age, and also with decreasing socioeconomic status. On average, both children and adults spend nearly eight waking hours of each day in a sedentary state. Nearly $120 billion healthcare costs per in the United States are attributed to this phenomenon [3].

On the bright side, data from the National Health Interview Survey suggest an overall trend toward increasing physical activity over the first decade and a half of the new millennium, with the percentage of individuals reporting no leisure-time moderate or vigorous physical activity decreasing from ~40% in 1998 to ~30% in 2015 [3].

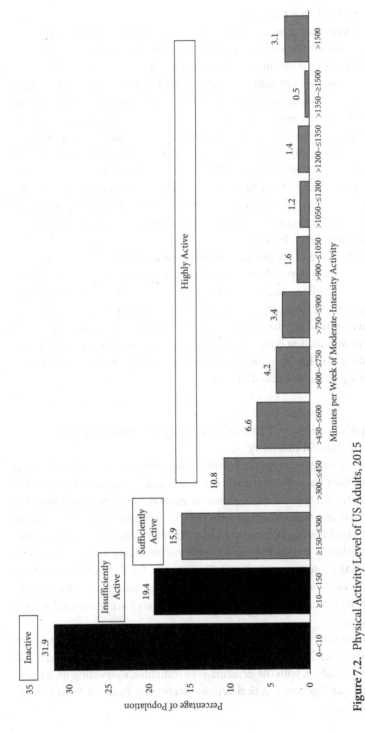

Figure 7.2. Physical Activity Level of US Adults, 2015

From 2018 Physical Activity Guidelines Advisory Committee Scientific Report, US Department of Health and Human Services [3].

Not so reassuring is the obesity trend, with nearly a 20% increase in the prevalence of that condition (defined as body mass index $\geq$ 30 kg/m^2) in US adults from 33.7% in 2007–2008 to 39.6% in 2015–2016 [45]. That figure is projected to eclipse 50% by the year 2030 [46].

Comorbidities

While showing no clear directionality of relationship, it should be noted that over the past several years the association or clustering of lifestyle risk factors such as tobacco use and poor diet with PI/sedentary lifestyle has been consistently demonstrated in the literature [47, 48] across multiple nations and cultures. As with PI alone, these lifestyle risk factor clusters seem more pronounced among lower socioeconomic status groups.

Perioperative Considerations

Surgical Consequences of Physical Deconditioning/Inactivity

Most orthopedic and spine, general, gynecologic and urologic, cardiothoracic and vascular operations confer major physical (and also psychosocial) stress that significantly challenge the organism's homeostatic and healing resilience and reserves. In order to repair the significant trauma that occurs during surgery, a catabolic state mediated largely by increased hypothalamic-pituitary-adrenal axis (and other endocrine) governance, and sympathetic nervous system activity ensues. In addition to these systemic and metabolic demands, additional mechanical challenges to basic physical functioning and activities of daily living may persist for weeks or months following major surgery.

As might be expected, the greater the individual's functional capacity prior to surgery, the better they are able to withstand the increased physiologic demands and psychological challenges of the postoperative period [49–51]. Conversely, deconditioning and PI have been shown to confer worsened surgical outcomes [52–55].

From a CRF standpoint, Ross et al [4] reported that 8 of 12 studies investigating the predictive ability of preoperative cardiopulmonary exercise testing showed a strong association between low CRF and postoperative complications. Sarcopenia (loss of skeletal muscle mass) has also been associated with increased postoperative morbidity and mortality as well as overall poor surgical outcomes [56].

Evidence for Prehabilitation

"Prehabilitation" is a neologism coined earlier this new millennium to describe a process of physical and psychological capacity enhancement in anticipation of an imminent significant stressor [57]. Early studies at the end of last century and into the first part of this one hailed primarily from the orthopedic realm, but by this decade, substantial interest in applying the concept multiple surgical disciplines began to manifest; recent reviews are summarized here.

Valkenet et al in 2011 published a systematic review of preoperative exercise therapy including seven total joint arthroplasty and five cardiac or major vascular surgical controlled trials [58]. There was significant heterogeneity in the interventions ranging from unsupervised home-based programs to those fully supervised by physical therapists, and some were specifically designed to target inspiratory muscle training. Among the cardiac/vascular trials, there was significant benefit from this latter intervention in terms of reducing postoperative pulmonary complications, and also hospital length of stay. No significant outcome differences were seen in the orthopedic studies reviewed.

Santa Mina et al in 2014 [59] published the results of a systematic review and meta-analysis of preoperative "total-body" exercise comprising various combinations of aerobic versus resistance training. Thirteen orthopedic and eight abdominopelvic papers ($n = 1,371$) were analyzed, with various outcomes measured; overall the authors reported, "the majority of studies found that total-body prehabilitation improved postoperative pain, length of stay [statistically significant with Hedges' g statistic $= -.039$, $p < 0.05$] and physical function, but it was not consistently effective in improving health-related quality of life for aerobic fitness in the studies that examined these outcomes."

Pouwels et al presented a more focused review in 2015 [60] of studies looking specifically at preoperative exercise in lung cancer patients scheduled for thoracic surgery. Eleven trials or cohort studies ($n = 916$; 277 patients undergoing intervention) with widely disparate programs with duration ranging from less than 1 week to 4 weeks, and with frequencies ranging from 1 to 10 sessions per week. Different and inconsistent results were seen, nonetheless overall the authors report that preoperative exercise "might have a beneficial effect on postoperative complications, mortality, length of hospital stay, physical fitness and quality of life" while admitting to the very limiting heterogeneity.

The same group in 2016 presented a larger and more diverse scoping review of systematic reviews of preoperative exercise trials across multiple specialties [61]; 21 reviews (212 primary studies) were examined, but the number of patients was not presented, and across the reviews there was considerable redundancy of primary studies. Again, the heterogeneity of patient populations, interventions, and outcome measurements precluded any definitive reporting of results, however the authors note that "it seems that preoperative exercise therapy exerts beneficial effects on physical fitness and postoperative outcome measures" based on the available data.

Moran et al [62] in 2016 performed a systematic review and meta-analysis of randomized controlled trials evaluating preoperative exercise in patients undergoing abdominal surgery. Nine trials ($n = 435$) with various interventions were included. Statistically significant reduction in postoperative complications (odds ratio = 0.59; 95% Confidence Interval: 0.38–0.91; $p = 0.03$) was seen; there was no significant effect shown on length of stay.

Wang et al [63] in 2016 performed a systematic review and meta-analysis of randomized controlled trials evaluating prehabilitation before total joint arthroplasty. Twenty-two studies ($n = 1,492$) were included, again with very heterogeneous interventions. Prehabilitation was associated with decreased postoperative pain during the first 4 weeks, and statistically significant improvements in various physical function indices up to the 3-month mark. No differences were seen for length of stay or total cost.

Moyer et al [64] in 2017 provided a much larger systematic review and meta-analysis of randomized controlled trials evaluating prehabilitation in total joint arthroplasty patients; 35 studies ($n = 2,956$) again with various interventions were included. Among total hip arthroplasty (THA) patients, significant improvements in postoperative pain and function were seen; among the total knee arthroplasty (TKA) patients comparable improvements in function but no improvement with pain were seen. Length of stay was significantly reduced in both groups.

Orange et al in 2018 [65] presented a mixed review incorporating six prior systematic reviews (55 studies, $n = 3,181$) supplemented with various other studies, with the goal of ascertaining whether prehabilitation should be recommended as part of standardized Enhanced Recovery After Surgery (ERAS) programs. The authors note that to date, only two studies of prehabilitation have been performed within the context of ERAS programs. Significant heterogeneity of patient populations, interventions, and measured outcomes were noted, obviating firm conclusions; however, the authors did state that prehabilitation "appears to be effective for improving physical fitness prior to elective intra-cavity surgery. Some studies have also reported an accelerated recovery of postoperative functional capacity, which is a central tenet of ERAS pathways." They note, however, that due to limited evidence of benefit in terms of complications and length of stay at present, and given the strong focus within the ERAS community on cost-effectiveness, at present more data showing positive benefit in these economic indicators would be required before prehabilitation could be routinely incorporated into ERAS programs.

Luther et al [66] in 2018 performed a systematic review of 16 studies (n = 2,591) investigating the effect of prehabilitation on patients undergoing intra-abdominal surgery, with the specific goal also of ascertaining "the collective impact of total body prehabilitation across four main domains (physical exercise . . . , nutritional and psychosocial optimisation and cessation of negative health behaviours)" on functional and clinical outcomes. Only three studies employing such a multimodal approach were identified (and are presented later). The authors reported that six of the studies showed positive benefit via varying interventions including preoperative exercise, nutritional supplementation, and smoking cessation; they also reported the conclusion that multimodal prehabilitation is more likely to yield consistent benefit.

Dr. Francesco Carli's group from McGill University has provided the only literature to date evaluating the effects of a multimodal prehabilitation strategy on postoperative outcomes. Their initial paper [67] compared outcomes of a 42-patient intervention group to a historical cohort comprising 45 patients; all patients were undergoing colorectal resection for cancer. In contradistinction to previous efforts by the group plagued by poor patient adherence, they deliberately reduced exercise frequency to 3 days per week, with only mild to moderate intensity for 30 minutes. In addition, nutritional counseling and protein supplementation were provided, as well as specific anxiolytic-focused psychology interventions. The median duration of prehabilitation was 33 days. Primary outcome was functional walking capacity as measured by the 6-minute walking test (6MWT). Statistically significant improvements in functional capacity were seen in the intervention group at preoperative and 1-month and 2-month postoperative visits.

In a follow-up trial [68], 38 colorectal cancer patients were randomized to multimodal prehabilitation, with 39 colorectal cancer patients in the control group; median duration of intervention was 24.5 days (compared to 20 days in the control group.) Again, statistically significant improvement was seen in the prehabilitation group in the same indices. Data from all of these patients and additional subsequent participants were then pooled and reanalyzed (n = 185), with similar findings reported [69]. Of note, compared to poor adherence rates seen by this group prior to these publications (in the context of much more rigorous regimen) adherence exceeded 75% in all three of these publications.

Fit for Surgery: A Plan

Overview

While weak to moderate evidence of benefit exists for various prehabilitation regimens in a multiplicity of settings, in general there has not yet been consistent evidence of economic outcomes benefit. When considering the costs involved in multiple formal physical therapy visits, the cost:benefit ratio may indeed be unfavorable. As such, we recommend and have prescribed informal and home-based regimens tailored to the individual and their resources, relying primarily on walking 3 days per week, beginning anywhere from 5–30 minutes at a session depending on the patient's baseline condition. In the exercise-naive we aim to initiate this aspect of our multimodal program no later than 4 weeks before the proposed operative date, based on data from the McGill group, as discussed earlier, indicating that significant benefit at least in functional capacity may be seen in even 1 month of mild to moderate exercise thrice weekly. For those rare individuals who already do exercise regularly, or display functional capacity at or above predicted levels on the 6MWT (based on the formula 868 meters – [age × 2.9] – 74.7 if female, from the McGill group) we then craft goals in approximation to the DHHS guidelines (150 minutes of moderate-intensity physical activity per week with resistance training 2d/week) adjusted for chronic conditions.

Optimize Sleep Prior to Exercise

There is increasing recognition of a bidirectional relationship between exercise and sleep [70, 71], such that while healthy sleep duration and architecture appear dependent at least in part on regular and sufficient physical activity, excessive physical activity (especially resistance training) may be counterproductive and even harmful without adequate restorative sleep. Exercise results in considerable short-term catabolism and often micro-injuries that require adequate sleep and especially slow-wave (delta-wave, NREM Stage 3) sleep [72, 73] to recover from.

While many if not most situations of sleep disturbance will be amenable to correction with the gradual introduction and optimization of physical activity, there remain many situations (e.g., untreated obstructive sleep apnea, severe post-traumatic stress disorder [PTSD] and related night terror scenarios, excessive caffeine or other stimulant intake) that may not respond favorably simply to initiation of, or increase in exercise. Careful evaluation of sleep hygiene issues (including both over-the-counter and prescribed pharmacotherapy), respectful and sensitive screening for PTSD and related conditions, and so forth, are critical for success and patient well-being, and such individualization is increasingly recognized as necessary for optimal benefit [74, 75]. Along these lines, in severe cases of sleep disturbance, careful consideration of a short course of rational slow wave sleep–facilitating pharmacotherapy may be indicated—it should be highlighted here that most drugs commonly prescribed today "for sleep" (e.g., z-hypnotics, benzodiazepines) are counterproductive in that regard as that they favor superficial sleep cycles at the expense of slow-wave sleep, and furthermore confer significant abuse and dependence liability.

The Necessity of the Biopsychosocial-Spiritual Approach

General Considerations

Although exercise may appear on the surface to constitute a solely physical issue, it has become quite clear over the past several decades that PI and related barriers to physical activity have tremendous psychosocial components and origins. Low self-efficacy, fear-avoidance behaviors, and many other cognitive/emotional distortions may actually play primary roles affecting both physical activity and inactivity states [76–78] and failure to address these issues may invalidate all other efforts toward facilitating activity.

Motivational Enhancement

Despite fairly broad assent among most of us to the reality that more physical fitness is something we need/in our best interest, there are tremendous complex and multifactorial barriers for most individuals in terms of initiating let alone perpetuating regular exercise. As discussed in greater detail in chapter 3, in the context of limited personal resources affecting prioritization of effort and activities, clear and salient goal enrichment, and enhancement of autonomy, competence, and relatedness (recognition of which is essential for intrinsic motivation, per self-determination theory) are required.

Toward both ends, motivational interviewing (MI) [79] may be of great value. Overcoming the ambivalence that almost always accompanies consideration of increasing physical activity is prerequisite to initiating let alone sustaining activity when it is neither enjoyable nor habitual, and hearing oneself vocalize rationale and intention are among the most important factors in increasing self-efficacy. The reader is referred to Clifford and Curtis's monograph *Motivational Interviewing in Nutrition and Fitness* [80] for an excellent and thorough treatment of the subject, with multiple practical examples of the technique.

Habit

While motivational enhancement and tailoring of interventions based on readiness to change/transtheoretical model stages may be beneficial in terms of initial activity adoption, sustained adherence based on these methods is poor [81]. Overcoming the inertia of sedentary/PI habits and cultivation of new and active habits requires considerable effort on the part of the individual, and informed support [82] on the part of the care team often spells the difference between success and failure.

Rational, individually tailored goal-setting forms the foundation of implementation intention, which is a key first step to bridging the intention-behavior gap. It is critical, as discussed in greater detail in chapter 11, that goals be specific/measurable, attainable, and also scheduled.

Behavioral "priming" of both motivational processes [83] (increasing self-efficacy) and also solidifying a cue-activity sequence [82] is essential to overcoming inertia and biopsychosocial barriers. Activity scheduling is absolutely necessary; however, careful identification of obstacles along with means of circumventing them are of inestimable value. For example, given that daily routine and/or circadian energy levels are highly relevant for most individuals, prioritizing a dedicated time for exercise when resources are maximal is crucial. Incorporating exercise into existing daily rituals may also be useful; for example, placing an exercise bicycle in front of the television and not allowing oneself to indulge in viewing without pedaling has been useful for many, as has implementing a daily 20 to 30 minute walk into a lunch break.

Finally, accountability both via family or peer group and also on a weekly basis with the preoperative care team is invaluable as well. As discussed in chapter 4, while pairing of extrinsic rewards (whether physical comforts or validation and praise) runs the risk of hampering cultivation of intrinsic motivation and habit formation, we have found that encouragement and positive feedback more often help to bolster self-efficacy and self-determination.

References

1 US Department of Health and Human Services. Physical Activity Guidelines for Americans. 2nd ed. Washington, DC: US Department of Health and Human Services; 2018. https://health.gov/paguidelines/secondedition/pdf/Physical_Activity_Guidelines_2nd_edition.pdf. Accessed November 22, 2018.

2 Fletcher GF, Landolfo C, Niebauer J, Ozemek C, Arena R, Lavie CJ. Promoting physical activity and exercise: JACC health promotion series. J Am Coll Cardiol. 2018;72:1622–39.

3 2018 Physical Activity Guidelines Advisory Committee. 2018 Physical Activity Guidelines Advisory Committee Scientific Report. Washington, DC: US Department of Health and Human Services; 2018.

4 Ross R, Blair SN, Arena R, et al. Importance of assessing cardiorespiratory fitness in clinical practice: a case for fitness as a clinical vital sign: a scientific statement from the American Heart Association. Circulation. 2016;134(24):e653–99. doi:10.1161/CIR.0000000000000461.

5 Lee IM, Shiroma EJ, Lobelo F, et al. Effect of physical inactivity on major noncommunicable diseases worldwide: an analysis of burden of disease and life expectancy. Lancet. 2012;380:219–29.

6 Lang C, Kalak N, Brand S, Holsboer-Trachsler E, Pühse U, Gerber M. The relationship between physical activity and sleep from mid adolescence to early adulthood. A systematic review of methodological approaches and meta-analysis. Sleep Med Rev. 2016;28:32–45.

7 Kelley GA, Kelley KS. Exercise and sleep: a systematic review of previous meta-analyses. J Evid Based Med. 2017;10:26–36.

8   Hillman CH, Erickson KI, Kramer AF. Be smart, exercise your heart: exercise effects on brain and cognition. Nat Rev Neurosci. 2008;9:58–65.

9   Fernandes J, Arida RM, Gomez-Pinilla F. Physical exercise as an epigenetic modulator of brain plasticity and cognition. Neurosci Biobehav Rev. 2017;80:443–56. doi: 10.1016/j.neubiorev.2017.06.012.

10 Cooney GM, Dwan K, Greig CA, et al. Exercise for depression. Cochrane Database Syst Rev. 2013;(9):CD004366. doi: 10.1002/14651858.CD004366.pub6.

11 Archer T, Josefsson T, Lindwall M. Effects of physical exercise on depressive symptoms and biomarkers in depression. CNS Neurol Disord Drug Targets. 2014;13: 1640–53.

12 Nilsen TI, Holtermann A, Mork PJ. Physical exercise, body mass index, and risk of chronic pain in the low back and neck/shoulders: longitudinal data from the Nord-Trondelag Health Study. Am J Epidemiol. 2011;174:267–73.

13 Yang H, Haldeman S. Behavior-related factors associated with low back pain in the US adult population. Spine. 2018;43:28–34.

14 Sharif K, Watad A, Bragazzi NL, Lichtbroun M, Amital H, Shoenfeld Y. Physical activity and autoimmune diseases: get moving and manage the disease. Autoimmun Rev. 2018;17:53–72.

15 Le H, Tfelt-Hansen P, Skytthe A, Kyvik KO, Olesen J. Association between migraine, lifestyle and socioeconomic factors: a population-based cross-sectional study. J Headache Pain. 2011;12:157–72.

16 Hagen K, Åsberg AN, Stovner L, et al. Lifestyle factors and risk of migraine and tension-type headache: follow-up data from the Nord-Trøndelag Health Surveys 1995–1997 and 2006–2008. Cephalalgia. 2018;38:1919–26.

17 Messier SP. Obesity and osteoarthritis: disease genesis and nonpharmacologic weight management. Rheum Dis Clin North Am. 2008;34:713–29.

18 Ouchi N, Parker JL, Lugus JJ, Walsh K. Adipokines in inflammation and metabolic disease. Nat Rev Immunol. 2011;11:85–97.

19 Tsukumo DM, Carvalho BM, Carvalho Filho MA, Saad MJ. Translational research into gut microbiota: new horizons on obesity treatment: updated 2014. Arch Endocrinol Metab. 2015;59:154–60.

20 Bleau C, Karelis AD, St-Pierre DH, Lamontagne L. Crosstalk between intestinal microbiota, adipose tissue and skeletal muscle as an early event in systemic low-grade inflammation and the development of obesity and diabetes. Diabetes Metab Res Rev. 2015;31:545–61.

21 Lugrin J, Rosenblatt-Velin N, Parapanov R, Liaudet L. The role of oxidative stress during inflammatory processes. Biol Chem. 2014;395:203–30.

22 Marseglia L, Manti S, D'Angelo G, et al. Oxidative stress in obesity: a critical component in human diseases. Int J Mol Sci. 2014;16:378–400.

23 Wu H, Ballantyne CM. Skeletal muscle inflammation and insulin resistance in obesity. J Clin Invest. 2017;127:43–54.

24 Irwin MR, Olmstead R, Carroll JE. Sleep disturbance, sleep duration, and inflammation: a systematic review and meta-analysis of cohort studies and experimental sleep deprivation. Biol Psychiatry. 2016;80:40–52.

25 Lavie CJ, Church TS, Milani RV, Earnest CP. Impact of physical activity, cardiorespiratory fitness, and exercise training on markers of inflammation. J Cardiopulm Rehabil Prev. 2011;31:137–45.

26 Gratas-Delamarche A, Derbré F, Vincent S, Cillard J. Physical inactivity, insulin resistance, and the oxidative-inflammatory loop. Free Radic Res. 2014;48:93–108.

27 Kuner R, Flor H. Structural plasticity and reorganisation in chronic pain. Nat Rev Neurosci. 2016;18:20–30.

28 Liepert J, Tegenthoff M, Malin JP. Changes of cortical motor area size during immobilization. Electroencephalogr Clin Neurophysiol. 1995;97:382–6.

29 Mischel NA, Subramanian M, Dombrowski MD, Llewellyn-Smith IJ, Mueller PJ. (In)activity-related neuroplasticity in brainstem control of sympathetic outflow: unraveling underlying molecular, cellular, and anatomical mechanisms. Am J Physiol Heart Circ Physiol. 2015;309:H235–43.

30 Silverman MN, Deuster PA. Biological mechanisms underlying the role of physical fitness in health and resilience. Interface Focus. 2014;4(5):20140040. doi: 10.1098/rsfs.2014.0040.

31 Flodin P, Martinsen S, Mannerkorpi K, et al. Normalization of aberrant resting state functional connectivity in fibromyalgia patients following a three month physical exercise therapy. Neuroimage Clin. 2015;9:134–9.

32 Ellingson LD, Stegner AJ, Schwabacher IJ, Koltyn KF, Cook DB. Exercise strengthens central nervous system modulation of pain in fibromyalgia. Brain Sci. 2016;6(1). pii: E8. doi: 10.3390/brainsci6010008.

33 Cobianchi S, Arbat-Plana A, Lopez-Alvarez VM, Navarro X. Neuroprotective effects of exercise treatments after injury: the dual role of neurotrophic factors. Curr Neuropharmacol. 2017;15:495–518.

34 Naugle KM, Fillingim RB, Riley JL 3rd. A meta-analytic review of the hypoalgesic effects of exercise. J Pain. 2012;13:1139–50.

35 Lima LV, Abner TSS, Sluka KA. Does exercise increase or decrease pain? Central mechanisms underlying these two phenomena. J Physiol. 2017;595:4141–50.

36 Booth FW, Roberts CK, Laye MJ. Lack of exercise is a major cause of chronic diseases. Compr Physiol. 2012;2:1143–211.

37 Shiri R, Falah-Hassani K. Does leisure time physical activity protect against low back pain? Systematic review and meta-analysis of 36 prospective cohort studies. Br J Sports Med. 2017;51:1410–8.

38 Geneen LJ, Moore RA, Clarke C, Martin D, Colvin LA, Smith BH. Physical activity and exercise for chronic pain in adults: an overview of Cochrane Reviews. Cochrane Database Syst Rev. 2017;4:CD011279. doi:10.1002/14651858.CD011279.pub3

39 Ortega E, García JJ, Bote ME, et al. Exercise in fibromyalgia and related inflammatory disorders: known effects and unknown chances. Exerc Immunol Rev. 2009;15:42–65.

40 Riddle DL, Stratford PW. Body weight changes and corresponding changes in pain and function in persons with symptomatic knee osteoarthritis: a cohort study. Arthritis Care Res (Hoboken). 2013;65:15–22.

41 Messier SP, Resnik AE, Beavers DP, et al. Intentional weight loss in overweight and obese patients with knee osteoarthritis: is more better? Arthritis Care Res (Hoboken). 2018;70:1569–75.

42 Schrepf A, Harte SE, Miller N, et al. Improvement in the spatial distribution of pain, somatic symptoms, and depression after a weight loss intervention. J Pain. 2017;18:1542–50.

43 Koltyn KF. Analgesia following exercise: a review. Sport Med. 2000;29:85–98.

44   Koltyn KF, Brellenthin AG, Cook DB, Sehgal N, Hillard C. Mechanisms of exercise-induced hypoalgesia. J Pain. 2014;15:1294–304.

45   Hales CM, Fryar CD, Carroll MD, Freedman DS, Ogden CL. Trends in obesity and severe obesity prevalence in us youth and adults by sex and age, 2007–2008 to 2015–2016. JAMA. 2018;319:1723–5.

46   Wang YC, McPherson K, Marsh T, Gortmaker SL, Brown M. Health and economic burden of the projected obesity trends in the USA and the UK. Lancet. 2011;378:815–25.

47   Schuit AJ, Van Loon AJ, Tijhuis M, Ocke M. Clustering of lifestyle risk factors in a general adult population. Prev Med. 2002;35:219–24.

48   Noble N, Paul C, Turon H, Oldmeadow C. Which modifiable health risk behaviours are related? A systematic review of the clustering of Smoking, Nutrition, Alcohol and Physical activity ('SNAP') health risk factors. Prev Med. 2015;81:16–41.

49   Cook JW, Pierson LM, Herbert WG, et al. The influence of patient strength, aerobic capacity and body composition upon outcomes after coronary artery bypass grafting. Thorac Cardiovasc Surg. 2001;49:89–93.

50   Santa Mina D, Guglietti CL, Alibhai SMH, et al. The effect of meeting physical activity guidelines for cancer survivors on quality of life following radical prostatectomy for prostate cancer. J Cancer Surviv. 2014;8:190–8.

51   Myers JN, Fonda H. The impact of fitness on surgical outcomes: the case for prehabilitation. Curr Sports Med Rep. 2016;15:282–9.

52   Mayo NE, Feldman L, Scott S, et al. Impact of preoperative change in physical function on postoperative recovery: argument supporting prehabilitation for colorectal surgery. Surgery. 2011;150:505–14.

53   Kassin MT, Owen RM, Perez SD, et al. Risk factors for 30-day hospital readmission among general surgery patients. J Am Coll Surg. 2012;215:322–30.

54   Lin HS, Watts JN, Peel NM, Hubbard RE. Frailty and post-operative outcomes in older surgical patients: a systematic review. BMC Geriatr. 2016;16:157.

55   Richardson K, Levett DZH, Jack S, Grocott MPW. Fit for surgery? Perspectives on preoperative exercise testing and training. Br J Anaesth. 2017;119(Suppl 1):i34–43.

56   Friedman J, Lussiez A, Sullivan J, Wang S, Englesbe M. Implications of sarcopenia in major surgery. Nutr Clin Pract. 2015;30:175–9.

57   Carli F, Zavorsky GS. Optimizing functional exercise capacity in the elderly surgical population. Curr Opin Clin Nutr Metab Care. 2005;8:23–32.

58   Valkenet K, van de Port IG, Dronkers JJ, de Vries WR, Lindeman E, Backx FJ. The effects of preoperative exercise therapy on postoperative outcome: a systematic review. Clin Rehabil. 2011;25:99–111.

59   Santa Mina D, Clarke H, Ritvo P, et al. Effect of total-body prehabilitation on postoperative outcomes: a systematic review and meta-analysis. Physiotherapy. 2014;100:196–207.

60   Pouwels S, Fiddelaers J, Teijink JA, Woorst JF, Siebenga J, Smeenk FW. Preoperative exercise therapy in lung surgery patients: a systematic review. Respir Med. 2015;109:1495–504.

61   Pouwels S, Hageman D, Gommans LN, et al. Preoperative exercise therapy in surgical care: a scoping review. J Clin Anesth. 2016;33:476–90.

62   Moran J, Guinan E, McCormick P, et al. The ability of prehabilitation to influence postoperative outcome after intra-abdominal operation: a systematic review and meta-analysis. Surgery. 2016;160:1189–201.

63 Wang L, Lee M, Zhang Z, Moodie J, Cheng D, Martin J. Does preoperative rehabilita-
    tion for patients planning to undergo joint replacement surgery improve outcomes?
    A systematic review and meta-analysis of randomised controlled trials. BMJ Open.
    2016;6(2):e009857. doi: 10.1136/bmjopen-2015-009857.

64 Moyer R, Ikert K, Long K, Marsh J. The value of preoperative exercise and educa-
    tion for patients undergoing total hip and knee arthroplasty: a systematic review and
    meta-analysis. JBJS Rev. 2017;5(12):e2. doi: 10.2106/JBJS.RVW.17.00015.

65 Orange ST, Northgraves MJ, Marshall P, Madden LA, Vince RV. Exercise
    prehabilitation in elective intra-cavity surgery: a role within the ERAS pathway?
    A narrative review. Int J Surg. 2018;56:328–33.

66 Luther A, Gabriel J, Watson RP, Francis NK. The impact of total body prehabilitation
    on post-operative outcomes after major abdominal surgery: a systematic review.
    World J Surg. 2018;42:2781–91.

67 Li C, Carli F, Lee L, et al. Impact of a trimodal prehabilitation program on functional
    recovery after colorectal cancer surgery: a pilot study. Surg Endosc. 2013;27:1072–82.

68 Gillis C, Li C, Lee L, et al. Prehabilitation versus rehabilitation: a randomized con-
    trol trial in patients undergoing colorectal resection for cancer. Anesthesiology.
    2014;121:937–47.

69 Minnella EM, Bousquet-Dion G, Awasthi R, Scheede-Bergdahl C, Carli F.
    Multimodal prehabilitation improves functional capacity before and after colorectal
    surgery for cancer: a five-year research experience. Acta Oncol. 2017;56:295–300.

70 Baron KG, Reid KJ, Zee PC. Exercise to improve sleep in insomnia: exploration of the
    bidirectional effects. J Clin Sleep Med. 2013;9:819–24.

71 Kline CE. The bidirectional relationship between exercise and sleep: implications for
    exercise adherence and sleep improvement. Am J Lifestyle Med. 2014;8:375–9.

72 Van Cauter E, Spiegel K, Tasali E, Leproult R. Metabolic consequences of sleep and
    sleep loss. Sleep Med. 2008;9(Suppl 1):S23–8.

73 Fullagar HH, Skorski S, Duffield R, Hammes D, Coutts AJ, Meyer T. Sleep and athletic
    performance: the effects of sleep loss on exercise performance, and physiological and
    cognitive responses to exercise. Sports Med. 2015;45:161–86.

74 Valenza MC, Rodenstein DO, Fernández-de-las-Peñas C. Consideration of sleep dys-
    function in rehabilitation. J Bodyw Mov Ther. 2011;15:262–7.

75 Nijs J, Kosek E, Van Oosterwijck J, Meeus M. Dysfunctional endogenous analgesia
    during exercise in patients with chronic pain: to exercise or not to exercise? Pain
    Physician. 2012;15(3 Suppl):ES205–13.

76 Bauman AE, Reis RS, Sallis JF, Wells JC, Loos RJ, Martin BW. Correlates of phys-
    ical activity: why are some people physically active and others not? Lancet.
    2012;380:258–71.

77 Vlaeyen JW, Linton SJ. Fear-avoidance and its consequences in chronic musculoskel-
    etal pain: a state of the art. Pain. 2000;85:317–32.

78 Crombez G, Eccleston C, Van Damme S, Vlaeyen JW, Karoly P. Fear-avoidance model
    of chronic pain: the next generation. Clin J Pain. 2012;28:475–83.

79 Miller WR, Rollnick S. Motivational Interviewing: Helping People Change. 3rd
    Edition. New York: Guilford Press; 2013.

80 Clifford D, Curtis L. Motivational Interviewing in Nutrition and Fitness.
    New York: Guilford Press; 2016.

81 Adams J, White M. Are activity promotion interventions based on the transtheoretical
    model effective? A critical review. Br J Sports Med. 2003;37:106–14.

82 Rebar AL, Dimmock JA, Jackson B, et al. A systematic review of the effects of non-conscious regulatory processes in physical activity. Health Psychol Rev. 2016;10:395–407.

83 St Quinton T. Promoting physical activity through priming the content of motivation. Front Psychol. 2017;8:1509. doi: 10.3389/fpsyg.2017.01509.

8

Preoperative Nutritional Management

Heath B. McAnally

Introduction

Malnutrition in the developed world generally comprises both excess of calories with poor macronutrient (carbohydrate—protein—fat) proportioning, and deficit of multiple micronutrients (vitamins, minerals, and phytonutrients). These excesses, deficits, and imbalances all confer health risks, and many are associated with the development of systemic inflammation and chronic pain.

In the perioperative context, malnutrition is also associated with suboptimal surgical outcomes; from a nutrient deficiency standpoint, compromised wound healing and increased incidence of infections are seen. From a caloric excess standpoint, obesity confers markedly increased perioperative morbidity and mortality. Most of the evidence-based literature supports the use of so-called immunonutrition preoperatively in populations at risk.

As with all of the lifestyle modification issues discussed in this book, enhancement of patients' intrinsic motivation, and thoughtful identification and replacement of maladaptive habits with better alternatives are of the essence.

Nutrition, Health, and Pain

Background/Overview of General Concepts of Nutrition and Malnutrition

Human beings require a relatively simple mixture of macronutrients (carbohydrates, proteins, and fats) and micronutrients (vitamins, minerals, and more recently recognized phytonutrients) for survival and vitality. There is considerable "buffering" built into our metabolic system in terms of the former elements, which are in a sense interchangeable in terms of energy currency and also to some extent structural/protein requirements. The final common denominator of macronutrient input into the Krebs cycle is acetyl coenzyme A, which may be derived from both fats and protein in addition to complex carbohydrates; similarly, the majority of amino acids can be synthesized from molecular building blocks derived from carbohydrates and fats. Exceptions to this flexibility include the nine essential amino acids, and the essential fatty acids linoleic acid, and alpha-linoleic acid.

Micronutrients are not interchangeable, and as such, specific deficiencies of these compounds are more prevalent in the developed world, where adequate food supplies are available. Conversely, the problem with macronutrients in these areas is typically excess, and both of these problems are discussed at greater length shortly.

Nutritional guidelines and recommended daily intake levels of all of these nutrients have been provided by several organizations; for the purposes of this effort we are relying primarily on the Dietary Reference Intakes (DRI) provided by the Institute of Medicine [1] for macronutrient recommendations; exceptions are referenced. For micronutrient recommendations, we are relying on the DRI and on information provided by Oregon State University's Linus Pauling Institute.

In general, authorities are in agreement in recommending a diet based on as many natural foods as possible (minimizing processed components) with a balance favoring multiple vegetables and fruits and also including protein and grain varieties, with healthy fats/oils. Conversely, limiting intake of saturated and *trans* fats, added sugars, and sodium are recommended. Furthermore, in areas of food plenty, in view of reducing chronic diseases associated with excess, overall caloric and also specific nutrient limitations have been recommended with the latter discussed individually later. Specific daily caloric intake requirements vary of course based on a person's energy expenditure; in general a 2,000 kilocalorie (kCal) daily intake is more than adequate, and in the increasingly sedentary West, often excessive. More targeted recommendations may be given based on estimated energy requirements (EERs) as demonstrated in the formulae shown in Figure 8.1.

Carbohydrates

Carbohydrates (CHOs) constitute the main energy source for cellular activity under most scenarios, and in particular are essential for brain function. Carbohydrates are normally ingested, and also synthesized (gluconeogenesis) to meet continuously fluctuating needs. Excess ingested CHO may be either stored as glycogen or converted into fat. Also, CHO may be converted to nonessential amino acids if dietary intake/supply of the latter is insufficient.

On average, 130 g of CHOs are required each day for brain function, and that number therefore constitutes the Recommended Dietary Allowance (RDA). Based on insufficient scientific evidence, and also the complexities of widely varying metabolic needs and interchangeability of macronutrients as discussed previously, a specific upper limit for overall CHOs has not been set. However,

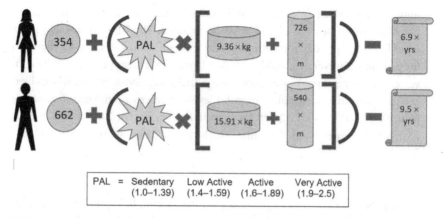

Figure 8.1. Estimated Energy Requirements for Adults
From the Institute of Medicine's Dietary Reference Intakes [1].
kg = weight in kilograms; m = height in meters; PAL = physical activity level; yrs = age in years.

limitation of daily simple/added sugars to ≤10% of daily caloric intake has been recommended. More recently, the concept of acceptable macronutrient distribution ranges (AMDR) has been proposed, with AMDR comprising a percentage of total energy intake (again, recognizing interchangeability with other energy sources and heterogeneity of requirements). The AMDR for CHO has been proposed at between 45% and 65% of daily energy requirements. An AMDR for fiber (largely CHO) has not been set due to its noncontributory nature from an energy standpoint and because on the high end there are no known adverse effects from any degree of consumption.

Excessive dietary CHO, especially in the context of low-fat diets, tends to result in an atherogenic lipoprotein constellation comprising hypertriglyceridemia, elevated LDL and decreased HDL profiles. In addition, more recently the measurement of glycemic index (GI) has gained attention in terms of shaping dietary recommendations; GI represents the increase in blood glucose levels experienced over the 2 hours following ingestion of a given amount of CHO compared to a reference CHO such as glucose (usually 50 g). Lower-GI CHOs (<55; reference = 100 from pure glucose) seem to translate to a more favorable/less atherogenic lipid milieu.

Protein
Protein serves as the main structural element of the body, as well as forming enzymes, hormones and neurotransmitters, membrane channels and carriers, and so forth. Proteins are chains of amino acids (AAs) produced by ribosomes based on mRNA templates transcribed from genomic DNA. Most of these AAs

may be synthesized from CHO and available nitrogen, however nine essential AAs cannot be derived and must be ingested. The RDA for protein is 0.8 g per kilogram per day for both men and women. No upper limit has been set for protein (however, it should be remembered that excess protein will be converted into other forms of energy storage including glycogen and fat, and excess nitrogen may accumulate harmful levels in cases of renal insufficiency or failure). Nonetheless an AMDR for protein has been set at 10% to 35% of daily energy requirements based on that which remains after subtracting CHO and fat AMDR.

Fats

Fats/lipids serve a variety of physiologic roles as well, being the primary component of cell membranes and many hormones, and of course also constitute a major source of energy storage. As introduced earlier, excess dietary CHO is transformed into various fats for such reserve. Within the body, fats/lipids essentially exist as either cholesterol and other steroid ring molecules, or as fatty acid (FA) chain molecules. There are different structural subtypes of FA based on hydrogen content and carbon double bonds, with saturated and monounsaturated FA (one to no double bonds, plentiful hydrogen moieties) synthesizable by the body and associated with chronic diseases in excess. *Trans* FA are a form of unsaturated FA rarely found in nature but commonplace in the Western diet due to industrial era mass production of more stable fat sources. Due to significant associations with cardiovascular disease among other things, most health organizations have called for the elimination of *trans* FA from manufacturing and from the human diet, with governmental regulations supporting this in many places.

Polyunsaturated FAs (PUFAs) represent a highly diverse and important family of molecules, some of which (in particular certain short chain PUFAs with so-called ω-3 and ω-6 PUFAs, based on placement of carbon double bonds) cannot be synthesized by humans and as such are labeled essential FAs (EFAs). Two of these molecules are linoleic acid (an ω-6 PUFA) and α-linoleic acid (an ω-3 PUFA).

The adult AMDR for fat has been proposed as 20% to 35% of daily energy requirements. Within that, the AMDR for linoleic acid has been recommended at 5%–10%, and for α-linoleic acid at 0.6%–1.2% of daily energy requirements. As per brief discussion earlier, elimination of *trans* FA (largely facilitated by regulation) has been advised; current recommendations are to keep saturated fats at less than 10% of daily caloric intake [2]. Historically, specific daily limitations on cholesterol have been recommended, more recent guidelines (including the DRI) have abandoned this approach in favor of a general recommendation to minimize intake based on insufficient evidence of a distinct cutoff for harms.

Micronutrients

Micronutrients (vitamins, minerals, and phytonutrients) as discussed earlier are not interchangeable nor for the most part synthesizable (Vitamin D being a notable exception), and dietary deficiencies often result in significant pathology and, in extreme cases, death. These compounds are too numerous and of limited specific perioperative relevance for the most part to discuss individually; recommended intakes are presented in Table 8.1. In our (HM, LF) VALERAS preoperative optimization program, specific recommendations for Vitamin D, Vitamin C, and magnesium are provided, as discussed in what follows.

Epidemiology of Malnutrition and of Obesity

The World Health Organization (WHO) recognizes that malnutrition may result from deficiencies, excesses, or imbalances in energy and/or nutrient intake [3]. Inadequate caloric intake is rare at present in the chronic pain population presenting for elective surgery. Specific macronutrient and micronutrient deficiencies are more common, and especially so among certain subgroups (e.g., the elderly, people with substance use disorders including alcoholism, etc.) but in the context of this book we focus epidemiologically on states of excessive intake with resultant obesity.

Both the National Institutes of Health (NIH) and WHO define overweight status as a BMI from 25 to 30 kg/m^2, and obesity as a BMI $\geq$30 kg/m^2. As highlighted in the previous chapter, there has been a nearly 20% increase in the prevalence of obesity in US adults from 33.7% in 2007–2008 to 39.6% in 2015–2016 [4], with that figure projected to eclipse 50% by the year 2030 [5].

Malnutrition and Pain

Malnutrition is increasingly recognized as a risk factor for chronic pain. Most of these mechanisms have to do with dietary contributions to a pro-inflammatory state, as discussed in what follows.

Obesity

One fairly obvious constellation of mechanisms whereby malnutrition (in the form of caloric excess) exerts pronociceptive effects is via the mediation of obesity. The prevalence of various chronic pain states (e.g., low back pain with or without radicular symptoms, appendicular pain, headaches, etc.) is significantly increased in the obese [6].

Table 8.1. Adequate/Recommended Dietary Intakes of Nutrients

Nutrient	Recommended Daily Intake (Adult Males/Females)	Nutrient	Recommended daily intake (Adult Males/Females)
Carbohydrates	45–65% EER/45–65% EER	Biotin	30 μg/30 μg
Fats, overall	20–35% EER/20–35% EER	Choline	550 mg/425 mg
Linoleic acid	5–10% EER/5–10% EER	Sodium	1.2–1.5 g/1.2–1.5 g
α-linoleic acid	0.6–1.2% EER/0.6–1.2% EER	Potassium	4.7 g/4.7 g
Protein	0.8 mg•kg^{-1}/0.8 mg•kg^{-1}	Chloride	1.8–2.3 g/1.8–2.3 g
Vitamin A	900 μg/700 μg	Calcium	1.0–1.2 g/1.0–1.2 g
Thiamine	1.2 mg/1.1 mg	Chromium	30–35 μg/20–25 μg
Riboflavin	1.3 mg/1.1 mg	Copper	900 μg/900 μg
Niacin	16 mg/14 mg	Fluoride	4 mg/3 mg
Vitamin B6	1.3–1.7 mg/1.3–1.5 mg	Iodine	150 μg/150 μg
Folate	400 μg/400 μg*	Iron	8 mg/8–18 mg**
Vitamin B12[†]	2.4 μg/2.4 μg	Magnesium	420 mg/320 mg
Vitamin C	90 mg/75 mg	Manganese	2.3 mg/1.8 mg
Vitamin D[‡]	15–20 μg/15–20 μg	Molybdenum	45 μg/45 μg
Vitamin E	15 mg/15 mg	Phosphorus	700 mg/700 mg
Vitamin K	120 mg/90 mg	Selenium	5 5μg/45 μg
Pantothenic acid	5 mg/5 mg	Zinc	11 mg/8 mg

EER = estimated energy requirement.

* while most nutrient recommendations are increased in pregnant and lactating women, folate in particular is markedly increased to 600 μg/day.

** 18 mg/day in premenopausal women.

[†] many individuals and especially chronic pain patients cannot adequately absorb Vit B12 enterally and will require sublingual or injectable supplementation.

[‡] 1 μg = 40 IU; many individuals and especially chronic pain patients are Vit D deficient and many authorities advise 1,000–5,000 IU/day.

Besides the long-held attribution of increased mechanical load on the muscu-loskeletal system, along with altered force vectors [7], recent evidence is revealing a host of other complex direct and downstream systemic pro-inflammatory effects of obesity. In the obese state adipocytes (and in particular visceral ones) increase secretion of a vast and surprising array of pro-inflammatory cytokines including tumor necrosis factor, interleukin-6, plasminogen activator inhibitor-1, and leptin [8]; conversely they decrease secretion of protective adipokines such as adiponectin, and in concert this altered milieu results in phenotypic switch of the immune system to a pro-inflammatory and thus pro-nociceptive state. Obesity (and associated poor diet) also alter the normal gut flora ("microbiome") in a reciprocal fashion [9, 10], and this alteration also confers a systemic inflam-matory state thought currently to be mediated predominantly by increased lip-opolysaccharide burden with resultant Toll-like receptor-4 (TLR-4) activation and cytokine cascade. A downward spiral of oxidative stress and further chronic inflammation ensues [11, 12]. Skeletal muscle also undergoes immune cell in-filtration and inflammatory myocyte changes [13]. Obesity is also strongly correlated with obstructive sleep apnea and other sleep disturbance states, which increase inflammation in their own right [14].

Pro-Inflammatory Diet

There is increasing evidence of a strong relationship between diet and a chronic inflammatory state, which is in turn increasingly recognized as a major contrib-utor to cardiovascular disease, the metabolic syndrome, many cancers, reac-tive airways disease, inflammatory bowel disease, and many other autoimmune states.

The most solid data come from lipid research, with considerable evidence linking excessive saturated FA and ω-6 PUFA with a systemically inflamed state. Both animal models and human cell culture lines have shown that exposure to saturated FA results in upregulated TLR-4 and nuclear factor κB (NFκB) ac-tivity with resultant inflammation [15]. Arachidonic acid is an ω-6 PUFA found in cell membranes and is the precursor to multiple inflammatory eicosanoids including various prostaglandins and leukotrienes. The ω-3 PUFAs can com-petitively substitute for ω-6 PUFAs within the lipid bilayer, and furthermore fa-cilitate the formation of resolvins, which are molecules that assist in terminating the inflammatory response. A 1:4 intake ratio for ω-3:ω-6 PUFAs has been recommended in terms of minimizing the pro-inflammatory burden of arachi-donic acid [15, 16], however the typical American diet currently reflects a ratio closer to 1:15–20. Multiple human studies have shown not only reduced inflam-matory biomarkers but also decreased inflammatory symptoms including pain with increased ω-3 PUFA consumption [15, 17, 18].

In terms of CHO, there is evidence that excess simple sugars or foods with high glycemic load (GI multiplied by the amount ingested) increase free radical and pro-inflammatory cytokine production [16]. Initial concerns regarding specifically disproportionate pathogenicity from fructose (which has seen exponential increase in Western food production over the past several decades, primarily in the form of high-fructose corn syrup) seem to have been unfounded, and the issue is more likely to simply be one of excessive sugars and calories [19]. The immunogenic and pro-inflammatory effects of excessive gluten (and other proteins within wheat and other grains, e.g., wheat germ agglutinin), once thought restricted to patients with celiac disease are now recognized as affecting a far larger segment of the population [20, 21]. Conversely, diets that are higher in whole grains have been demonstrated to result in reduced inflammatory marker and cytokine levels [22].

Malnutrition by inadequate micronutrient intake is increasingly recognized as pro-inflammatory as well, with deficiencies of several micronutrients (e.g., Vitamin D [23], magnesium [24], numerous trace elements [25]) apparently predisposing to a systemically inflamed state that is reversible with replenishment. Along those lines, many phytonutrients such as polyphenols and carotenoids have clearly demonstrated beneficial antioxidant and anti-inflammatory effects [15], and diets lacking in sufficient quantity and variety of vegetables and fruit may favor a pro-inflammatory state by omission or under-representation of these compounds.

Intestinal Microbiome Alteration and Leaky Gut Syndrome

This decade has seen increasing recognition of the vital role that commensal intestinal bacteria play in terms of maintaining not only gut health but also that of the entire human organism. These microbiota help maintain the integrity of the intestinal lumen, competitively inhibit pathogens, and interact positively with gut-associated lymphoid tissue and other immune system components. Observational studies have shown significant changes in the composition of the intestinal microbiome (IM) within obese individuals [26, 27] and prospective/interventional studies examining the effects of dietary change on the IM composition show significant consistent alterations [26–28].

One of many consequences of this population shift, and perhaps the one with the most far-reaching consequences is an increase in permeability of the intestinal wall from various mechanisms including protective mucus attrition and a weakening of luminal endothelial tight junctions [26, 29]. This increased permeability (referred to as "leaky gut syndrome") appears to facilitate diffusion of endotoxin (lipopolysaccharide) into the bloodstream, which may lead to varying

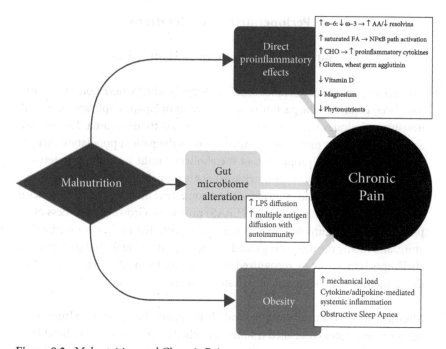

Figure 8.2. Malnutrition and Chronic Pain

ω-3/6 = Omega-3/6 fatty acids; AA = arachidonic acid; CHO = sugars; LPS = lipopolysaccharide;
NFkB = nuclear factor kB

degrees of toxemia ranging from subclinical inflammation to full-blown sepsis. This increased permeability also allows for diffusion of larger peptides (which may be antigenic) into the circulation, which may not only elicit an inflammatory response but also result in adaptive autoimmunity given cross-reactivity between these dietary (or bacterial) antigens and components of the body (Figure 8.2). Several autoimmune conditions including inflammatory bowel diseases, systemic lupus erythematosus, multiple sclerosis, and even Type I diabetes mellitus have been postulated as originating out of such disturbance [30].

Interactions with Physical Inactivity
Physical inactivity (PI) has been shown to be an independent risk factor for chronic pain, as discussed at length in the previous chapter, and malnutrition is frequently observed in concert with PI [31]. This may be due to inadequate energy reserves, overweight/obese status with resultant difficulties in mobility, or other psychosocial confounding variables.

Perioperative Considerations

Surgical Consequences of Malnutrition

Appreciation for the importance of adequate perioperative nutritional status may have been greater in the past prior to the advent of laparoscopic and minimally invasive techniques with correspondingly reduced tissue trauma. Nonetheless, as surgery becomes more commonplace, and as the patient population includes a continually greater proportion of metabolically unfit individuals, interest in preoperative optimization of nutritional status remains high, especially within the general surgical field, as evidenced by consistent inclusion of these issues in Enhanced Recovery After Surgery (ERAS) protocols. Growing awareness of the prevalence of malnutrition, however, is also manifested in the orthopedic literature, and finally the disturbing trend of obesity, with its manifold perioperative challenges is increasingly recognized as a major problem affecting every surgical discipline and anesthesia, and also postoperative care.

Malnutrition, Compromised Wound Healing, and Perioperative Infection

Surgery constitutes controlled trauma, and elicits a complex yet predictable sequence of defensive and restorative functions, beginning with at least a local acute inflammatory response. Under normal circumstances, within a matter of hours to days (see chapter 10, Figure 10.3 for a graphic representation of timeline) a proliferative phase ensues, with increased fibroblast and other reparative cell activity working to reestablish tissue structural and functional integrity. Together these stages (as well as a subsequent maturation phase) generally require considerable systemic catabolic activity in order to provide both energy and also raw materials for the inflammatory response and focused anabolism that follows.

Daily energy requirements for adequate wound healing often increase on the order of 20%–30% (with recommended intake of 30–35 kCal/kg/day) [32, 33]; protein requirements also escalate significantly (with recommended intake of 1.25–1.5 g/kg/day [33]). If these demands are not met by daily ingestion, the body's reserves are tapped, which may significantly prolong wound healing, or predispose to dehiscence/breakdown, and infection depending on preoperative health status. Certain AAs, namely arginine, cysteine, and methionine, are thought to be particularly important in the proliferative phase with high use related to collagen synthesis [32]; arginine and glutamine are also thought to play a significant role in immunocompetence [32, 34] as discussed further in what follows. Adequate vitamin C, iron, and zinc levels are also required for many anabolic processes including RNA transcription and translation, specifically collagen synthesis, and also immune response. Deficiencies in any of these micronutrients may lead to inadequate healing and chronic wound status.

Systemic Inflammation

As discussed at some length previously, malnutrition may result in a systemically inflamed state either by direct mediation of specific nutrients, or by alteration of the IM, or by the mediation of obesity. Regardless of the specific etiologies, this phenotypic alteration is ultimately coordinated and executed by cytokine activity under the control of the immune system (including central nervous system components, e.g., microglia) and related local tissue defense components. Such cytokine activity—and perturbation thereof—plays an important role not only in immunodefense/infection but also in wound healing and other organ function/dysfunction [35]. While it is still not broadly appreciated that such perturbation occurs much more commonly outside of the context of infection, it is increasingly recognized within the surgical literature that "recent systemic inflammatory condition may predispose to infection and adversely influence outcome" [36], with particular attention to this phenomenon within the colorectal surgical discipline, where inflammatory bowel disease has been implicated [37].

Perioperative Challenges of Obesity

No discussion of perioperative nutritional considerations would be complete without at least a brief treatment of the significant and growing issue of the anesthetic and surgical consequences of obesity. Obesity confers airway and respiratory (primarily oxygenation rather than ventilation) challenges owing to functional restrictive lung disease and decreased functional residual capacity often to levels below that of closing capacity. Increased circulatory system pathology, including systemic and pulmonary hypertension, contributes to perioperative morbidity and mortality. Technical challenges of intraoperative positioning and the surgical procedure itself abound. Postoperative issues of renal/fluid, electrolyte, and nutrition management often complicated by diabetes are increased. Surgical site infections and pressure ulcers are more prevalent in the obese [38]. From an orthopedic standpoint, increased postoperative hip prosthetic dislocations, and total knee arthroplasty implant failures and other complications are seen [39].

Due to the typical time constraints we work under, we (HM, LF) do not routinely address weight loss as part of our VALERAS preoperative optimization program. When more time is available, for example, when surgery has been postponed indefinitely until the patient's BMI is acceptable to the surgeon, we then work with the patient on a highly individualized basis addressing issues of not only nutrition but also, of course, physical activity and, frequently of equal importance, disordered sleep (given that sleep disturbance of any etiology can markedly dysregulate not only autonomic nervous system and cortisol activity but also leptin and ghrelin balance, leading to intractable weight gain). Along those lines, a high index of suspicion for obstructive sleep apnea, especially in the overweight and obese is always advised given the tremendous and increasing prevalence of this condition, and its potentially lethal consequences amplified by anesthetic and postoperative analgesic depression of respiratory drive and also airway musculature function.

Preoperative Nutritional Assessment

The importance of preoperative nutritional optimization is emphasized by recommendations in both the United States (The Joint Commission [41]) and the United Kingdom (National Institute for Health and Care Excellence [42]) for nutritional screening upon admission to care facilities.

Historically, clinical judgment based on morphometrics and other clinical indicators have directed laboratory evaluation of nutritional status focusing primarily on leukocyte count (e.g., < 1,500 cells/mm^3), transferrin levels (e.g., <200 mg/dL), albumin levels, and more recently prealbumin. Traditionally, a serum albumin level < 3.5 g/dL (and especially < 3.0) has been considered an indicator of malnutrition sufficient enough to confer worsened outcomes [43] and to warrant preoperative nutritional intervention; more recently, it has been noted that albumin levels are highly variable based on numerous other pathophysiologic states and its use as a sole biomarker has fallen out of favor [44]. Serum prealbumin has a much shorter half-life and thus theoretically more accurately reflects metabolic status; it has recently been examined as an alternate prognostic measure, with some studies showing correlation between levels <10–15 mg/dL with poor postoperative outcomes [45–47].

With increasing appreciation of the unreliability of single variable analysis, several nutritional assessment tools have been developed over the past few decades; the Subjective Global Assessment (SGA) is perhaps the most widely used instrument at present, however the arguably less cumbersome Nutritional Risk Screening (NRS-2002) [48] is the best-validated instrument at present [44] and is shown in Figure 8.3.

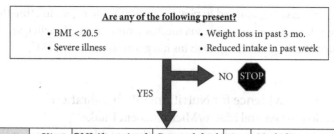

Score	> 5% wt. loss over	BMI, if associated with "impaired general condition"	Past week food intake as % of normal	Age	Morbidity status
1 for each of the following:	3 mo.		50%–75%	≥70	Mild: chronic conditions e.g., COPD, ESRD; hip fracture
2 for each of the following:	2 mo.	18.5–20.5	25%–50%		Moderate: major surgery, CVA or MI, major infection
3 for each of the following:	1 mo.	<18.5	0%–25%		Severe: APACHE score > 10 in ICU pts, severe head injury

If score ≥ 3, proceed with nutritional evaluation

Figure 8.3. Nutritional Risk Screening (NRS-2002)

Adapted from [48].

APACHE = Acute Physiologic Assessment and Chronic Health Evaluation; BMI = body mass index, kg/m^2; COPD = chronic obstructive pulmonary disease; CVA = cerebrovascular accident; ESRD = end-stage renal disease; ICU = intensive care unit.

Immunonutrition

The concept of providing supplemental nutrients specifically intended to enhance immune system performance has become increasingly popular; while various specific components have been evaluated, the most common and enduring ones are the AA arginine and ω-3 PUFAs.

Arginine is significantly involved in cell growth and proliferation, and is believed to play a crucial role in maintaining immune cell and particularly lymphocyte integrity and function [49]. In the absence of adequate dietary intake, arginine is sufficiently synthesized under normal conditions and thus is not considered an essential AA, however it is rapidly depleted under conditions of increased metabolic stress such as surgery [50] and is thus classified as a semi-essential or conditionally essential amino acid. A similarly important perioperative role for the AA glutamine has also been proposed, but is not backed by the same degree of evidence, and as such is not discussed here.

The ω-3 PUFAs are believed to play a significant role in modulating the postoperative inflammatory response via mechanisms described earlier, and in particular their role in generating resolvins has garnered attention [51].

Evidence for Nutritional Prehabilitation

Optimization of General Macro/Micronutrient Intake

Much of the literature examining preoperative nutritional support in the malnourished has to do with special populations such as oncologic surgical patients, or with specific interventions such as total parenteral nutrition (TPN; not relevant to the scope of this work) or with immunonutrition (IN; discussed separately in the next section.) Few investigations, let alone systematic reviews/meta-analyses, have reported on general nutritional optimization for the malnourished surgical population outside of the context of IN.

Zhong et al in 2015 [52] performed a systematic review and meta-analysis of randomized controlled trials (RCTs) evaluating outcomes benefits of various preoperative nutritional interventions in malnourished surgical patients (various specialties). Secondary analysis comparing specific IN (components not defined in this report) to "standard nutritional support" was carried out. In total, 15 trials (n = 3,831) were included; infectious complications (relative risk [RR] = 0.58; 95% Confidence Interval [95CI] = 0.50–0.68), noninfectious complications (RR = 0.74; 95CI = 0.63–0.88), and length of stay (LOS; -2.6 days; 95CI = -0.16 to -5.13 days) were all significantly reduced in the nutritional support group compared to the control group, and there was additional statistically significant benefit in terms of infectious complications seen in the IN group. No significant difference in mortality or costs was seen.

Brennan et al in 2018 [53] performed a meta-analysis of preoperative nutritional support in Crohn's disease patients undergoing abdominal surgery; this population is generally quite malnourished due to malabsorptive issues and other intestinal pathology. Two of five studies included in the analysis limited the preoperative intervention to enteral nutrition (with the other three comprising TPN) and among this group, postoperative complications occurred significantly less frequently (21.9%) in the nutritionally supported group compared to the control group (73.2%; odds ratio = 0.09, 95CI = 0.06–0.13).

Gillis et al in 2018 [54] performed a meta-analysis of preoperative nutritional support in patients undergoing elective colorectal surgery; six of the nine trials included comprised enteral nutritional support only, with three trials investigating a multimodal prehabilitation approach as discussed in chapter 7. Median duration of supplementation was generally between 2 and 4 weeks. Pooled data including all nine trials revealed statistically significant decrease in postoperative complications with nutritional support (+/- multimodal prehabilitation) with RR = 0.79; 95CI = 0.64–0.98. Length of stay was also significantly reduced.

Specific macronutrient augmentation comprising protein supplementation (1.2 g/kg/day of whey protein isolate) has been incorporated into the McGill University group's multimodal prehabilitation protocol as discussed in chapter 7; while their two prospective trials have demonstrated significant outcomes benefits, it is of course impossible to tease out the contribution of nutrition versus exercise.

Recently, the practice of immediate preoperative CHO loading has become popular especially in the field of general surgery, and has in fact entered many ERAS protocols [55]. This practice, commonly consisting of administration of a CHO-rich beverage containing 100 g the night before surgery, and 50 g two hours prior to surgery, appears to improve postoperative insulin sensitivity and with that, various subjective indicators of well-being. Of greater interest perhaps is an apparent reduction in LOS, with a Cochrane systematic review supporting this phenomenon [56]. At present, however, the application of these findings to the chronic pain population remains obscure.

Immunonutrition

Multiple systematic reviews and meta-analyses of IN were performed at the beginning of this decade, and key papers are summarized briefly here.

Marik et al in 2010 performed a meta-analysis of 21 trials ($n = 1,918$) of IN in patients with gastrointestinal cancers undergoing excision. Both arginine and fish oil products together significantly reduced the risk of infections and other wound complications, as well as LOS [57]. Benefits were not seen with either component in isolation.

Drover et al in 2011 [58] performed a meta-analysis of 35 trials (25 gastrointestinal and 10 other specialty trials) evaluating arginine supplementation. Overall analysis of 28 studies reporting infectious complications showed significant reduction in the arginine group compared to controls (RR = 0.59; 95CI = 0.50–0.70). A subgroup analysis comparing a specific commercial product (Impact; contains arginine, ω-3 PUFA, and nucleotides) to other heterogeneous formulae showed benefit only in the commercial product group.

Marimuthu et al in 2012 [59] performed a meta-analysis of 26 trials ($n = 2,496$) with a specific goal of determining the effect of combinations of two or more IN components compared to standard care in an open abdominal surgical population. Statistically significant reductions in both infectious and noninfectious complications and also in LOS were seen.

One systematic review and meta-analysis was performed by Hegazi et al in 2014 [60]; they repeated pooled analysis of many of the previously reviewed studies but limited the scope strictly to preoperative IN intervention (whereas the reviews discussed earlier included data from both preoperative and post-operative supplementation.) Eight RCTs ($n = 561$) comparing IN to standard enteral nutrition supplementation, and 9 RCTs ($n = 895$) of IN versus no supplementation were analyzed. No significant differences were seen in the former, however the latter analysis did show statistically significant reductions in infectious complications (odds ratio = 0.49; 95CI = 0.30–0.83) and LOS (mean difference—2.22 days; 95CI = -1.45 to -2.99) when comparing IN to no supplementation at all.

Cost-Benefit Evaluation

Walzer et al performed a systematic review of studies reporting economics outcomes for preoperative nutritional supplementation. Overall, 34 studies were reviewed and it was concluded that "medical nutrition interventions offer value for money in the different healthcare settings" [61]. When the focus was narrowed to enteral nutrition supplementation (and dietitian wages) for malnutrition, excluding studies based on cancer, pancreatitis, and other conditions, a span of comparative outcomes was seen ranging from cost savings to a fairly significant incremental cost-effectiveness ratio of €26,962/quality-adjusted life year.

Preoperative Nutritional Optimization: A Practical Plan

A Suggested Approach

Among other practical obstacles, human nature coupled with the uncontrolled availability of food sources in the West precludes any realistic attempt at rigorous construction of an ideal preoperative nutritional regimen. As such, we remain limited for the most part to extrapolation of preclinical data supplemented with intermittent discrete evidence-based approaches such as supplementation with arginine. From a public health standpoint, it is clear that the vast majority will benefit from improvements in food choices as discussed throughout this chapter, and application of those principles to the perioperative context is both reasonable and rational.

Basic principles of caloric intake optimization and macronutrient proportioning, and limitation of processed/convenience foods and simple sugars should be discussed with all patients. Detailed education regarding specific nutrients (e.g., saturated fats, phytonutrients, etc.) are typically overwhelming and not beneficial to most patients; tailoring such input according to patient interest is strategic. We focus on the following highlights with all patients:

- elimination of soda pop/soft drinks and other sweetened beverages (which contribute nearly half of all added sugars in US diets [2], beginning as early as possible in the process—ideally, 8–10 weeks preoperatively.

- minimization of fast foods/junk foods; significant alteration of purchasing patterns (discussed in greater detail in chapter 11) is the key.
- supplementation with a multivitamin, additional magnesium (avoiding carbonate, chloride, gluconate, and oxide anions due to increased risk of gastrointestinal upset), and ω-3 PUFA.
- supplementation with curcumin (1,000–2,000 mg/day) + piperine; discontinue 7 days preoperatively.
- for anticipated major surgery, supplementation with arginine 5–10 g/day beginning 7–14 days preoperatively (available very economically as a bulk powder).

As discussed briefly earlier, we do not routinely address specific issues of overweight/obesity status in our (HM, LF) VALERAS preoperative optimization program; however, when we do a comprehensive assessment and plan evaluating sleep disorders including but not limited to obstructive sleep apnea, nutritional and physical activity, and also psychosocial factors are used.

Motivational Enhancement

The barriers to nutritional improvement are in many ways even more complex than those opposing consistent and adequate physical activity given the ubiquitous function of reward that food represents. On the other hand, however, we find that reticence barriers and perceived inability/decreased self-efficacy seem to be less with instituting dietary change than with instituting exercise. As with all lifestyle modification efforts, enhancement of patients' motivation for change is of the essence, and toward that end, motivational interviewing (MI) [62] may be of great value. Overcoming ambivalence and progressing along stages of change from precontemplation to action may be best facilitated by hearing oneself vocalize rationale and intention. The reader is referred to Clifford and Curtis's monograph *Motivational Interviewing in Nutrition and Fitness* [63] for an excellent and thorough treatment of the subject, with multiple practical examples of the technique.

Habit and Dietary Change

While motivational enhancement may be beneficial in terms of initiating dietary change, sustaining it requires safeguarding against established deleterious habits in moments of weakened resolve or absent-mindedness. As is well-known essentially to every adult in Western society, "most lapses in diet adherence are precipitated by temptation from palatable food" [64]. The concepts of ego fatigue (failure of resolve when biopsychosocial resources are taxed) and delay discounting (choosing immediate gratification despite cognitive dissonance due to reduced salience of future consequences), discussed in chapters 3 and 4, are worth reviewing in this context. In general, a two-pronged approach involving both implementation of prevention tactics (e.g., restricting or eliminating availability of and access to junk food) and also bolstering resistance mechanisms (e.g., attaching a reinforcing photograph to the refrigerator, or a smartphone alarm system) when prevention is insufficient [64] is most effective.

Simple elimination of an undesirable habit is extraordinarily difficult, and replacement of action/behavior in the context of a stable cue is always preferable [65]. If possible, identification of reinforcing reward is beneficial [66] but not as critical as maintaining consistency of new routine(s) [65, 67].

Finally, enlisting both motivational and practical support from family and peers is invaluable. The difficulty in avoiding lapses to poor food choices (or cigarettes, or alcohol) is magnified tremendously when associates, roommates, family members, and others indulge in tempting and habitual behaviors. Conversely, encouragement as well as accountability from both supportive family and peer groups (and on a weekly basis with the preoperative care team) is invaluable. As discussed in chapter 4, while pairing of extrinsic rewards (whether physical comforts or validation and praise) runs the risk of hampering cultivation of intrinsic motivation and habit formation, we have found that encouragement and positive feedback more often help to bolster self-efficacy and self-determination.

References

1 Otten JJ, Hellwig JP, Meyers LD, eds. Institute of Medicine. Dietary Reference Intakes: The Essential Guide to Nutrient Requirements. Washington, DC: National Academies Press; 2006.

2 US Department of Health and Human Services and US Department of Agriculture. 2015–2020 Dietary Guidelines for Americans. 8th ed. December 2015. http://health.gov/dietaryguidelines/2015/guidelines/. Accessed November 27, 2018.

3 World Health Organization. The Double Burden of Malnutrition: Policy Brief. Geneva: World Health Organization; 2017.

4 Hales CM, Fryar CD, Carroll MD, Freedman DS, Ogden CL. Trends in obesity and severe obesity prevalence in US youth and adults by sex and age, 2007–2008 to 2015–2016. JAMA. 2018;319:1723–25.

5 Wang YC, McPherson K, Marsh T, Gortmaker SL, Brown M. Health and economic burden of the projected obesity trends in the USA and the UK. Lancet. 2011;378:815–25.

6 Narouze S, Souzdalnitski D. Obesity and chronic pain: systematic review of prevalence and implications for pain practice. Reg Anesth Pain Med. 2015;40:91–111.

7 Messier SP. Obesity and osteoarthritis: disease genesis and nonpharmacologic weight management. Rheum Dis Clin North Am. 2008;34:713–29.

8 Ouchi N, Parker JL, Lugus JJ, Walsh K. Adipokines in inflammation and metabolic disease. Nat Rev Immunol. 2011;11:85–97.

9   Tsukumo DM, Carvalho BM, Carvalho Filho MA, Saad MJ. Translational research into gut microbiota: new horizons on obesity treatment: updated 2014. Arch Endocrinol Metab. 2015;59:154–60.

10 Bleau C, Karelis AD, St-Pierre DH, Lamontagne L. Crosstalk between intestinal microbiota, adipose tissue and skeletal muscle as an early event in systemic low-grade inflammation and the development of obesity and diabetes. Diabetes Metab Res Rev. 2015;31:545–61.

11 Lugrin J, Rosenblatt-Velin N, Parapanov R, Liaudet L. The role of oxidative stress during inflammatory processes. Biol Chem. 2014;395:203–30.

12 Marseglia L, Manti S, D'Angelo G, et al. Oxidative stress in obesity: a critical component in human diseases. Int J Mol Sci. 2014;16:378–400.

13 Wu H, Ballantyne CM. Skeletal muscle inflammation and insulin resistance in obesity. J Clin Invest. 2017;127:43–54.

14 Irwin MR, Olmstead R, Carroll JE. Sleep disturbance, sleep duration, and inflammation: a systematic review and meta-analysis of cohort studies and experimental sleep deprivation. Biol Psychiatry. 2016;80:40–52.

15 Totsch SK, Waite ME, Sorge RE. Dietary influence on pain via the immune system. Prog Mol Biol Transl Sci. 2015;131:435–69.

16 Ricker MA, Haas WC. Anti-inflammatory diet in clinical practice: a review. Nutr Clin Pract. 2017;32:318–25.

17 Prego-Dominguez J, Hadrya F, Takkouche B. Polyunsaturated fatty acids and chronic pain: a systematic review and meta-analysis. Pain Physician. 2016;19:521–35.

18 Abdulrazaq M, Innes JK, Calder PC. Effect of ω-3 polyunsaturated fatty acids on arthritic pain: a systematic review. Nutrition. 2017;39–40:57–66.

19 Della Corte KW, Perrar I, Penczynski KJ, Schwingshackl L, Herder C, Buyken AE. Effect of dietary sugar intake on biomarkers of subclinical inflammation: a systematic review and meta-analysis of intervention studies. Nutrients. 2018;10(5). pii: E606. doi: 10.3390/nu10050606.

20 de Punder K, Pruimboom L. The dietary intake of wheat and other cereal grains and their role in inflammation. Nutrients. 2013;5:771–87.

21 Leonard MM, Sapone A, Catassi C, Fasano A. Celiac disease and nonceliac gluten sensitivity: a review. JAMA. 2017;318:647–56.

22 Lefevre M, Jonnalagadda S. Effect of whole grains on markers of subclinical inflammation. Nutr Rev. 2012;70:387–96.

23 Gonçalves de Carvalho CM, Ribeiro SM. Aging, low-grade systemic inflammation and vitamin D: a mini-review. Eur J Clin Nutr. 2017;71:434–40.

24 Nielsen FH. Effects of magnesium depletion on inflammation in chronic disease. Curr Opin Clin Nutr Metab Care. 2014;17:525–30.

25 Mocchegiani E, Costarelli L, Giacconi R, et al. Micronutrient-gene interactions related to inflammatory/immune response and antioxidant activity in ageing and inflammation. A systematic review. Mech Ageing Dev. 2014;136–37:29–49.

26 Cox AJ, West NP, Cripps AW. Obesity, inflammation, and the gut microbiota. Lancet Diabetes Endocrinol. 2015;3:207–15.

27 Weiss GA, Hennet T. Mechanisms and consequences of intestinal dysbiosis. Cell Mol Life Sci. 2017;74:2959–77.

28 Chassaing B, Vijay-Kumar M, Gewirtz AT. How diet can impact gut microbiota to promote or endanger health. Curr Opin Gastroenterol. 2017;33:417–21.

29 Chan YK, Estaki M, Gibson DL. Clinical consequences of diet-induced dysbiosis. Ann Nutr Metab. 2013;63 Suppl 2:28–40.

30 Mu Q, Kirby J, Reilly CM, Luo XM. Leaky gut as a danger signal for autoimmune diseases. Front Immunol. 2017;8:598. doi: 10.3389/fimmu.2017.00598.

31 Noble N, Paul C, Turon H, Oldmeadow C. Which modifiable health risk behaviours are related? A systematic review of the clustering of Smoking, Nutrition, Alcohol and Physical activity ("SNAP") health risk factors. Prev Med. 2015;81:16–41.

32 Wild T, Rahbarnia A, Kellner M, Sobotka L, Eberlein T. Basics in nutrition and wound healing. Nutrition. 2010;26:862–6.

33 National Pressure Ulcer Advisory Panel, European Pressure Ulcer Advisory Panel and Pan Pacific Pressure Injury Alliance. Prevention and Treatment of Pressure Ulcers: Quick Reference Guide. Perth, Australia: Cambridge Media; 2014.

34 Molnar JA, Vlad LG, Gumus T. Nutrition and chronic wounds: improving clinical outcomes. Plast Reconstr Surg. 2016;138(3 Suppl):71S–81S.

35 Hsing CH, Wang JJ. Clinical implication of perioperative inflammatory cytokine alteration. Acta Anaesthesiol Taiwan. 2015;53:23–8.

36 Lowry SF. The stressed host response to infection: the disruptive signals and rhythms of systemic inflammation. Surg Clin North Am. 2009;89:311–26.

37 De Magistris L, Paquette B, Orry D, et al. Preoperative inflammation increases the risk of infection after elective colorectal surgery: results from a prospective cohort. Int J Colorectal Dis. 2016;31:1611–17.

38 Leonard KL, Davies SW, Waibel BH. Perioperative management of obese patients. Surg Clin North Am. 2015;95:379–90.

39 Mihalko WM, Bergin PF, Kelly FB, Canale ST. Obesity, orthopaedics, and outcomes. J Am Acad Orthop Surg. 2014;22:683–90.

41 The Joint Commission. PC.02.01.03 EP 7. In Comprehensive Accreditation Manual for Hospitals: The Official Handbook. Oak Brook, IL: Joint Commission Resources; 2010.

42 National Institute for Health and Care Excellence. NICE Quality Standard [Q24] Nutrition Support in Adults. https://www.nice.org.uk/guidance/qs24/chapter/quality-statement-1-screening-for-the-risk-of-malnutrition. Accessed November 29, 2018.

43 Gibbs J, Cull W, Henderson W, Daley J, Hur K, Khuri SF. Preoperative serum albumin level as a predictor of operative mortality and morbidity: results from the National VA Surgical Risk Study. Arch Surg. 1999;134:36–42.

44 Torgersen Z, Balters M. Perioperative nutrition. Surg Clin North Am. 2015;95:255–67.

45 Tempel Z, Grandhi R, Maserati M, et al. Prealbumin as a serum biomarker of impaired perioperative nutritional status and risk for surgical site infection after spine surgery. J Neurol Surg A Cent Eur Neurosurg. 2015;76:139–43.

46 Yu PJ, Cassiere HA, Dellis SL, Manetta F, Kohn N, Hartman AR. Impact of preoperative prealbumin on outcomes after cardiac surgery. JPEN J Parenter Enteral Nutr. 2015;39:870–4.

47 Guan J, Holland CM, Schmidt MH, Dailey AT, Mahan MA, Bisson EF. Association of low perioperative prealbumin level and surgical complications in long-segment spinal fusion patients: a retrospective cohort study. Int J Surg. 2017;39:135–40.

48 Kondrup J, Rasmussen HH, Hamberg O, Stanga Z; Ad Hoc ESPEN Working Group. Nutritional risk screening (NRS 2002): a new method based on an analysis of controlled clinical trials. Clin Nutr. 2003;22:321–36.

49 Bansal V, Ochoa JB. Arginine availability, arginase, and the immune response. Curr Opin Clin Nutr Metab Care. 2003;6:223–8.

50 Zhu X, Herrera G, Ochoa JB. Immunosuppression and infection after major surgery: a nutritional deficiency. Crit Care Clin. 2010;26:491–500.

51 Evans DC, Martindale RG, Kiraly LN, Jones CM. Nutrition optimization prior to surgery. Nutr Clin Pract. 2014;29:10–21.

52 Zhong JX, Kang K, Shu XL. Effect of nutritional support on clinical outcomes in perioperative malnourished patients: a meta-analysis. Asia Pac J Clin Nutr. 2015;24:367–78.

53 Brennan GT, Ha I, Hogan C, et al. Does preoperative enteral or parenteral nutrition reduce postoperative complications in Crohn's disease patients: a meta-analysis. Eur J Gastroenterol Hepatol. 2018;30:997–1002.

54 Gillis C, Buhler K, Bresee L, et al. Effects of nutritional prehabilitation, with and without exercise, on outcomes of patients who undergo colorectal surgery: a systematic review and meta-analysis. Gastroenterology. 2018;155:391–410.

55 Ljungqvist O. Preoperative fasting and carbohydrate treatment. In Feldman LS, Delaney CP, Ljungqvist O, Carli F, eds., The SAGES/ERAS Society Manual of Enhanced Recovery Programs for Gastrointestinal Surgery (pp. 41–49). Cham, Switzerland: Springer; 2015.

56 Smith MD, McCall J, Plank L, Herbison GP, Soop M, Nygren J. Preoperative carbohydrate treatment for enhancing recovery after elective surgery. Cochrane Database Syst Rev. 2014;(8):CD009161. doi: 10.1002/14651858.CD009161.pub2.

57 Marik PE, Zaloga GP. Immunonutrition in high-risk surgical patients: systematic review and analysis of the literature. JPEN J Parenter Enteral Nutr. 2010;34:378–86.

58 Drover JW, Dhaliwal R, Weitzel L, Wischmeyer PE, Ochoa JB, Heyland DK. Perioperative use of arginine-supplemented diets: a systematic review of the evidence. J Am Coll Surg. 2011;212:385–99.

59 Marimuthu K, Varadhan KK, Ljungqvist O, Lobo DN. A meta-analysis of the effect of combinations of immune modulating nutrients on outcome in patients undergoing major open gastrointestinal surgery. Ann Surg. 2012;255:1060–8.

60 Hegazi RA, Hustead DS, Evans DC. Preoperative standard oral nutrition supplements vs immunonutrition: results of a systematic review and meta-analysis. J Am Coll Surg. 2014;219:1078–87.

61 Walzer S, Droeschel D, Nuijten M, Chevrou-Séverac H. Health economics evidence for medical nutrition: are these interventions value for money in integrated care? Clinicoecon Outcomes Res. 2014;6:241–52.

62 Miller WR, Rollnick S. Motivational Interviewing: Helping People Change. 3rd ed. New York: Guilford Press; 2013.

63 Clifford D, Curtis L. Motivational Interviewing in Nutrition and Fitness. New York: Guilford Press; 2016.

64 Appelhans BM, French SA, Pagoto SL, Sherwood NE. Managing temptation in obesity treatment: a neurobehavioral model of intervention strategies. Appetite. 2016;96:268–79.

65 Lally P, Wardle J, Gardner B. Experiences of habit formation: a qualitative study. Psychol Health Med. 2011;16:484–9.

66 Duhigg C. The Power of Habit: Why We Do What We Do in Life and Business. New York: Random House; 2014.

67 Lally P, Gardner B. Promoting habit formation. Health Psychol Rev. 2013;7(Suppl 1): S137–58.

9

Preoperative Management of Tobacco

Heath B. McAnally

Introduction

Despite significant reductions in prevalence in the United States over the past half-century, smoking (and the use of other tobacco products) continues to constitute the most common chemical dependency (aside from caffeine, perhaps) and the leading preventable cause of morbidity and mortality in the developed world.

It is well documented that the use of tobacco products increases overall health risks and, in the context of this work, perioperative complications. Less well recognized but also supported by the literature is an independent association with chronic pain in general after adjusting for common comorbid health risks, and also with worsened postoperative pain control. Conversely, there is evidence that preoperative tobacco cessation results in substantial improvements in outcomes.

In this chapter we briefly review basic and clinical science underpinning these phenomena, the descriptive epidemiology and available outcomes data pertinent to the issue, and what the current literature has to say about preoperative tobacco cessation and support, both biologic/pharmacologic and behavioral. As with previous chapters addressing some of these related but distinct modifiable risk factors, recognizing the complex issues surrounding tobacco use, we highlight the importance of both motivational enhancement and habit alteration.

General Concepts Related to Tobacco Use

Nicotine (and Other Tobacco Component) Biology

Nicotine, a parasympathomimetic, is an alkaloid found in tobacco and its chief active compound. Its effects are complex, with direct stimulation of nicotinic acetylcholine receptors in the brain including the mesolimbic system and also secondary release of other neurotransmitters (e.g., dopamine, beta-endorphin) likely responsible for its relaxing and rewarding properties [1]. Conversely, it also acts as an indirect sympathetic stimulant, eliciting adrenal release of norepinephrine and epinephrine and also cortisol. Users report a paradoxical relaxant/calming effect with concomitant alertness/mental clarity and arousal.

Cigarette smoke, however, contains far more than nicotine, and among the often-cited 2,000–4,000 chemical compounds contained therein, over 70 of them are carcinogenic [2], with many more exerting other harmful effects. Pertinent to the perioperative setting is carbon monoxide (CO), which competitively binds hemoglobin at its oxygen binding sites with a 200-fold greater affinity, forming carboxyhemoglobin (COHb), which in essence cannot bind and deliver oxygen, resulting in tissue hypoxia. Typical human COHb levels in industrialized nations is less than 3%, while greater than half of smokers show levels in excess of 6% with some as high as 18% [3].

Tobacco: Epidemiology

An estimated 15% of Americans currently smoke cigarettes [4], with another 5% using other forms of tobacco. Paralleling that prevalence and bearing witness to its extreme health risks, one in five American deaths (nearly 500,000 annually) are attributed to tobacco use [5]—a figure greater than that attributed to motor vehicle accidents, alcohol and other substance abuse, suicides, and HIV combined [6].

The prevalence of smoking among surgical patients is double that of the general populace, at 30% [7, 8] and the prevalence of smoking among chronic pain patients has been reported generally as being somewhere between two and three times that of the national rate [9].

Tobacco: An Addictionology Perspective

While there exists the occasional if not rare part-time smoker who is able to "quit whenever they like," universal anecdotal evidence as well as the literature attest to the overwhelming addictive potential of tobacco. It is widely accepted that nicotine constitutes the primary component within tobacco, with considerable reinforcing properties including both positive/hedonic reward, and also negative/withdrawal consequences once dependent. Withdrawal typically begins within several hours and peaks usually within 1 to 3 days; it may last for weeks to months. Both physical and psychological distress, ranging from mild irritability to severe anxiety, often render absence intolerable.

As with most drugs of abuse, from a neurobiologic standpoint there seems to be enhanced activity within the mesolimbic dopaminergic system leading to a positive reinforcement scenario also mediated in part via glutamanergic, GABAergic, opioid peptide, and serotonergic systems [10]. Withdrawal phenomena involve perturbations in the new/adjusted "allostatic setpoints" of these neurotransmitters, and also seem to involve the stress-cortisol system and the dynorphin-kappa opioid system; also as with opioids, the habenula seems to be one of if not the primary regions of the brain involved [11].

Tobacco and Pain

The literature increasingly supports a contributory if not causal role for tobacco in much chronic pain. After adjusting for common comorbid risk factors, smoking (and other forms of tobacco use) has been associated with increased incidence, prevalence, chronicity, and severity of pain in numerous populations and disease states [12–15].

Tobacco and Pain: Disease-Specific Evidence
Low Back Pain
Numerous studies have confirmed strong association between smoking and chronic low back pain; Shiri et al [13] reviewed 40 cross-sectional and cohort studies and found an odds ratio (OR) of 1.79 (95% Confidence Interval [95CI] 1.27–2.50). Frequently cited mechanisms for this include increased breakdown of the annulus fibrosis with increased discogenic pain and herniation [16, 17], and increased inflammatory activity leading to spondyloarthritis [18]; among post-spine surgical patients who smoke, there is also increased fusion failure rate, as discussed later.

Arthritis
Both osteoarthritis and rheumatoid arthritis have been linked to cigarette smoking as well [19, 20]. The data for osteoarthritis are mixed, with associations ranging from negative to positive; it is possible that decreased obesity rates in smokers may be protective. On the other hand, smoking increases matrix metalloproteinase activity [21] which is a well-characterized contributor to the disease state.

Sugiyama et al [20] performed a meta-analysis of studies investigating smoking as a risk factor for rheumatoid arthritis; overall odds ratios ranged from 1.76 to 1.89 depending on former versus current smoking status, and among seropositive patients, the risk was even more pronounced (OR 2.46–3.91 depending on former versus current smoking status).

Fibromyalgia
The prevalence of smoking is higher in patients with fibromyalgia compared to a control population [22]. Symptom severity also correlates with tobacco use [23, 24]. Given that the pathophysiology of fibromyalgia has yet to be clearly determined, it is difficult to draw any firm conclusions as to the pathologic link between smoking and fibromyalgia. However, as discussed elsewhere in this section, smoking results in a systemic inflammatory state, and furthermore smoking is associated with disordered sleep architecture [25], a well-known risk factor for the development of fibromyalgia.

Ischemic/Neuropathic Pain Syndromes
Given the well-established pathophysiologic link between smoking and vascular pathology, and also hypoxia, it is not surprising that ischemic and also neuropathic pain syndromes occur with greater prevalence and severity in smokers. Peripheral vascular disease as well as more acutely life-threatening coronary and mesenteric ischemic syndromes are all increased in smokers; the association between smoking and these painful states is so axiomatic as to be banal.

Among patients with diabetes, smoking is an independent risk factor for the development of diabetic peripheral neuropathy [26]—certainly the most common of the systemic neuropathic pain syndromes seen in the United States. Smoking has also been shown to be a significant risk factor for the development of postherpetic neuralgia [27] and lumbar radicular syndromes, namely, sciatica [28].

Tobacco and Pain Pathophysiology: Biologic Considerations
Pain is a subjective experience varying widely between and even within individuals in relation to a consistent noxious stimulus; this variability and the ethical and moral limitations on human experimental data confer some difficulty in unequivocally explaining mechanisms behind the association between tobacco use and chronic pain. From a general systemic pathologic standpoint, vasoconstrictive and hypoxic effects are easily invoked in the case of ischemic and neuropathic pain states.

More common nociceptive pain states (e.g., chronic low back pain, osteoarthritis) are also much more common in smokers, and this phenomenon has been attributed to numerous factors as shown in Figure 9.1, including bone and connective tissue breakdown; increased inflammatory chemokines, cytokines, and other mediators such as leukotrienes; withdrawal and induced hyperalgesia (akin to opioid-induced hyperalgesia); and altered pain processing [29–31].

Tobacco and Pain Pathophysiology: Psychosocial Considerations
A bidirectional or reciprocal association between tobacco use and affective disorders such as anxiety and depression has been well documented [32]. These

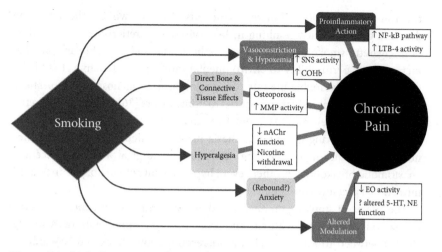

Figure 9.1. Links Between Smoking and Chronic Pain
5-HT = serotonin; COHb = carboxyhemoglobin; EO = endogenous opioid; LTB-4 = leukotriene B4; MMP = matrix metalloproteinase; NE = norepinephrine; SNS = sympathetic nervous system.

conditions of course have also been well characterized as independent risk factors for, and also sequela of chronic pain. Specific pain-related anxiety correlates with cigarette dependence even after controlling for both general anxiety trait and reported pain severity [33], demonstrating the complexity and interconnectivity of these factors. Similarly, the expectancy of efficacy of tobacco in perceived reduction of both affective dysregulation states and even pain itself is a significant driver of continued use [34].

In addition, nicotine withdrawal, which often begins within a matter of hours and may persist for many weeks is associated with depression, anxiety, insomnia, and irritability.

Social factors such as education and socioeconomic status, social and family support systems, and access to healthcare all play a role as well in both tobacco use and in chronic pain as well as coping mechanisms including smoking [35].

Rationale and Evidence for Preoperative Tobacco Cessation

Perioperative Risks/Complications

Airway and Respiratory Complications
The anesthesiology literature is replete with warnings about increased airway irritability and bronchoconstriction as a result of smoking. Smoking decreases

tracheal ciliary motility and increases mucous secretions while at the same time decreasing its elasticity, resulting in hyperviscous secretion buildup. In addition, cigarette smoke disrupts protective bronchial and bronchiolar epithelia, increasing its permeability to environmental (and smoke) irritants. The literature shows nearly double the rate of laryngospasm, bronchospasm, aspiration, and reintubation in smokers compared to nonsmokers [36], and any anesthetist with more than a few months of practice can attest to the difficulties in smooth extubations following general anesthesia in these patients. The frequent phenomenon of "bucking on the tube" may result in surgical wound dehiscence/anastomotic breakdown or other severe hyperdynamic circulatory or increased intracranial pressure consequences.

The effects of smoking on airway and alveolar function in general are otherwise well established, with chronic bronchitis and emphysema rates widely cited at between 10% and 15%, but more recently shown to exceed 30% among smokers with at least 25 years' smoking history [37]. Resultant disruptions in both pulmonary mechanics, gas exchange, and ventilation-perfusion matching during general anesthesia compound both intraoperative and postoperative risks. These concerns are accentuated during operations involving increased abdominal pressures (e.g., laparoscopic operations) or those with additional restrictive effects (e.g., Trendelenburg positioning).

Also observed within the perioperative setting (as well as without), the risk of respiratory superinfections is increased [36]. Besides increased viscous secretion burden/decreased clearance, which may provide a hospitable milieu for respiratory pathogens, alveolar macrophage and other immune cell function is dramatically reduced [38].

Cardiovascular and Cerebrovascular Complications

Tobacco users consistently display elevations in vascular resistance, heart rate, and blood pressure owing to nicotinic stimulation of catecholaminergic release. Over the long term, chronic use results in elevated "set points" for these parameters by carotid body and aortic autoregulation [39].

Intraoperative hyperdynamic circulation may result from airway irritability as discussed previously, and in addition, the greater baseline cardiac workload coupled with decreased oxygen transport, and greater atherosclerotic plaque burden all combine to dramatically increase supply-demand mismatch. The highly powered study by Turan et al (discussed in greater detail later) showed significantly greater odds of both perioperative myocardial infarction and cardiac arrest in smokers compared to nonsmokers; cerebrovascular accident risk was also markedly increased [40].

Hematologic Complications

Smoking results in polycythemia, increased platelet reactivity, stimulation of the coagulation cascade, and impairment of fibrinolysis [41]. Smoking also confers significant vascular endothelial disruption and dysfunction. When compounded by the general procoagulant effect of surgery [42], the result is frequently increased thrombosis, both arterial and venous. While currently supported by scant literature, a recent very large ($n > 1 \times 10^6$) study [43] showed increased risk of postoperative deep venous thrombosis (DVT) in smokers.

Given the already disproportionate rate of that potentially fatal (in the context of pulmonary embolus) complication in orthopedics, which discipline also serves a disproportionate number of chronic pain patients, as noted previously, increased awareness and concern on the part of the perioperative care team is warranted, especially in view of the fact that perioperative hypercoagulability may last up to 3 months.

Wound Infections and Dehiscence

Postoperative infections and wound breakdown occur much more frequently in smokers [40, 44], likely owing to a combination of mechanisms including impaired perfusion as discussed earlier, and immune system dysregulation.

Both innate immune system components (e.g., macrophages and natural killer cells) and also adaptive system cell lines (e.g., T-cells and B-cells) are affected by smoking; interestingly while there appears to be upregulation in the context of autoimmune states, immunosuppression occurs in the context of microbial infections, and the reasons for this paradoxical response remain unclear [45].

Arthroplasty and Spinal Fusion Failure

Smoking confers catabolic effects via increased cortisol activity, inhibition and even apoptosis of osteoblasts, calcitonin inhibition, and in females, decreased estrogen activity. Together, these activities result in imbalance of bone resorption at the expense of formation, leading to osteopenia and osteoporosis.

The arthroplasty literature contains multiple reports both retrospective and prospective showing that tobacco use is associated with significantly increased risk of prosthetic complications including deep infection, aseptic implant loosening, and overall necessity for revision [46]. Periprosthetic infection, a major cause of implant failure in its own right, is always a significant concern in these operations given the ability of bacteria to adhere to the nonperfused/indefensible hardware, and as discussed previously, smoking compromises the immune response.

In a recent meta-analysis of six cohort studies ($n = 8,181$) evaluating hip arthroplasty complications as a function of smoking, Teng et al [47] found that the risk of all-cause revisions was markedly and significantly increased in smokers (risk ratio [RR] = 2.58; 95CI: 1.27–5.22); the risks of both infectious and aseptic failures were comparable (RR = 3.71; 95CI: 1.86–7.41, and RR = 3.05, 95% CI: 1.42–6.58, respectively.)

Complications, however, are not limited to arthroplasty; a recent systematic review of anterior cruciate ligament repair operations showed significantly worsened anterior translation and subjective outcome indices in smokers, undoubtedly owing to suboptimal healing of the graft or bone plugs [48].

Similarly, increased rates of spinal fusion pseudo-arthrosis have been noted for over 20 years [49], and this has been attributed to diminished revascularization of cancellous bone graft [50]. A recent meta-analysis of investigations examining the effect of smoking on lumbar fusions (40 studies, n = 7,516) showed a twofold rate of either nonunion or delayed union (RR = 2.2; 95CI: 1.9–2.6) [51]. Of even greater concern (given the presence of the spinal cord) are similar data showing increased cervical fusion failure rates in smokers [52].

Outcomes Data

Postoperative Morbidity and Mortality

Over 300 studies over the past 70 years have been performed investigating the association between cigarette smoking and surgical outcomes [53]; there is overwhelming concordance in terms of evidence linking current or recent smoking to increased postoperative morbidity and mortality [40, 54, 55]; see Table 9.1.

The Danish Health and Medicines Authority and the National Institute of Public Health recently provided a large meta-analysis [54] based on international data comprising 107 studies (n > 530,000). Positive smoking history was associated with a statistically significantly increased risk of overall postoperative morbidity (RR = 1.52; 95CI: 1.33–1.74); however, in this analysis increases in cardiovascular complications and also mortality (RR = 1.13; 95CI: 0.98–1.31) did not meet criteria for statistical significance. The authors admit that the quality of the data overall are fairly low, with "diverse and ambiguous definitions of smoking status . . . only 27 of the included studies indicated how long time before the surgery the patients should have ceased smoking to be categorized as ex- or nonsmokers." In addition, they note that most of the studies were very small and did not include adjustment for confounding variables.

Hawn et al [55] performed a retrospective analysis of nearly 400,000 patients using the Veterans Affairs Surgical Quality Improvement Program database. A little more than one-third of this population (34.5%) were current smokers, with another 18% former smokers. Analyses were stratified by current versus former smokers compared to never-smoking controls, and in all morbidity and

Table 9.1. Adverse Postoperative Outcomes Associated with Smoking

Outcome	Odds Ratio Associated with Smoking (95% Confidence Interval)
Unplanned Tracheal Intubation	1.57 (1.10–2.25)
Pneumonia	1.80 (1.11–2.92)
Myocardial Infarction	2.09 (1.80–2.43)
Cardiac Arrest	1.87 (1.58–2.21)
Cerebrovascular Accident	1.53 (1.31–1.79)
Surgical Site Infection	1.05 (0.78–1.42)
Sepsis	1.38 (1.11–1.72)
Any major morbidity	1.55 (1.29–1.87)
30-day mortality	1.30 (1.15–1.46)

Data from the National Surgical Quality Improvement Program Database, 2005–2008 [40].

mortality outcomes (with the exceptions of DVT and urinary tract infections) current smokers statistically significant increases in risk, with 29% increased risk of death within 30 days of the operation (95CI: 20%–39%) and 55% increased risk within one year (95CI: 50%–61%). In most complications, and in all mortality analyses, former smokers exhibited statistically significantly increased risk compared to never-smoking controls, but decreased risk compared to current smokers.

Turan et al [40] performed a large (n = 635,265) retrospective analysis of patient outcomes by smoking status using the American College of Surgeons National Surgical Quality Improvement Program Database from 2005–2008; 26.5% of this cohort were current smokers (defined as smoking within 1 year of the operative admission). Over 80,000 currently smoking noncardiac surgical patients were matched to never-smokers based on multiple factors including age, gender, alcohol use, American Society of Anesthesiologists Physical Status Classification, and many specific disease conditions (e.g., diabetes, renal failure, heart failure.) They were also matched by procedure and whether the operation was emergent.

Smoking increased the risks of myocardial infarction by 80% (95CI: 11%–292%); stroke by 73% (95CI: 18%–253%); pneumonia by 209% (95CI: 80%–243%) and septic shock by 55% (95CI: 29%–87%). Overall mortality was increased by 38% (95CI: 11%–72%).

Economic Outcomes

While the contribution of smoking to postoperative complications is incontrovertible, few studies have examined disposition and economic outcomes specifically. The Danish meta-analysis discussed earlier [54] did no analyses of length of stay nor costs, but did find that smoking was associated with increased incidence of admission to an intensive care unit (RR = 1.60; 95CI: 1.14–2.25). The VA study [55] showed statistically significant increase in hospital length of stay by a mean of 0.4 days for current smokers compared to nonsmokers.

Nearly 15 years ago at the time of this writing, it was estimated that pulmonary complications, the majority of which were associated with positive smoking status, increased perioperative incident costs by over $50,000 [56].

Evidence Supporting Preoperative Tobacco Cessation

There is ample evidence in the literature to support the efficacy of preoperative smoking cessation efforts on both successful abstinence and cessation, and also in achieving improved postoperative outcomes. When compared to general population cessation rates (<10% success rate among those attempting to quit in any given year; [57]) it appears that the perioperative period is associated with increased patient readiness to change, and numerous recommendations for capitalizing on this "teachable moment" have been made.

Effect on Cessation

Zaki et al [58] performed a systematic review of four randomized controlled trials (RCTs; $n = 610$) investigating the effects of various cessation methods applied between 1 and 14 weeks preoperatively; follow-up ranged from 3 weeks to 12 months. All four trials included both behavioral counseling and pharmacotherapy comprising either nicotine replacement therapy [NRT] or bupropion. At the 3- to 6-month mark, 24.2% of patients in the pooled intervention groups had successfully discontinued smoking, compared to 17.4% in the nonintervention group (again, perhaps highlighting the increased readiness to change conferred by the perioperative period). The pooled odds ratio for intervention was 1.58 with 95CI: 1.02–2.45. However, at the 12-month mark, analyzed by only one of the trials, no difference was seen.

Cropley et al [7] also performed a systematic review of RCTs (nine studies; $n = 1,507$) and found a mean quit rate of 55% among patients receiving a smoking intervention (behavioral counseling, pharmacotherapy, or combined approach) compared to 26.5% in controls.

Thomsen et al, in a Cochrane review [59] investigated thirteen RCTs (total n = 2,010) examining the efficacy of various smoking cessation support interventions on both quit rates and postoperative complications. One trial evaluated nicotine replacement therapy (NRT), one evaluated varenicline, and 10 evaluated behavioral interventions. Among the latter, eight also offered NRT in combination.

The pure NRT trial [60] relied only on nicotine lozenges offered the night before surgery (in concert with a two-minute brief counseling provided at the preoperative visit) and not surprisingly did not show any benefit in terms of either cessation rates nor in outcomes.

The varenicline trial [61] provided the drug 1 week prior to the operation, continuing for 12 weeks postoperatively, and also provided one 15-minute counseling session at the preoperative visit and another at the postoperative visit. Participants were instructed to quit smoking 24 hours before the operation. This study did not show statistically significant cessation at the time of surgery, nor as would be expected any difference in complications. However, at 12-month follow-up, abstinence rates were statistically higher in the varenicline group, with 36.4% abstinence versus 25.2% in the placebo control group (RR = 1.45; 95CI: 1.01–2.07).

Among the behavioral intervention trials, two were deemed "intensive" and offered four to eight weekly counseling sessions, either in person or by telephone. These investigations also offered NRT, and one offered the services of a QuitLine. Pooled analysis of these two studies (n = 210) revealed impressive success in cessation at the time of surgery, with a nearly 11-fold increase in quit rate (95CI: 4.55–25.46) compared to an assumed quit rate in the control group; complication rates were also significantly lower (RR 0.42; 95CI: 0.27–0.65) in the intervention group. Within this group, abstinence rates remained significantly increased (2.96; 95CI: 1.57–5.55) at the 12-month mark.

The behavioral trials deemed nonintensive (generally comprising one or two counseling sessions) showed very modest benefit in terms of cessation rate at the time of surgery, with no sustained abstinence improvements at 12 months; there were also no decreases seen in postoperative complication rates.

Effect on Outcomes

As discussed above, the Cochrane review [59] showed that postoperative complication rates were significantly attenuated in patients who participated in intensive preoperative counseling (coupled with pharmacotherapy.)

A large systematic review and meta-analysis (140 studies; n = 479,150) of the impact of smoking cessation on postoperative outcomes showed significant benefit in terms of postoperative healing and decreased wound infection rates [62]. Patients were stratified according to never-smoker status, former smokers (roughly half of the studies defined this as having quit within 1 year prior to the operation with a median of 4 weeks; the other half did not define duration of cessation), and current smokers. Those who discontinued tobacco use preoperatively had increased risks of healing complications compared to never-smokers, but significantly improved outcomes compared to current smokers (OR = 0.69; 95CI: 0.56–0.85).

Mills et al [63] performed another systematic review and meta-analysis of the effects of preoperative smoking cessation on postoperative outcomes; 21 studies including 6 RCTs were included (raw data not available in the report). The RCTs investigated heterogeneous interventions including strict pharmacotherapy, behavioral counseling, and combination therapy; preoperative duration of intervention ranged from 1 day to 8 weeks. Pooled data revealed overall relative risk reduction of 41% (95CI: 15–59%) for successful quitters, and also of interest, the authors report that each week of cessation increased the magnitude of effect by 19%, with a significant breakpoint at the 4-week mark.

Similarly, Wong et al [64] in another systematic review and meta-analysis (25 studies; n = 21,381) showed that preoperative cessation of at least 4 weeks was necessary to achieve significant reductions in postoperative respiratory complications (RR = 0.77; 95CI: 0.61–0.96) and at least 3 weeks' abstinence was required to achieve significant reduction in postoperative infectious complications (RR = 0.69; 95CI: 0.56–0.84).

Optimal Duration of Preoperative Cessation

Historic literature and preoperative practice guidelines advocated against cessation any later than roughly 1 month preoperatively due to concerns for increased airway irritability from short-term mucolysis and return of ciliary function. More recent recommendations note that this practice may not be in the patient's best interest [65, 66], noting that improved outcomes may be seen with even as little as 1 day of preoperative abstinence. Such short-term benefit is thought to be a function of improved oxygen delivery with reduced carboxyhemoglobin concentration, as it requires several weeks of abstinence to see improvements in wound healing and pulmonary and cardiovascular functional improvements, and several months to see restoration of immunocompetence [66].

As noted previously [59, 63, 64] and elsewhere [67] the breakpoint for evidence of benefit seems to lie at least 4 if not 8 weeks prior to surgery. While further investigations have the potential to refine the data, from a pragmatic standpoint it seems clear that at least 4 weeks of cessation in the context of elective surgery should be mandatory, and the longer the better.

Perioperative Tobacco Cessation
Support Considerations

Despite the overwhelming evidence of benefit to the patient from successful abstinence, only roughly 40% of surgeons and 70% of anesthesiologists routinely
advise preoperative tobacco cessation [68]. While there are likely numerous
reasons for this oversight, unfamiliarity with outcome and efficacy data as
presented previously, and also unfamiliarity with support options undoubtedly
play a role. As such, our recommendations for preoperative optimization of this
highly significant problem are presented in what follows.

Pharmacotherapy

Nicotine Replacement Therapy (NRT)

Approximately 1–2 mg of nicotine are absorbed from a cigarette, and daily intake
for smokers averages around 38 mg [69]. FDA-approved nicotine replacement
vehicles include transdermal patches with multiple dose strengths available
ranging from 7 mg to 21 mg; gum (2 mg, 4 mg); lozenges (2 mg, 4 mg); nasal
spray (0.5 mg per spray) and inhalers (4 mg per cartridge).

While the benefits of reducing airway and pulmonary complications from
smoking (not to mention elimination of the thousands of other toxic chemicals
in cigarettes) are incontrovertible, the preoperative use of NRT remains contro-
versial (especially in the fields of orthopedic and plastic surgery) due to concerns
for harmful vasoconstrictive and other pharmacodynamic effects on bone and
wound healing, implant incorporation and arthrosis, and so forth. This is unfor-
tunate given that the efficacy of NRT (in concert with behavioral interventions)
in achieving short-term smoking cessation approaches 60% [7, 70, 71] and there
is a well-documented history of safety of NRT in the general populace [71, 72].
Solid preclinical and clinical evidence exists showing potential improvement in
wound and bone healing with NRT at best, and at worst, markedly reduced risk
when compared to cigarettes [73]; such harm reduction strategy surely deserves
consideration given the scope of the problem.

Varenicline

Varenicline, a new partial nicotinic receptor agonist has recently become available for use in tobacco cessation support; it appears to be at least equally efficacious compared to NRT, and more effective then bupropion [71]. To date,
however, only one study showing perioperative benefit from the institution of
varenicline exists, as reviewed earlier [61].

Given the potential for significant adverse psychiatric effects, patients should
be extensively counseled prior to a trial, and if the practitioner is unfamiliar/

uncomfortable with the use of this agent, referral back to the patient's primary care provider, or behavioral health provider (if applicable) in consideration of varenicline institution is never unwarranted.

Bupropion

Equally sparse data showing perioperative benefit from the addition of bupropion exist [74]; while theoretically beneficial from numerous standpoints (e.g., tobacco abstinence support, antidepressant benefit, neuropathic pain improvement) and backed by evidence of efficacy in increasing cessation rates [71], perioperative institution of bupropion must be approached with extreme caution. The high rate of antidepressant (including tramadol) pharmacotherapy in the chronic pain population renders concomitant elevated risks of seizure and serotonin syndrome, and as such we do not generally advise it unless careful risk:benefit ratio analysis is favorable.

Electronic Cigarettes and Other "Vaping" Devices

While electronic nicotine delivery systems contain fewer toxins carcinogens than do cigarettes [75], and while the data do seem to support their efficacy in terms of supporting smoking cessation [76], lack of standardization of devices and unproven safety lead us to advise patients to avoid these devices in favor of the adjuncts discussed previously.

Behavioral Support

As introduced previously, intensive tobacco cessation counseling comprising at least weekly sessions for several weeks seems to deliver the highest yield outcomes in terms of both incidence and duration of abstinence. Such counseling may of course be delivered by "higher echelon" doctorate-level or masters-level professionals as well as by physicians and other providers and, increasingly, by individuals with varying levels of training including telephonic "QuitLine" staff, or certified Tobacco Treatment Specialists. Given the magnitude of the scope of the problem and the generally limited resources available, it is incumbent on all parties involved in healthcare to participate in this public health effort. Along those lines, the US Public Health Service's "5 As" clinical practice guideline [77] recommends that every clinician should

- Ask all patients about smoking status
- Advise all smokers to quit
- Assess readiness to quit
- Assist interested patients (commensurate with scope of practice)
- Arrange for follow-up

Motivational Enhancement

Simply advising people to stop smoking, or even bludgeoning them with warnings about adverse consequences, and so on, doesn't typically work. There is usually such significant "delay discounting" phenomenon involved such that the threat of remote cancer, COPD, heart attack, and stroke is not clearly perceived as relevant. As discussed previously, tobacco is highly addictive, and furthermore is not typically regularly consumed without complex underlying biopsychosocial incentives (e.g., anxiolysis/stress management, peer acceptance, and community). Assisting patients' insight and understanding of their reasons for smoking is key to facilitating cessation, and while formal cognitive-behavioral therapy toward that end can certainly be very effective, motivational interviewing (MI) techniques may be at least as beneficial and more accessible. Motivational interviewing was initially developed as a tool for alcohol use disorder counseling but rapidly showed significant utility in addressing multiple problem behaviors, including smoking. The simple (not easy!) application of its principles and techniques may be synergistic with other counseling methods [78], which probably bears special relevance to the perioperative setting, given the potentially enhanced openness to more directive input leveraged by the "teachable moment" of surgery. The efficacy of MI in assisting with smoking cessation has not been widely evaluated specifically in the context of the perioperative setting; however, in general it has proven to be more effective than brief advice or usual care [79]. The classic text by Miller and Rollnick [80] is replete with examples of application to smoking cessation counseling, and readers are directed to that source for further exposure and instruction.

Addressing Habit

As with all addictive behaviors, smoking involves a significant component of habit. As discussed in much greater detail in chapter 4, habitual behavior develops with conditioned association between an action and a reward, and almost always also includes conditioning to an independent but associated cue (e.g., the experience of stress, being in a certain place or encountering a certain individual, etc.).

Understanding the cue, action, and reward components and sequence is important in breaking/replacing undesirable habits, and may be effectively achieved by application of MI, as discussed earlier. We have found in clinical practice, however, that even simple inquiry as to both smoking reward and cue often yields fairly consistent and intervention-inviting information (e.g., many people smoke primarily for perceived anxiolytic benefit, and common cues include workplace stress, driving in traffic, and various domestic triggers). (Conversely, simple inquiry/discussion also generally reveals consistent competing desire to quit smoking for health and economic reasons.)

In our experience as well as in much of the habit literature (see chapter 4) we have found that elimination of undesirable habits proceeds most effectively with both cue-action sequence interruption and with substitution of a different action suitable for achieving the same desired reward. In terms of the former, altering the environment (e.g., storing cigarettes or better yet the cigarette lighter in the freezer) often provides suitable disruption to allow for increased mindfulness of behavior. In terms of rewarding activities substitution, NRT or other psychosocially pleasant pursuits are of inestimable value. Taking a 10–20 minute walk if feasible is often a highly effective and of course very beneficial substitute as well that may facilitate improved exercise habit. Implementation intention activities such as setting a quit date, and also committing to carrying out different cigarette procurement means (e.g., instead of buying discounted cartons, purchasing one cigarette pack at a time, and throwing away an increasing proportion of unsmoked cigarettes) may be beneficial as well.

Combined Approach

Data from the general population [71] as well as the perioperative arena [59] favor combined behavioral counseling in concert with pharmacotherapy. Success rates practically double with such dual therapy, and if at all possible it should be used. However, given the concerns that many surgeons still have regarding NRT at least, frank discussion of the options must occur in cases where the surgeon's considerations are uncertain. In some cases, a truncated course one to four weeks prior to surgery may be negotiated of pharmacotherapy terminating.

Abstinence (Biomarker) Monitoring

Finally, although in general for some reason patients do not engage in the same sort of deceptive/self-deceptive underestimation or denial of cigarette use as they do for alcohol, qualitative and quantitative biomarker testing may be useful not only for establishing and verifying compliance with abstinence but also in many cases for providing additional incentive for tobacco avoidance [81]. A handful of assays have been used with some regularity over the years; these and a few other uncommon tests are discussed briefly in what follows.

Cotinine
Cotinine is the main active metabolite of nicotine, and has a plasma half-life of roughly 20 hours [82]. As such, it is fairly reliable as a biomarker for any degree of regular smoking, and may be assayed via blood, urine or saliva;

either point-of-care immunoassay methods or greater accuracy and greater cost spectroscopic methods may be used. It has very good sensitivity (reported at 96%–97% with cutoff values of 25–50 ng/mL in urine) with lower specificity (reported between 85%–99%) [82, 83]). Specificity is increasingly diminishing as NRT (including electronic cigarette) use increases, and as with all of these methods, it does not distinguish active smoking from secondhand smoke exposure. Nonetheless, given its convenience and good sensitivity, it remains perhaps the most widely used method at least in the perioperative arena for confirming abstinence, and given that many surgeons still remain unwilling to operate on patients using NRT it is likely to maintain its place of prominence.

Carboxyhemoglobin and Carbon Monoxide

Carbon monoxide (CO) and carboxyhemoglobin (COHb) are ubiquitously elevated in smokers in dose-dependent fashion, as is true also of cotinine. However, these methods have the advantage of distinguishing smoking from NRT (or smokeless tobacco products). Both methods also correlate well with each other, and show relatively good sensitivity (86%–90%) and specificity (89%–92%) at cutoff values of 8 ppm exhaled CO, and 1.6% COHb [83]. The decreased sensitivity lies mainly in the short half-lives of both CO and COHb (2–3 hours, and 4–6 hours respectively), and the imperfect specificity is due primarily to multiple other environmental sources of CO and also the fact that a small amount is always physiologically present and active.

While exhaled CO is an extremely economical means of monitoring (once upfront costs of the monitoring device are absorbed) many payers still do not reimburse for this, rendering the more expensive and invasive serum COHb the only viable option in some small practices.

Other Biomarkers

Thiocyanate has been used in the past as a tobacco biomarker, but shows very poor sensitivity and specificity [83], with the latter property owing to multiple other sources; it is not widely used today.

Anabasine and anabatine, two alkaloids found in tobacco, may be assayed in both urine and plasma and have the advantage of distinguishing tobacco use from NRT, not being found in the latter. Reported sensitivity for tobacco use is only 79% (at a cutoff value of 2 ng/mL), but at that level specificity is 100% [84]. In theory at least, the combination of cotinine (with its excellent sensitivity) and anabasine/anatabine (with its excellent specificity) would represent the ideal monitoring method; at present, however, the latter is not available via most laboratories, and remains cost-prohibitive and is not reimbursed by most payers.

References

1 Pomerleau OF. Nicotine and the central nervous system: biobehavioral effects of cigarette smoking. Am J Med. 1992;93(1A):2S–7S.

2 International Agency for Research on Cancer. Tobacco smoking. IARC Monographs 100E. World Health Organization: Lyon, France; 2012.

3 Wald NJ, Idle M, Boreham J, Bailey A. Carbon monoxide in breath in relation to smoking and carboxyhaemoglobin levels. Thorax. 1981;36:366–9.

4 Phillips E, Wang TW, Husten CG, et al. Tobacco product use among adults—United States, 2015. MMWR Morb Mortal Wkly Rep. 2017;66:1209–15.

5 Schroeder SA. Tobacco control in the wake of the 1998 master settlement agreement. N Engl J Med. 2004;350:293–301.

6 Centers for Disease Control and Prevention (CDC). Smoking-attributable mortality, years of potential life lost, and productivity losses—United States, 2000–2004. MMWR Morb Mortal Wkly Rep. 2008;57:1226–8.

7 Cropley M, Theadom A, Pravettoni G, Webb G. The effectiveness of smoking cessation interventions prior to surgery: a systematic review. Nicotine Tob Res. 2008;10:407–12.

8 American College of Surgeons. Statement on the Effects of Tobacco Use on Surgical Complications and the Utility of Smoking Cessation Counseling. 2014. https://www.facs.org/about-acs/statements/71-tobacco-use#ref5. Accessed November 19, 2018.

9 Fishbain DA, Lewis JE, Bruns D, Meyer LJ, Gao J, Disorbio JM. The prevalence of smokers within chronic pain patients and highest pain levels versus comparison groups. Pain Med. 2013;14:403–16.

10 Watkins SS, Koob GF, Markou A. Neural mechanisms underlying nicotine addiction: acute positive reinforcement and withdrawal. Nicotine Tob Res. 2000;2:19–37.

11 Antolin-Fontes B, Ables JL, Görlich A, Ibañez-Tallon I. The habenulo-interpeduncular pathway in nicotine aversion and withdrawal. Neuropharmacology. 2015;96:213–22.

12 Zvolensky MJ, McMillan K, Gonzalez A, Asmundson GJ. Chronic pain and cigarette smoking and nicotine dependence among a representative sample of adults. Nicotine Tob Res. 2009;11:1407–14.

13 Shiri R, Karppinen J, Leino-Arjas P, Solovieva S, Viikari-Juntura E. The association between smoking and low back pain: a meta-analysis. Am J Med. 2010;123(1):87.e7–35. doi: 10.1016/j.amjmed.2009.05.028.

14 Pisinger C, Aadahl M, Toft U, Birke H, Zytphen-Adeler J, Jørgensen T. The association between active and passive smoking and frequent pain in a general population. Eur J Pain. 2011;15:77–83.

15 Holley AL, Law EF, Tham SW, et al. Current smoking as a predictor of chronic musculoskeletal pain in young adult twins. J Pain. 2013;14:1131–9.

16 Jhawar BS, Fuchs CS, Colditz GA, Stampfer MJ. Cardiovascular risk factors for physician-diagnosed lumbar disc herniation. Spine J. 2006;6:684–91.

17 Tian W, Qi H. Association between intervertebral disc degeneration and disturbances of blood supply to the vertebrae. Chin Med J. 2010;123:239–43.

18 Wendling D, Prati C. Spondyloarthritis and smoking: towards a new insight into the disease. Expert Rev Clin Immunol. 2013;9:511–16.

19 Amin S, Niu J, Guermazi A, et al. Cigarette smoking and the risk for cartilage loss and knee pain in men with knee osteoarthritis. Ann Rheum Dis. 2007;66:18–22.

20 Sugiyama D, Nishimura K, Tamaki K, et al. Impact of smoking as a risk factor for developing rheumatoid arthritis: a meta-analysis of observational studies. Ann Rheum Dis. 2010;69:70–81.

21 Perlstein TS, Lee RT. Smoking, metalloproteinases, and vascular disease. Arterioscler Thromb Vasc Biol. 2006;26:250–6.

22 Goesling J, Brummett CM, Meraj TS, Moser SE, Hassett AL, Ditre JW. Associations between pain, current tobacco smoking, depression, and fibromyalgia status among treatment-seeking chronic pain patients. Pain Med. 2015;16:1433–42.

23 Weingarten TN, Podduturu VR, Hooten WM, Thompson JM, Luedtke CA, Oh TH. Impact of tobacco use in patients presenting to a multidisciplinary outpatient treatment program for fibromyalgia. Clin J Pain. 2009;25:39–43.

24 Pamuk ON, Dönmez S, Cakir N. The frequency of smoking in fibromyalgia patients and its association with symptoms. Rheumatol Int. 2009;29:1311–14.

25 Deleanu OC, Pocora D, Mihălcuţă S, Ulmeanu R, Zaharie AM, Mihălţan FD. Influence of smoking on sleep and obstructive sleep apnea syndrome. Pneumologia. 2016;65:28–35.

26 Ziegler D, Papanas N, Vinik AI, Shaw JE. Epidemiology of polyneuropathy in diabetes and prediabetes. Handb Clin Neurol. 2014;126:3–22.

27 Boogaard S, Heymans MW, de Vet HC, et al. Predictors of persistent neuropathic pain--a systematic review. Pain Physician. 2015;18:433–57.

28 Shiri R, Karppinen J, Leino-Arjas P, et al. Cardiovascular and lifestyle risk factors in lumbar radicular pain or clinically defined sciatica: a systematic review. Eur Spine J. 2007; 16:2043–54.

29 Shi Y, Weingarten TN, Mantilla CB, Hooten WM, Warner DO. Smoking and pain: pathophysiology and clinical implications. Anesthesiology. 2010; 113:977–92.

30 Smith HS. Smoking-induced nociception. Pain Physician. 2011;14:E1–4.

31 Parkerson HA, Zvolensky MJ, Asmundson GJ. Understanding the relationship between smoking and pain. Expert Rev Neurother. 2013;13:1407–14.

32 Fluharty M, Taylor AE, Grabski M, Munafò MR. The association of cigarette smoking with depression and anxiety: a systematic review. Nicotine Tob Res. 2017;19:3–13.

33 Ditre JW, Zale EL, Kosiba JD, Zvolensky MJ. A pilot study of pain-related anxiety and smoking-dependence motives among persons with chronic pain. Exp Clin Psychopharmacol. 2013;21:443–49.

34 Copeland AL, Brandon TH, Quinn EP. The Smoking Consequences Questionnaire-Adult: measurement of smoking outcome expectancies of experienced smokers. Psychol Assess. 1995; 7:484–94.

35 Ditre JW, Brandon TH, Zale EL, Meagher MM. Pain, nicotine, and smoking: research findings and mechanistic considerations. Psychol Bull. 2011;137:1065–93.

36 Schwilk B, Bothner U, Schraag S, Georgieff M. Perioperative respiratory events in smokers and nonsmokers undergoing general anaesthesia. Acta Anaesthesiol Scand. 1997;41:348–55.

37 Løkke A, Lange P, Scharling H, Fabricius P, Vestbo J. Developing COPD: a 25 year follow up study of the general population. Thorax. 2006;61:935–9.

38 Khullar D, Maa J. The impact of smoking on surgical outcomes. J Am Coll Surg. 2012;215:418–26.

39 Gourgiotis S, Aloizos S, Aravosita P, et al. The effects of tobacco smoking on the incidence and risk of intraoperative and postoperative complications in adults. Surgeon. 2011;9:225–32.

40   Turan A, Mascha EJ, Roberman D, et al. Smoking and perioperative outcomes. Anesthesiology. 2011;114:837–46.

41   Csordas A, Bernhard D. The biology behind the atherothrombotic effects of cigarette smoke. Nat Rev Cardiol. 2013;10:219–30.

42   Lison S, Weiss G, Spannagl M, Heindl B. Postoperative changes in procoagulant factors after major surgery. Blood Coagul Fibrinolysis. 2011;22:190–6.

43   Sweetland S, Parkin L, Balkwill A, Green J, Reeves G, Beral V. Smoking, surgery, and venous thromboembolism risk in women: United Kingdom cohort study. Circulation. 2013;127:1276–82.

44   Neumayer L, Hosokawa P, Itani K, El-Tamer M, Henderson WG, Khuri SF. Multivariable predictors of postoperative surgical site infection after general and vascular surgery: results from the patient safety in surgery study. J Am Coll Surg. 2007;204:1178–87.

45   Qiu F, Liang CL, Liu H, et al. Impacts of cigarette smoking on immune responsiveness: Up and down or upside down? Oncotarget. 2017;8:268–84.

46   Duchman KR, Gao Y, Pugely AJ, Martin CT, Noiseux NO, Callaghan JJ. The effect of smoking on short-term complications following total hip and knee arthroplasty. J Bone Joint Surg Am. 2015;97:1049–58.

47   Teng S, Yi C, Krettek C, Jagodzinski M. Smoking and risk of prosthesis-related complications after total hip arthroplasty: a meta-analysis of cohort studies. PLoS One. 2015;10(4):e0125294. doi: 10.1371/journal.pone.0125294.

48   Novikov DA, Swensen SJ, Buza JA 3rd, Gidumal RH, Strauss EJ. The effect of smoking on ACL reconstruction: a systematic review. Phys Sportsmed. 2016;44:335–41.

49   Hadley MN, Reddy SV. Smoking and the human vertebral column: a review of the impact of cigarette use on vertebral bone metabolism and spinal fusion. Neurosurgery. 1997;41:116–24.

50   Glassman SD, Anagnost SC, Parker A, Burke D, Johnson JR, Dimar JR. The effect of cigarette smoking and smoking cessation on spinal fusion. Spine. 2000;25: 2608–15.

51   Pearson RG, Clement RG, Edwards KL, Scammell BE. Do smokers have greater risk of delayed and non-union after fracture, osteotomy and arthrodesis? A systematic review with meta-analysis. BMJ Open. 2016;6(11):e010303. doi:10.1136/bmjopen-2015-010303.

52   Berman D, Oren JH, Bendo J, Spivak J. The effect of smoking on spinal fusion. Int J Spine Surg. 2017;11:29. doi: 10.14444/4029.

53   Tønnesen H. Surgery and smoking at first and second hand: time to act. Anesthesiology. 2011;115:1–3.

54   Grønkjær M, Eliasen M, Skov-Ettrup LS, Tolstrup JS, Christiansen AH, Mikkelsen SS, et al. Preoperative smoking status and postoperative complications: a systematic review and meta-analysis. Ann Surg. 2014;259:52–71.

55   Hawn MT, Houston TK, Campagna EJ, et al. The attributable risk of smoking on surgical complications. Ann Surg. 2011;254:914–20.

56   Dimick JB, Chen SL, Taheri PA, Henderson WG, Khuri SF, Campbell DA Jr. Hospital costs associated with surgical complications: a report from the private-sector National Surgical Quality Improvement Program. J Am Coll Surg. 2004;199: 531–7.

57   Babb S, Malarcher A, Schauer G, Asman K, Jamal A. Quitting smoking among adults—United States, 2000–2015. MMWR Morb Mortal Wkly Rep. 2017;65:1457–64.

58 Zaki A, Abrishami A, Wong J, Chung FF. Interventions in the preoperative clinic for long term smoking cessation: a quantitative systematic review. Can J Anaesth. 2008;55:11–21.

59 Thomsen T, Villebro N, Møller AM. Interventions for preoperative smoking cessation. Cochrane Database Syst Rev. 2014;(3):CD002294. doi:10.1002/14651858. CD002294.pub4.

60 Warner DO, Kadimpati S. Nicotine lozenges to promote brief preoperative abstinence from smoking: pilot study. Clin Health Promot. 2012; 2:85–8.

61 Wong J, Abrishami A, Yang Y, et al. A perioperative smoking cessation intervention with varenicline. A double-blind, randomized placebo-controlled trial. Anesthesiology. 2012;117:755–64.

62 Sørensen LT. Wound healing and infection in surgery. The clinical impact of smoking and smoking cessation: a systematic review and meta-analysis. Arch Surg. 2012;147:373–83.

63 Mills E, Eyawo O, Lockhart I, Kelly S, Wu P, Ebbert JO. Smoking cessation reduces postoperative complications: a systematic review and meta-analysis. Am J Med. 2011;124:144–54.

64 Wong J, Lam DP, Abrishami A, Chan MT, Chung F. Short-term preoperative smoking cessation and postoperative complications: a systematic review and meta-analysis. Can J Anaesth. 2012;59:268–79.

65 Myers K, Hajek P, Hinds C, McRobbie H. Stopping smoking shortly before surgery and postoperative complications: a systematic review and meta-analysis. Arch Intern Med. 2011;171:983–9.

66 Katznelson R, Beattie S. Perioperative smoking risk. Anesthesiology. 2011;114:734–6.

67 Theadom A, Cropley M. Effects of preoperative smoking cessation on the incidence and risk of intraoperative and postoperative complications in adult smokers: a systematic review. Tob Control. 2006;15:352–8.

68 Warner DO; American Society of Anesthesiologists Smoking Cessation Initiative Task Force. Feasibility of tobacco interventions in anesthesiology practices: a pilot study. Anesthesiology. 2009;110:1223–8.

69 Benowitz NL, Jacob P 3rd. Daily intake of nicotine during cigarette smoking. Clin Pharmacol Ther. 1984;35:499–504.

70 Stead LF, Perera R, Bullen C, Mant D, Hartmann-Boyce J, Cahill K, Lancaster T. Nicotine replacement therapy for smoking cessation. Cochrane Database Syst Rev. 2012;11:CD000146. doi: 10.1002/14651858.CD000146.pub4.

71 Cahill K, Stevens S, Perera R, Lancaster T. Pharmacological interventions for smoking cessation: an overview and network meta-analysis. Cochrane Database Syst Rev. 2013;(5):CD009329. doi: 10.1002/14651858.CD009329.pub2.

72 Moore D, Aveyard P, Connock M, Wang D, Fry-Smith A, Barton P. Effectiveness and safety of nicotine replacement therapy assisted reduction to stop smoking: systematic review and meta-analysis. BMJ. 2009;338:b1024. doi:10.1136/bmj.b1024.

73 Nolan MB, Warner DO. Safety and efficacy of nicotine replacement therapy in the perioperative period: a narrative review. Mayo Clin Proc. 2015;90:1553–61.

74 Myles PS, Leslie K, Angliss M, Mezzavia P, Lee L. Effectiveness of bupropion as an aid to stopping smoking before elective surgery: a randomised controlled trial. Anaesthesia. 2004;59:1053–8.

75 Goniewicz ML, Knysak J, Gawron M, et al. Levels of selected carcinogens and toxicants in vapour from electronic cigarettes. Control. 2014;23:133–9.

76 Hartmann-Boyce J, McRobbie H, Bullen C, Begh R, Stead LF, Hajek P. Electronic cigarettes for smoking cessation. Cochrane Database Syst Rev. 2016;9:CD010216. doi: 10.1002/14651858.CD010216.pub3.

77 Anonymous. A clinical practice guideline for treating tobacco use and dependence: 2008 update. A U.S. Public Health Service report. Am J Prev Med. 2008;35:158–76.

78 Miller WR, Rose GS. Toward a theory of motivational interviewing. Am Psychol. 2009;64:527–37.

79 Lindson-Hawley N, Thompson TP, Begh R. Motivational interviewing for smoking cessation. Cochrane Database Syst Rev. 2015;(3):CD006936. doi: 10.1002/14651858.CD006936.pub3.

80 Miller WR, Rollnick S. Motivational Interviewing: Helping People Change. 3rd ed. New York: Guilford Press: 2013.

81 Shi Y, Ehlers S, Hinds R, Baumgartner A, Warner DO. Monitoring of exhaled carbon monoxide to promote preoperative smoking abstinence. Health Psychol. 2013;32:714–17.

82 Marrone GF, Shakleya DM, Scheidweiler KB, Singleton EG, Huestis MA, Heishman SJ. Relative performance of common biochemical indicators in detecting cigarette smoking. Addiction. 2011;106:1325–34.

83 Jarvis MJ, Tunstall-Pedoe H, Feyerabend C, Vesey C, Saloojee Y. Comparison of tests used to distinguish smokers from nonsmokers. Am J Public Health. 1987;77:1435–8.

84 Jacob P, Hatsukami D, Severson H, Hall S, Yu L, Benowitz NL. Anabasine and anatabine as biomarkers for tobacco use during nicotine replacement therapy. Cancer Epidemiol Biomarkers Prev. 2002;11:1668–73.

10

Preoperative Management of Chronic Opioid Therapy

Heath B. McAnally and Beth Darnall

Introduction

As introduced in chapter 1, the literature increasingly supports an association between chronic preoperative opioid use and:

- worsened postoperative pain control and patient satisfaction
- increased medical complications,
- compromised surgical outcomes,
- prolonged length of stay (LOS), and
- increased financial costs.

Conversely, there is evidence (as well as considerable anecdotal support and face validity) that preoperative opioid reduction may result in substantial improvements in outcomes.

In this chapter we briefly review basic and clinical science underpinning these phenomena, the descriptive epidemiology and available outcomes data pertinent to the issue, and what the current literature has to say about preoperative opioid weaning. In keeping with the general theme of the book, we emphasize once again both the intricate and intertwined relationship of chronic pain and chronic opioid use with a host of other pertinent contributors, some more biologic and others more psychosocial in nature. As with previous chapters addressing some of these related but distinct modifiable risk factors, recognizing the complex behavioral issues surrounding chronic opioid use, we highlight the importance of both motivational enhancement and habit alteration. Finally, the somewhat perennially murky distinction between poorly defined categories of opioid dependence and addiction is discussed briefly, along with the complicated issue of perioperative medication-assisted treatment for opioid use disorder.

General Concepts Related to Chronic Opioid Therapy

Opioid Biology and Pharmacology: Analgesic Perspective

Opioids constitute a chemically heterogeneous group of compounds that are defined by their ability to bind and activate endogenous opioid receptors located in various organs but most notably the brain and spinal cord. Three such receptor classes have been well characterized, and the best understood is the mu-opioid receptor (MOR), which seems to be responsible for the majority of the effects commonly attributed to opioids, including analgesia, euphoria, respiratory depression, and constipation.

The biology of the endogenous opioid system, and the pharmacology of these naturally derived and also synthetic agents are well described elsewhere for those desiring greater detail [1]; suffice it to say for the purposes of this effort that opioids effect a blunting of the central nervous system's (CNS) transmission and perception of nociceptive messages by actions at the dorsal horn of the spinal cord, and in the mesencephalon and rhombencephalon. Their analgesic effects include both affective and pain-consciousness alteration, but also purer physiologic modulation, well evidenced by downregulation of sympathetic nervous system activity and other stress responses in unconscious, for example, anesthetized, patients.

As with all pharmacologic agents, there is significant interpersonal variability in response to opioids, and both genetic and situational factors seem to play a role. One of the more notable and pertinent dynamic considerations (especially in the context of our focus on preoperative optimization) is the phenomenon of tolerance. Depending on a number of factors, opioid tolerance develops at different rates and degrees in different individuals, and may result from pharmacokinetic changes (i.e., altered metabolism), and also from pharmacodynamic ones (i.e., alterations in receptor expression and function).

Despite this unpredictability of effect, and despite recent dramatic change in practice guidelines and prescribing patterns, opioids remain one of the most widely relied-on modalities for treating moderate to severe pain both acute and chronic, and comprise the most "broad-spectrum" analgesics in the current pharmacotherapeutic armamentarium.

Opioid Biology and Pharmacology: Addictionology Perspective

Opioids are well-known euphorigenic agents, and this hedonic reward (in addition to analgesic benefits in many cases) confers significant abuse and dependence liability. The euphoria caused by opioids seems to be mediated primarily by the MOR; as with all drugs of abuse, at one point it was almost universally accepted that dopaminergism in the mesolimbic pathway (primarily involving the ventral tegmental area and nucleus accumbens) conferred the pleasurable effects responsible for dependence and addiction. It is now recognized that the role of dopamine in the development of addiction has much more to do with registering learning traces in the striatum (and other areas such as the nucleus accumbens) in response to differences between predicted and experienced reward [2, 3]—that is, marking/signaling a disproportionately reinforcing outcome [4].

A widely accepted principle of addictionology is that substances that exert more rapid effect (as well as more intense pleasurable effect) have a greater propensity for abuse and dependence [5, 6]. This "rate of rise" phenomenon is in one sense a factor of bioavailability; intravenous administration of a substance confers much more rapid effect than oral administration, and drug abusers have long known that crushing and snorting, smoking, or injecting their drug of choice results in a much more profound "high" than simply swallowing the agent. However, the ultimate issue at stake is transport into the CNS, which is a factor of both concentration gradient (plasma level), lipophilicity, and active transport across the blood-brain barrier (BBB).

This latter consideration may explain in large part the disproportionate addictive potential of oxycodone (see [7] for a comprehensive review), as that agent demonstrates a rate of access through the BBB, and brain concentration many times that of morphine [8–10]—which appears to correlate with markedly increased phasic dopaminergism in the nucleus accumbens compared to morphine [11]. As such, our (HM) practice pattern is to both avoid postoperative oxycodone prescriptions greater than 7 days in duration and also to immediately discontinue oxycodone in any patient using it chronically; if legitimate pain issues exist we transition immediately to an alternative opioid for weaning, with oxymorphone being the final fallback agent if necessary due to patient-reported allergies; oxymorphone is the most potent active metabolite of oxycodone and therefore cannot possibly confer allergic phenomena in patients who are accustomed to using oxycodone.

Opioid addictiveness, however, has to do with much more than simple hedonic reward; many factors including drug availability, cost, adverse effect profile, and perceived/actual risk all affect abuse and the development of addiction [12]. In addition, it is well known that while the initial stages of drug addiction are characterized by the pursuit of pleasure or reward, in latter stages (and certainly once tolerance has set in) continued use despite intentions to the contrary have much more to do with the avoidance of withdrawal phenomena [13], and this withdrawal avoidance phase is mediated in large part by the kappa-opioid receptor (KOR) system [14–16]. Again, oxycodone exhibits disproportionately strong KOR agonism [17, 18], likely explaining its extraordinary withdrawal scourge and contributing to its unparalleled addictive potential (Figure 10.1).

Individual factors ranging from genetics to personality disorders have all been implicated as risk factors for the development of opioid dependence and addiction; robust (and plentiful) literature supports psychological risk factors including other substance use disorders and anxiety as the most important predictors [19–21].

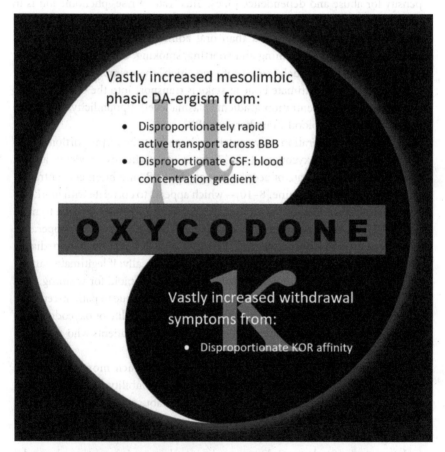

Figure 10.1. Oxycodone's Unparalleled Addictive Potential

BBB = blood-brain barrier; CSF = cerebrospinal fluid; DA = dopamine; κ, KOR = kappa opioid receptor; μ = mu opioid receptor.

Chronic Pain, Chronic Opioid Use, and Hyperalgesia

Chronic pain is not just acute pain lasting longer. Besides persistence of local or systemic inflammation, we understand currently that neurogenic and glial-mediated inflammation [22] and maladaptive neural plasticity in the spinal cord and brain often underlie and perpetuate the chronic pain experience [23–25] long after an original physical insult has resolved. Chronic pain may thus be better conceptualized as a pathologic deviation from the normal physiologic process and protective role of pain, rather than simple temporal extension of nociception.

Chronic opioid use (COU) is also now understood to contribute to chronic pain and in many cases may be the sole biologic mediator (Figure 10.2). Functional neuroimaging studies suggest shared neuroanatomic alterations [26, 27] and at the cellular level, opioid-induced hyperalgesia (OIH) occurs as a result of altered receptor function, direct inflammatory effects on microglia, and long-term potentiation/maladaptive plasticity effects on the spinal cord and brain [28, 29].

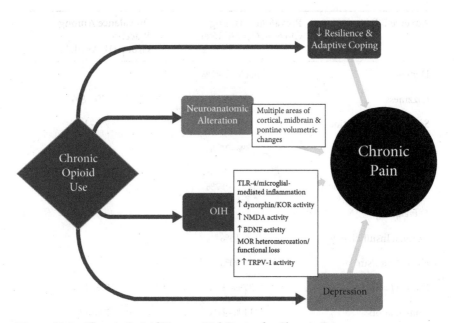

Figure 10.2. Chronic Opioid Use as a Risk Factor for Chronic Pain

BDNF = brain-derived neurotrophic factor; KOR = kappa opioid receptor; MOR = mu opioid receptor; NMDA = n-methyl-d-aspartate; TLR-4 = toll-like receptor 4; TRPV-1 = transient receptor potential/vanilloid receptor-1.

From a psychosocial standpoint, COU has been shown to independently predict the development of depression [30, 31], which is strongly associated with chronic pain. While literature evidence is lacking, it is also widely observed that COU is associated with decreased self-efficacy and resilience, which also amplify and perpetuate chronic pain.

Other Adverse Effects of Chronic Opioid Therapy

Opioid-related adverse drug effects (ORADE) are manifold and involve most physiologic systems. Some specific ORADE and their reported prevalence ranges are provided in Table 10.1.

Many recent reviews [32, 33] have established clear, statistically significant risk increases for these outcomes compared to placebo, and a thorough discussion of the issue may be found in [34].

Table 10.1. Prevalence of ORADE with COU [34]

Adverse Effect	Prevalence Among Chronic Opioid Users	Prevalence Among Placebo Group (IF Available)
Depression	8.4%–20.1%	
Dizziness	18%–22%	5%–8%
Somnolence/Sedation	18%–29%	7%–14%
Opioid Abuse and Dependence	3%–26%	
Respiratory Depression • *Sleep-disordered breathing*	0.3%–17% • *75%–85%*	• *10%–26%*
Adrenal Insufficiency	10%	
Hypogonadism	90%	
Nausea	27%–32%	9%–12%
Constipation	11%–41%	7%–11%
Urinary Retention	10%–18.1%	
Pruritis	2%–15 %	7%

Rationale for and Against Opioid Therapy in Chronic Pain

In situations involving severe acute pain, evidence (and practice consensus) favors consideration of opioid therapy, after careful consideration of the risk:benefit ratio and establishment of the inadequacy of more conservative options. From a preventive standpoint, it is apparent that one risk factor (of many) for the chronification of pain is inadequate treatment of severe acute pain [35, 36].

Conversely, the evidence increasingly supports the avoidance of opioid therapy in chronic noncancer pain (CNCP) for the most part, with the understanding that in certain cases, opioid therapy may improve functional outcomes and quality of life. Over 20 systematic reviews and meta-analyses have been performed in the past 15 years [37], showing no evidence of long-term benefit stacked against considerable evidence of long-term harms. Accordingly, recent clinical practice guidelines from professional societies and government agencies [38–40] have essentially unanimously advocated against chronic opioid therapy in CNCP in general, with allowance for individualized therapeutic decision-making.

Rationale for Preoperative Opioid Weaning

Surgery-Specific ORADE Associated with Preop COU

As many as two-thirds [41] of patients seeking elective operations (range: 33%–70% [42]) present with COU; available data show as much as a ninefold increase in COU among ambulatory surgery patients compared to the general populace [43]. Undoubtedly due to tolerance (and possibly additive distress from OIH [44, 45]), these patients demonstrate increased postoperative opioid requirements [46–48], which, as might be expected, confers an increased incidence of ORADE; see Table 10.2. Besides the usually encountered adverse effects of respiratory depression, ileus, nausea, and vomiting, all of which may increase morbidity and LOS, ORADE specific to the postoperative environment are also frequently seen, and are discussed briefly in what follows.

Increased Postoperative Pain
Disproportionately increased severity of postoperative pain owing to both biologic (e.g., hyperalgesia/central sensitization and tolerance) and psychosocial contributors (e.g., pain catastrophizing, anxiety, decreased resilience) are associated with preoperative COU [44, 49]. In addition, this increased pain not infrequently requires greater postoperative opioid doses to control, which in turn

Table 10.2. Adverse Outcomes Associated with Preoperative Chronic Opioid Use

Adverse Outcomes Associated with Preoperative Chronic Opioid Use
• ↑ risk of usual ORADE (respiratory depression, ileus, nausea/vomiting) due to increased postoperative opioid requirements • ↑ severity and duration of postoperative pain • ↑ infection (surgical site and other) rate • ↑ arthroplasty and intervertebral body fusion failures • ↑ length of stay and readmissions • ↑ persistent postoperative opioid use • ↑ rate of postoperative disability

ORADE = opioid-related adverse drug effect

increases the risk of other ORADE. Preoperative COU is also well documented as an independent risk factor for increased duration of postoperative pain [44, 46, 50–54].

Increased Wound Complications

Increased postoperative wound dehiscence has been associated with postoperative COU [55]. Wound-healing activities comprise normal sequelae of the inflammatory response to injury, and typically begin within days of insult, as shown in Figure 10.3.

Whether by immunosuppression [56, 57] or glial inflammation with increased activity of nuclear factor κB, interleukin-1, tumor necrosis factor-α, and so forth [58–60] possibly disrupting normal "resoleomics" [61], chronic opioid exposure has been shown in both in vitro and animal models to impair angiogenesis and fibroblast activity, delaying wound healing [62–65].

While the clinical relevance of opioid-related immunosuppression has been called into question repeatedly in the literature over the past decade [57, 66], the surgical literature shows compelling evidence that surgical site infections [67, 68] are increased with preoperative COU.

Increased Arthroplasty Complications

Several recent orthopedic publications [50, 53, 69–71] have highlighted increases in arthroplasty complications including arthrofibrosis and periprosthetic failures. A particularly large study of over 12,700 total knee arthroplasty patients with preoperative COU required significantly higher revision rates than nearly 20,000 controls [72]. In another recent large observational study [73], over 5,000 patients with preoperative COU were found to experience a statistically significant increased incidence of periprosthetic joint infection after total

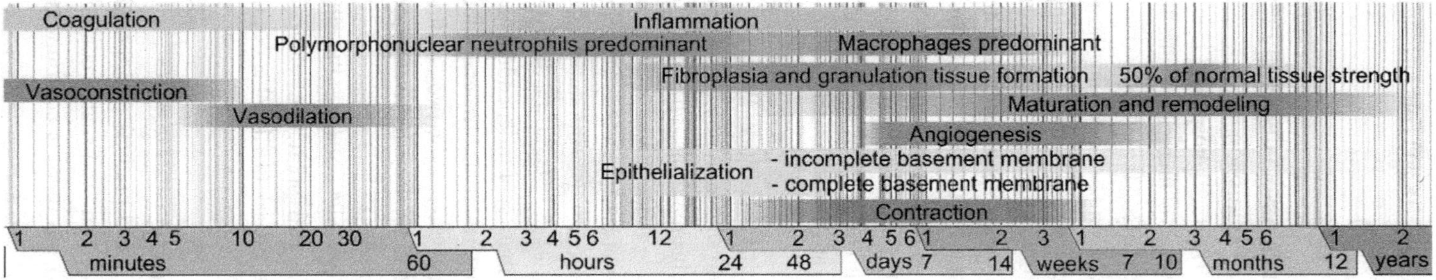

Figure 10.3. Normal Inflammatory Response to Injury

By Mikael Häggström, used with permission.—Own work (from the template Logarithmic time scale—milliseconds to years.svg), Public Domain, https://commons.wikimedia.org/w/index.php?curid=11587593

joint arthroplasty compared to over 18,000 controls (adjusted odds ratio 1.53, $p = .005$).

Other Adverse Outcomes Associated with Preoperative COU

Increased Length of Stay and Readmission

As highlighted in chapter 1 [50, 53, 74–76], hospital LOS is increased by an average of 1–2 days, not insignificant in terms of financial ramifications (with an average of $2,100/day hospitalization cost in 2015 in the United States), patient inconvenience, or increased risk of complications simply from being hospitalized (e.g., hospital-acquired infection). Increased postoperative pain requiring parenteral opioid administration certainly contributes to increased LOS, however other ORADE such as severe nausea, ileus, and respiratory depression may all delay discharge as well.

Readmission rates are also statistically significantly increased in patients engaging in preoperative COU; as also discussed in greater detail in chapter 1, available data show an association of preoperative chronic pain and COU with readmission [68, 74, 76–78] with odds ratios generally in the range of 1.5- to 2-fold increased risk of readmission.

Increased Incidence of Chronic Postsurgical Pain

Preoperative COU has also been shown in numerous investigations to be a risk factor for the development of chronic postsurgical pain (CPSP) [44, 50–54]. In the context of surgery, however, preoperative COU is almost always associated with CNCP; elective operations at least are rarely complicated by strictly recreational or non-pain-related addiction. Despite statistical adjustment for preoperative CNCP, innate complexities and diagnostic difficulties for both COU and CNCP render unequivocal attribution of independent and significant predictor variable status tenuous. This uncertainty is further confounded by considerable overlap in shared comorbidities between the two conditions (e.g., tobacco use, pro-inflammatory diet, malnutrition, sleep deprivation, sedentary lifestyle, anxiety/catastrophization, PTSD, etc.).

While recognizing these inevitable academic difficulties, from a pragmatic standpoint, consideration of shared predictive relationship (both COU and preoperative CNCP increasing the risk of CPSP) is not unreasonable given the strong degree of covariance.

Postoperative Chronic Opioid Use

Not surprisingly, preoperative COU predicts postoperative COU [47, 79, 80]. As with the strong direct association (and shared comorbidities) between preoperative COU and CNCP, so too there is confounding between CPSP and postoperative COU.

Nonetheless, while unlikely to ever be rigorously demonstrated by either prospective or retrospective investigation, common sense and ubiquitous observation support the supposition that the dependence-conferring and addictive properties of opioids render it much more difficult to discontinue postoperative COU in the context of habitual preoperative use.

Perhaps strengthening the argument for a direct and independent link between preoperative and postoperative COU are recent data from opioid-naive surgical patients showing that short-term prolonged duration (greater than 1 to 2 weeks generally) of postoperative exposure to opioid therapy independently increases the risk of dependence [81, 82].

Disability

Numerous reports, mostly from the spine surgical patient population over the past decade have shown that preoperative COU is independently associated with a higher degree of disability postoperatively, both in terms of subjective and objective function assessments, and also public assistance claims [41, 83–87.] As discussed in previous sections, teasing out the relationships between both preoperative and postoperative pain and opioid use (and other confounding comorbidities) is difficult at best, but there is strong face validity/plausibility to the association, given that chronic opioid use is associated with depression [31], which is strongly associated with disability [88, 89]; chronic opioid use is also likely to represent a higher degree of external locus of control and to be associated with and also confer reduced self-efficacy [42].

Evidence Supporting Preoperative Opioid Reduction

The data on postoperative complications associated with preoperative COU are consistent with the well-documented bigger picture of harms reviewed elsewhere [34]. Conversely, as might be expected, in the context of increasing global awareness of the general inadvisability of COU in CNCP, a growing body of literature supports opioid weaning and discontinuation [90–94].

Frank et al [94] recently performed a systematic review of investigations studying the success and health benefits of COU reduction or cessation, including 67 studies ($n = 12,546$ patients) examining a wide variety of interventions ranging from traditional interdisciplinary pain and behavioral health modalities with or without buprenorphine, to more alternative or unorthodox techniques including acupuncture and ketamine-assisted detoxification. Among the different approaches used, mean discontinuation (not clearly defined nor distinguished from reduction) rates ranged from around 20% for ketamine-assisted, strictly behavioral, and "other outpatient programs" to around 90% for interdisciplinary pain and buprenorphine-assisted treatment programs. Thirty-six of the studies examined pain severity outcomes; eight were judged as fair-quality, with all reporting improved pain after opioid dose reduction. Seventeen studies examined functional outcomes; five were judged as fair-quality, and all reported improved functional outcomes after opioid dose reduction. Twelve studies examined quality of life (QOL) outcomes; three were judged as fair-quality and all reported improved QOL after opioid dose reduction. The authors concluded that "several types of interventions may be effective to reduce or discontinue [COU] and that pain, function, and quality of life may improve with opioid dose reduction" [94].

At present there exists less evidence showing that preoperative opioid reduction results in reduction of complications/improvement of outcomes; to our knowledge only one such investigation has been published [85], but it demonstrated remarkable and encouraging findings paralleling our own clinical experience. In this study, 41 patients undergoing total knee or hip arthroplasty and who were engaging in preoperative COU weaned down to at least 50% of their baseline opioid dose prior to surgery. Comparison groups included 41 opioid-naive patients, and 41 patients with preoperative COU who did not wean their dose. The cohort that weaned demonstrated "substantially improved clinical outcomes that were comparable to patients who did not use [preoperative] opioids at all" [85] with significantly ($p < 0.005$) increased postoperative functionality as assessed by Western Ontario and McMaster Universities Arthritis Index (WOMAC), University of California Los Angeles (UCLA) Activity and Short Form 12 (SF12v2) Physical Component Scores.

In our clinical experience, whether in the general or preoperative setting, attrition is common, and published reports [92, 95] indicate that the majority of patients invited (or directed) into opioid tapering and discontinuation do not succeed. Patients frequently look for other sources of opioids, either via sanctioned prescription or by illicit traffic. However, exceptions to these dismal statistics exist [90, 91, 96, 97], and success is enhanced by first eliciting patients' trust, enhancing motivation, and providing an effective biopsychosocial-spiritual replacement milieu that increases self-efficacy.

How to Wean Patients and Influence Outcomes

In view of the grim statistics of the "opioid epidemic" (among other accumulating understanding of harms), interest in opioid weaning has burgeoned. There is, however, no consensus method nor protocol (nor will there likely ever be) for so complex a process with considerable inherent heterogeneity of patients' a priori and in-process intention and commitment, and resilience. Evidence-based methodology is lacking, and a Cochrane review [98] of five prospective trials ($n = 278$) incorporating a variety of adjunctive therapies concluded, "Based on the available evidence, we do not know the best method of reducing opioids in adults with chronic pain conditions." Another recent systematic review [99] concludes, "finding a plan that an individual patient can embrace with a significant degree of personal engagement might be more important than following a specific protocol." Having said that, the authors caution (and our experience corroborates the concern) that the literature does not yet support long-term benefits seen with patient-directed (not to be confused with patient-centered, as discussed later) weaning; gentle but consistent motivational enhancement is advised.

Recommendations from the Literature

Withdrawal Symptom Palliation

As reviewed in the literature [100, 101] many of the symptoms of acute opioid withdrawal are well-controlled with the use of adjunctive pharmacotherapeutic agents (e.g., clonidine, substitution methadone or buprenorphine), alternative techniques such as auricular acupuncture, and more recently electronic/neurostimulation devices. In general, however, when psychosocial risk assessment supports a more protracted weandown, often gentle reduction over time is sufficient to obviate physical withdrawal.

Psychological withdrawal is a distinct issue, however, and increased perception of pain is one of the most widely cited obstacles. Reassurance that many studies have shown either no increase or even decrease in pain with opioid reduction (see Berna et al [99] for an excellent review) in conjunction with significant improvements in function and quality of life is very beneficial. We underscore that patient fears and nocebic responses to opioid weaning must be addressed specifically because they oppose opioid analgesia and undermine taper response [102].

Weaning Protocols

Suggested rates of opioid tapering vary widely in the scant literature and in clinical practice. Perhaps the most frequently recommended slope is to target a 10% weekly reduction in dose [39, 40], and in most situations our experience has been that physiologic withdrawal distress ranges from easily controlled to nonexistent with that gentle approach. That said, preventing nocebic responses and catastrophizing about the taper is paramount. As such, national prescription opioid tapering research has adopted the conservative approach of 5% reduction in opioid doses for the first few dose decrements, which helps patients extinguish fear about the taper and to gain confidence early in the process. These methods were applied with good success in a community-based outpatient setting wherein patients received no other intervention other than a 4-month patient-centered opioid tapering program [103]. Careful attention was directed to addressing patient fears and concerns about the taper, and the taper pace was adjusted to meet the needs of the individual. Using these methods, the researchers reported overall that patients reduced their opioid doses by about 50% over 4 months, from almost 300 daily morphine milligram equivalents (MME) to about 150 MME, with four patients achieving opioid cessation and 16 patients reducing below 90 MME in the study timeframe.

Even less guidance for preoperative-specific opioid weaning exists at present. The Johns Hopkins Health System has developed a Perioperative Pain Program focusing on the use of preoperative education including the use of perioperative multimodal analgesia (including behavioral techniques) that targets a 10%–25% reduction in opioid dose over the 4-week period preceding surgery [104]. The aforementioned study by Nguyen et al [85], showing statistically equivalent outcomes (compared to opioid naivete) for a reduction in preoperative opioid dose by at least 50% comprises the only published data at present indicating any sense of target; in our 10-week program we have found it easy and well accepted to achieve that degree of reduction for the most part, as discussed later.

Cautions and "Patient-Centered" Approaches

The recent proliferation of both advisory and regulatory-level pressure to reduce opioid consumption in the United States has resulted in significant patient distress in many situations involving COU. As noted recently by an expert group including Dr. Jane Ballantyne,

> allostatic opponent process involved in development of opioid dependence can cause worsening pain, functional status, sleep, and psychiatric symptoms over time, and significant fluctuation of pain and other affective symptoms due to their bidirectional dynamic interaction with opioid dependence ("affective dynamism"). These elements of complex persistent dependence (CPD), the gray area between simple dependence and addiction, can lead to escalating and labile opioid need, often generating aberrant behaviors. Opioid tapering, a seemingly logical intervention in this situation, may lead to worsening of pain, function, and psychiatric symptoms due to development of protracted abstinence syndrome. [105]

In other words, the complexities of dependence—whether extending into frank addiction/OUD or into the aforementioned "gray area" of CPD may render overly aggressive weaning a proposition with risks outweighing benefits in some situations—some patients may become suicidal due to increasing psychiatric destabilization and despair over increased pain experience.

As such, there is an increasing call for "patient-centered" opioid management in the context of COU, and we emphasize that guidelines and practice patterns must remain flexible to prevent increasing suffering and harms in the most vulnerable patients. Indisputably, some patients benefit from opioid therapy, and not all patients should be tapered. Mandating opioid tapering in blanket fashion across populations serves to disregard the individual considerations that constitute best practices in pain medicine.

Our Experience

Opioid reduction/abstinence in the context of COU, let alone CPD or OUD is unlikely to occur in the absence of viable and palatable alternatives to managing both pain and psychosocial distress. In our clinical experience,

> Simply removing opioids without providing effective substitute coping mechanisms will invariably lead to noncompliance and dropout. A systematic, rigorous (e.g., weekly visit) program of opioid reduction/withdrawal palliation needs to be coupled with basic preoperative counseling addressing the replacement of multifactorial "wellness-killers" (e.g., poor self-valuation and esteem, unaddressed psychopathology, poor sleep, poor nutrition, sedentary lifestyle, tobacco use) with proactive steps supporting personal responsibility for health and wellness. [42]

Just as pain is a biopsychosocial condition, we must approach opioid reduction from a biopsychosocial perspective and with proper supports in place to attend to the whole person needs, and patients' fears surrounding the destabilization of their current pain care plan.

Biopsychosocial Opioid Weaning: Resume Course

Toward that end, as introduced in the preface of the book, beginning 5 years ago at the time of this writing, we (HM) developed a systematic 12-session individualized program addressing health reclamation related to common areas of deficit associated with chronic pain and COU. Led by a health coach and embedded within a followup visit, the Resume Cours© (RC) program begins with more "somatically focused" issues met with fairly universal acceptance (e.g., sleep improvement, postural and ergonomic improvement) before proceeding to more contentious topics such as diet, exercise, and finally "psychiatric" issues such as anxiety and pain catastrophizing. At every visit, gentle encouragement for replacement of opioids with other analgesic means—most importantly via biopsychosocial lifestyle modifications—is given.

We have found (unpublished data [97]) that both weaning and discontinuation rates and success are significantly greater when attempted in this supported context: median reduction of MME in the RC group was -95% of initial, compared to -38.5% in the usual care group (Mann-Whitney $U = 2521$, Z-score 1.93, $p = 0.0268$.) Thirty percent of RC participants successfully discontinued COU compared to 15.6% in the usual care group (t-statistic 1.78, $p = 0.076$).

Of course, participation in the RC program may self-select for individuals with greater self-efficacy/internal locus of control and openness to pursuit of alternative strategies, but that has not been our anecdotal experience.

Patient-Centered Opioid Weaning: The EMPOWER Study

Our (BD) current multisite Patient-Centered Outcomes Research Institute–funded EMPOWER study (Effective Management of Pain and Opioid-Free Ways to Enhance Relief) is establishing patient-centered methods for voluntary opioid reduction in community-based settings. This randomized controlled trial is comparing usual care versus therapist-led group sessions versus peer-led group sessions in an evaluation of chronic pain management and opioid reduction. Results of the trial will be posted at https://www.pcori.org/research-results/2017/comparing-cognitive-behavioral-therapy-peer-led-support-groups-patients.

PREOP Reduction: My Surgical Success and VALERAS

As discussed in chapter 5, "My Surgical Success" is a Stanford University–owned, digital, perioperative behavioral pain medicine program developed by Dr. Beth Darnall. The refined web-based "My Surgical Success" program includes three 15-minute skills-based learning modules, a downloadable personalized plan, and a relaxation audiofile "app." An early randomized controlled clinical trial comparing "My Surgical Success" to a digital health education control group was conducted in 68 opioid-naive women undergoing surgery for breast cancer. Women who received "My Surgical Success" stopped postsurgical opioid use 5 days sooner than controls [106]. Interestingly, this intervention does not specifically guide patients to reduce opioid use, it simply provides them with self-regulatory pain management options. Second phase studies of "My Surgical Success" are currently underway in diverse patient populations at Stanford University Hospital.

Within the VALERAS program, we (HM, LF) have chosen to target a 50%–100% reduction in MME, based on the data from Nguyen et al [85], and within a 10-week period such a goal is generally easy to achieve with a minimum of physiologic withdrawal symptoms if any. The close support of weekly refocusing on other health improvements seems to bolster motivation and adherence; pilot data are not yet available.

Anecdotally we find that individuals who choose to engage in the VALERAS program bring with them a high inherent degree of motivation likely augmented by the perceptible reality of a concrete event (postoperative pain and outcome.) In some cases the surgeon may have rendered the operation contingent on opioid weaning (as well as other factors, e.g., tobacco cessation), adding to the incentive.

Enhancing Motivation and Reshaping Habit in Preoperative Opioid Weaning

Motivation and Opioid Weaning

Patient motivation in opioid weaning is obviously critical, and enhancing it (per motivational interviewing (MI) strategies/tactics—originally designed for addiction—is of the essence. The following (entirely fabricated) scenario is presented along with two disparate approaches to introducing the subject of opioid weaning with patients—one directive (and confrontational) and the other informed by MI principles.

Mr. Smith is a 53 y.o. male with a primary pain complaint of chronic low back pain with radiation of pain into the left lumbosacral region and proximal posterior thigh (and secondarily chronic right shoulder pain) both of which he attributes to a workplace injury six years ago when he was struck by a moving pallet/ forklift while he was bent over applying a delivery label to a shrink-wrapped pallet. He immediately straightened up and attempted to dive out of the closing gap between the two pallets, twisting his trunk and falling to the left, but his right leg became entangled and he experienced an immediately painful "pop" in the lumbosacral region without any immediate neurologic features.

He underwent initial workup in a local urgent care clinic that afternoon and lumbar plain films were performed, showing no fracture or misalignment. He was given a prescription of oxycodone/acetaminophen, and physical therapy was advised. Within a week he began to complain of painful paresthesias in an L5 distribution and a footdrop, and MRI showed a left L5/S1 foraminal herniation (as well as a left paramedian L4/5 bulge with annular tear) and he underwent minimally invasive microdiscectomy at left L5/S1. He reported initial improvement in symptoms but by 4 weeks postop he reported no benefit and continued to request escalating doses of opioid analgesics.

Further evaluation based on his worsening presentation included another MRI this time with gadolinium, which showed no evidence of infection but re-extrusion of further disc material into the subarticular zone and foramen on the left, and the decision was made based on his anatomy (which included significant facet arthropathy) to proceed with left L5/S1 transforaminal lumbar interbody fusion. He initially reported good improvement in both low back pain and left leg pain for roughly 9 months following this operation, but remained incapable by his estimation of performing his former work duties and within 2 years had filed for permanent disability. He has remained on chronic opioid therapy since. Other pertinent history includes self-reported "ADD" and tobacco use. He admits to "1 or 2 beers" per day.

Over the past year he has reported progressive low back pain without neurologic features, and his surgeon has offered him extension of his fusion to include the L4/5 level owing to progressive disc-osteophyte complex with central stenosis to 8 mm and facet arthropathy at that level conferring Grade I spondylolisthesis which is stable on dynamic imaging.

His surgeon has referred him to you for management of his pain postoperatively given his significant opioid consumption (oxycodone extended-release 60 mg b.i.d. with oxycodone immediate-release 1 5mg 4–6x/day.) He also uses temazepam 30 mg and zolpidem 10 mg nightly.

EXAMPLE A: DIRECTIVE APPROACH

MD: So, Mr. Smith, your surgeon wants me to prescribe narcotics for you after your operation because she's afraid you're going to need far more than she's comfortable prescribing and she's also worried you might overdose. Frankly I share her concerns, and I'm going to reduce your dose by at least 50% before your operation so you don't run into so much trouble afterward.

MR. S: What the [expletive] are you talking about? I'm barely able to get out of bed and you want to give me *less* pain pills?

MD: That's right. A colleague of mine at the University has been studying this sort of thing for several years now and the plan we use here is the same one they use there: we're going to reduce your dose by 10% per week—most of the national guidelines go by that formula.

MR. S: I don't think you understand, pal—YOU try living with this pain, and then let me see you talk about taking your own [expletive] pills away!

MD: Actually, I understand pretty well. This sort of resistance on your part is what we call a red flag for addiction. Also you should know we don't prescribe oxycodone for this sort of thing—it's the most addictive narcotic out there, and also makes people hurt worse—more than any of the other narcotics . . .

MR. S: Now you're calling me an addict? I don't have to put up with this . . .

MD: . . . and you know you need to stop smoking, too, right? Your fusion is much more likely to fail if you don't, and actually I'm surprised she even offered to operate on you again—she's usually much smarter than that . . . .

EXAMPLE B: MOTIVATIONAL
INTERVIEWING—INFLUENCED APPROACH

MD: I see you're going back to the operating room –how do you feel about that? Any specific concerns on your part?

MR. S: Yeah, it ain't something I wanna do, but I can't take this pain any more.

MD: You sure have been through a lot. I know you're what we call an "ORV— an Operation Room Veteran" but it doesn't necessarily get easier over time, does it?

MR. S: Tell me about it! I thought the first operation was bad, but I couldn't get out of bed for a month after the second one. I don't know what I'm gonna do. . . . Doc tells me I'm gonna hurt even more this time and these pain pills just ain't cuttin' it!

MD: I hear you. Would you like to know a little more about our plan for helping you get through this in the best possible shape?

MR. S: For real!

MD: OK. I hesitate to bring it up, but hopefully this analogy makes sense a bit. I see you got sideswiped by a forklift and almost got crushed to death, right? *[Patient nods and blinks a few times and flinches.]* You must have some pretty good reflexes to dodge that train! By the way—do you think about that event much these days?

MR. S: Every day. I used to be quick and strong, like you said, but it all got taken away from me when that [expletive] tried to kill me. *[MD nods.]* I think about how my life would be now—I know I could be manager by now if that didn't happen.

MD: I'm sorry. Can I say a couple things about that though? *[Patient nods.]* We have this saying in medicine, and we used to say it in the military too: "What doesn't kill me makes me stronger."

MR. S: Yeah, I heard that too. My brother was infantry—got a Purple Heart in Iraq.

MD: Sounds like your plans got sideswiped that day and you got stuck between a rock and a hard place—or a forklift and a pallet, right? *[Patient nods and grimaces.]* That's a huge setback and I'm hearing it pretty much wrecked your life, right? *[Patient nods and swears.]* I know it might not sound legitimate, but have you considered that maybe the drugs are like the pallet that the pain is pushing you into? Does that make sense? Neither one is your friend?

MR. S: I know this [expletive reference to opioids] ain't helping no more. I'm sick of feeling like I need them all the time and knowing they quit working a long time ago, but I can't stop using them. I've tried a dozen times and I get so sick and also I hurt worse. . . . I feel trapped by the pain and the pills both.

MD: I think I'm hearing you say you feel stuck between a rock and a hard place again with the pain and the pills? *[Patient nods.]* Sounds like you come from some pretty good stock. Your brother managed to get out of that battle alive and while it sounds like his life has been changed forever, he may be stronger as a person in some ways—is that accurate?

MR. S: That's what my brother keeps telling me. He's like, "Look, I lost my leg in Fallujah, and I got off the narcotics after they showed me they was keeping my brain thinking my foot was still burning." He talks about some other crazy [expletive] mirror [expletive] trick they used on him at Walter Reed too that he swears made him stop feeling his leg that got blown off. Also they gave him a new leg. He still got nightmares though.

MD: He sounds like a pretty serious warrior. I'm sure he's made a lot more sacrifices for the greater good than what little I'm hearing about. And just like you managed to get out of that death trap yourself six years ago, I'd like to show you a way out of the one you're in right now. I'm guessing you've got the same strength inside that he does if you dig deep—I'm not saying it will be easy or fun or that there won't be some pain involved . . .

MR. S: Well, I'm hurting all the time anyway—you're telling me you've got another plan?

MD: Yes. We've been doing this for several years here, based on research and similar programs around the country, and our own experience. What we've found over the past 6 years actually is that by reducing "narcotic" usage before the operation (and we switch out oxycodone for something a whole lot cleaner) if we give it a couple months to work out, we recalibrate the system in a way that makes the drugs work a whole lot better after surgery—kind of like someone cutting back from drinking a "fifth" every day. And just like that situation, we don't do things "cold-turkey" or without support. We'll help you replace your oxycodone with other ways and other skills for controlling your pain that will benefit you and work a whole lot better in the long run. Interested in hearing more?

MR. S: I don't guess I got a whole lot to lose, really by trying . . .

   [5-minute discussion about opioid-induced hyperalgesia, oxycodone in particular being the worst offender, weaning plan, etc.]

MD: Couple other things, if you don't mind talking about it just a bit—do you ever have nightmares about that forklift?

Habit and Opioid Weaning

While COU incontrovertibly includes a significant component of habit, practical implementation of habit management science related to the issue lacks any literature guidance outside the context of OUD rehabilitation programs. Borrowing from that realm, however (e.g., identification of relapse triggers), our experience has been that frank discussion of the often unrecognized component of habit, along with an in-depth exploration of reward (e.g., analgesia and/or distress relief), cues (e.g., pain and/or stress) and established routine (e.g., going to the medicine cabinet) is invaluable. Such inventory allows for what may otherwise be inaccessible opportunity to practice replacement of alternate means of alleviating or transcending the pain experience, while facilitating optimization of other factors contributing to the pain state—including OIH.

Perioperative Management of Medication-Assisted Treatment for Opioid Use Disorder

While the vast majority of patients engaging in COU are undoubtedly physically (and even psychologically) opioid-dependent, and would experience withdrawal distress on abrupt cessation, the number of patients who exhibit significant psychosocial compromises as a result of their continued use (either prescribed or illicit) and who essentially meet the traditional definition of addiction—now generally referred to as opioid use disorder (OUD)—is increasing in the Western world. Concomitantly, there has been a tremendous increase in the use of FDA-approved opioid dependence maintenance agents (methadone, buprenorphine) or antagonists (naltrexone) in the management of OUD. All of these pose significant perioperative difficulties, and weaning of maintenance agents deserves special consideration, as these patients are at elevated risk of relapse to illicit opioid use with increased risk of overdose.

Naltrexone

Naltrexone is perhaps most frequently used in the form of an intramuscular injection which exerts roughly 30 days of MOR blockade; in the context of elective surgery there is really no viable strategy other than to schedule the operation at least 30 days after the most recent injection. It should be borne in mind that the patient who has been treated for any length of time with naltrexone is no longer opioid-tolerant, but rather opioid-naive and at potentially increased risk of ORADE given what may be a cavalier attitude on the part of either the patient or providers who might use or prescribe excessive doses, respectively, based on history.

Methadone

Methadone is only legally prescribed/administered for the maintenance of addiction, or "medication-assisted treatment" (MAT) of opioid use disorder (OUD) under the auspices of a federally licensed treatment facility. It is also used frequently in chronic pain management, but rarely by non-pain-medicine specialists, and its perioperative management is not discussed in this chapter other than to highlight that weaning is typically exceptionally difficult and may increase the risk of relapse to illicit opioid use.

Buprenorphine

Buprenorphine (with or without combination naloxone coingredient) is an increasingly used outpatient MAT option with several advantages over methadone, including vastly improved safety profile. Besides the aforementioned risk of increased relapse risk with weaning/discontinuation, its perioperative management is also challenging owing to its unique pharmacology, with very long half-life and dissociation kinetics (conferring extreme tenacity at the MOR) and what has generally been thought to be partial agonist effect. Buprenorphine has often been described as an opioid receptor "blocker" when in fact it is a profoundly potent opioid agent, and in fact it is increasingly recognized that one of the main concerns related to its preoperative use—that of marked difficulty in achieving adequate postoperative analgesia—may be not so much due to receptor occupancy as simple opioid tolerance. Recent work has shown that other potent opioids such as hydromorphone and sufentanil can easily displace buprenorphine [107], and an interesting study [108] found no difference in supplemental opioid analgesic requirements among patients receiving their usual buprenorphine or methadone dosing postoperatively. Even more surprising perhaps was the finding that patients who did not receive their usual buprenorphine dose postoperatively required more opioids than those who did receive their usual dose. Furthermore, as has been noted by anyone involved in perioperative care for any length of time, it is difficult to manage pain in *any* opioid-tolerant or dependent patient regardless of the agent they are accustomed to. As per a recent suggestion in the literature [109] it is possible that buprenorphine has simply "gotten a bad rap."

Accordingly, the literature increasingly supports continuation of preoperative buprenorphine through the perioperative and postoperative phase [109–111], especially if the projected postoperative opioid requirement is low [112]. Common practice, however, also supported by the literature [111, 113, 114] is to wean to discontinuation 72 hours preoperatively. This must be evaluated carefully on a case-by-case basis, weighing the risk of relapse to illicit opioid use (with amplified overdose risk)—especially in facilities where regional anesthetic expertise is sufficient to meet almost any postoperative analgesic needs.

References

1   McAnally HB. Understanding the agent, part I: opioid biology and basic pharmacology. In McAnally HB, Opioid Dependence: A Clinical and Epidemiologic Approach (pp. 23–47). Cham, Switzerland: Springer; 2017.

2   Hollerman JR, Schultz W. Dopamine neurons report an error in the temporal prediction of reward during learning. Nature Neurosci. 1998;1:304–9.

3   Montague PR, Hyman SE, Cohen JD. Computational roles for dopamine in behavioural control. Nature. 2004;431:760–7.

4   Wise RA. Dopamine, learning and motivation. Nat Rev Neurosci. 2004;5:483–94.

5   de Wit H, Bodker B, Ambre J. Rate of increase of plasma drug level influences subjective response in humans. Psychopharmacol. 1992;107:352–8.

6   Marsch LA, Bickel WK, Badger GJ, et al. Effects of infusion rate of intravenously administered morphine on physiological, psychomotor, and self-reported measures in humans. J Pharmacol Exp Ther. 2001;299:1056–65.

7   Remillard D, Kaye AD, McAnally H. Oxycodone's unparalleled addictive potential: is it time for a moratorium? Curr Pain Headache Rep. 2019;23. https://doi.org/10.1007/s11916-019-0751-7. (E-pub ahead of print.)

8   Villesen HH, Foster DJ, Upton RN, Somogyi AA, Martinez A, Grant C. Cerebral kinetics of oxycodone in conscious sheep. J Pharm Sci. 2006;95:1666–76.

9   Boström E, Simonsson US, Hammarlund-Udenaes M. In vivo blood-brain barrier transport of oxycodone in the rat: indications for active influx and implications for pharmacokinetics/pharmacodynamics. Drug Metab Dispos. 2006;34:1624–31.

10 Boström E, Hammarlund-Udenaes M, Simonsson US. Blood-brain barrier transport helps to explain discrepancies in in vivo potency between oxycodone and morphine. Anesthesiology. 2008;108:495–505.

11 Vander Weele CM, Porter-Stransky KA, Mabrouk OS, et al. Rapid dopamine transmission within the nucleus accumbens: dramatic difference between morphine and oxycodone delivery. Eur J Neurosci. 2014;40:3041–54.

12 Cicero TJ, Ellis MS, Paradis A, Ortbal Z. Determinants of fentanyl and other potent μ opioid agonist misuse in opioid-dependent individuals. Pharmacoepidemiol Drug Saf. 2010;19:1057–63.

13 Koob GF, Volkow ND. Neurocircuitry of addiction. Neuropsychopharmacol. 2010;35:217–38.

14 Wee S, Koob GF. The role of the dynorphin-kappa opioid system in the reinforcing effects of drugs of abuse. Psychopharmacology. 2010;210:121–35.

15 Butelman ER, Yuferov V, Kreek MJ. κ-opioid receptor/dynorphin system: genetic and pharmacotherapeutic implications for addiction. Trends Neurosci. 2012;35:587–96.

16 Ruan X, Mancuso KF, Kaye AD. Revisiting oxycodone analgesia: a review and hypothesis. Anesthesiol Clin. 2017;35(2):e163–e174. doi:10.1016/j.anclin.2017.01.022.

17 Ross FB, Smith MT. The intrinsic antinociceptive effects of oxycodone appear to be kappa-opioid receptor mediated. Pain. 1997;73:151–7.

18 Nielsen CK, Ross FB, Lotfipour S, Saini KS, Edwards SR, Smith MT. Oxycodone and morphine have distinctly different pharmacological profiles: radioligand binding and behavioural studies in two rat models of neuropathic pain. Pain. 2007;132:289–300.

19 Martins SS, Fenton MC, Keyes KM, Blanco C, Zhu H, Storr CL. Mood/anxiety disorders and their association with non-medical prescription opioid use and prescription opioid use disorder: longitudinal evidence from the National Epidemiologic Study on alcohol and related conditions. Psychol Med. 2012;42:1261–72.

20 Katz C, El-Gabalawy R, Keyes KM, Martins SS, Sareen J. Risk factors for incident nonmedical prescription opioid use and abuse and dependence: results from a longitudinal nationally representative sample. Drug Alcohol Depend. 2013;132:107–13.

21 McAnally HB. Opioid dependence risk factors and risk assessment. In McAnally HB, Opioid Dependence: A Clinical and Epidemiologic Approach (pp. 233–264). Cham, Switzerland; Springer: 2017.

22 Ji RR, Berta T, Nedergaard M. Glia and pain: is chronic pain a gliopathy? Pain. 2013;154(Suppl 1):S10–28.

23 Latremoliere A, Woolf CJ. Central sensitization: a generator of pain hypersensitivity by central neural plasticity. J Pain. 2009;10:895–926.

24 Apkarian AV, Hashmi JA, Baliki MN. Pain and the brain: specificity and plasticity of the brain in clinical chronic pain. Pain. 2011;152(3 Suppl):S49–64.

25 Kuner R, Flor H. Structural plasticity and reorganisation in chronic pain. Nat Rev Neurosci. 2017;18(2):113. doi: 10.1038/nrn.2017.5.

26 Wanigasekera V, Lee MC, Rogers R, Hu P, Tracey I. Neural correlates of an injury-free model of central sensitization induced by opioid withdrawal in humans. J Neurosci. 2011;31:2835–42.

27 Younger JW, Chu LF, D'Arcy NT, Trott KE, Jastrzab LE, Mackey SC. Prescription opioid analgesics rapidly change the human brain. Pain. 2011;152:1803–10.

28 Roeckel LA, Le Coz GM, Gavériaux-Ruff C, Simonin F. Opioid-induced hyperalgesia: cellular and molecular mechanisms. Neuroscience. 2016;338: 160–82.

29 Weber L, Yeomans DC, Tzabazis A. Opioid-induced hyperalgesia in clinical anesthesia practice: what has remained from theoretical concepts and experimental studies? Curr Opin Anaesthesiol. 2017;30:458–65.

30 Scherrer JF, Salas J, Lustman PJ, Burge S, Schneider FD, Residency Research Network of Texas (RRNeT) Investigators. Change in opioid dose and change in depression in a longitudinal primary care patient cohort. Pain. 2015;156:348–55.

31 Scherrer JF, Salas J, Copeland LA, et al. Prescription opioid duration, dose, and increased risk of depression in 3 large patient populations. Ann Fam Med. 2016;14:54–62.

32 Kalso E, Edwards J, Moore R, McQuay HJ. Opioids in chronic non-cancer pain: systematic review of efficacy and safety. Pain. 2004;112:372–80.

33 Furlan A, Chaparro LE, Irvin E, Mailis-Gagnon A. A comparison between enriched and nonenriched enrollment randomized withdrawal trials of opioids for chronic noncancer pain. Pain Res Manag. 2011;16:337–51.

34 McAnally HB. Understanding the agent, part II: adverse effects. In McAnally HB, Opioid Dependence: A Clinical and Epidemiologic Approach (pp. 49–71). Cham, Switzerland: Springer; 2017.

35 Sinatra R. Causes and consequences of inadequate management of acute pain. Pain Med. 2010;11:1859–71.

36 Pak DJ, Yong RJ, Kaye AD, Urman RD. Chronification of pain: mechanisms, current understanding, and clinical implications. Curr Pain Headache Rep. 2018;22(2):9. doi: 10.1007/s11916-018-0666-8.

37 McAnally HB. Best practices education, part II: evidence for and against opioid therapy. In McAnally HB, Opioid Dependence: A Clinical and Epidemiologic Approach (pp. 149–173). Cham, Switzerland: Springer; 2017.

38 Washington Agency Medical Directors Group. Interagency Guideline on Opioid Dosing for Chronic Non-Cancer Pain. 2010. http://www.agencymedicaldirectors.wa.gov/Files/OpioidGdline.pdf

39 Dowell D, Haegerich TM, Chou R. CDC guideline for prescribing opioids for chronic pain—United States, 2016. MMWR. 2016;65:1–49.

40 Manchikanti L, Kaye AM, Knezevic NN, et al. Responsible, safe, and effective prescription of opioids for chronic non-cancer pain: American Society of Interventional Pain Physicians (ASIPP) guidelines. Pain Physician. 2017;20(2S):S3–92.

41 Tye EY, Anderson J, Faour M, et al. Prolonged preoperative opioid therapy in patients with degenerative lumbar stenosis in a workers' compensation setting. Spine (Phila Pa 1976). 2017;42(19):E1140–E1146. doi:10.1097/BRS.0000000000002112

42 McAnally HB. Rationale for and approach to preoperative opioid weaning: a preoperative optimization protocol. Perioperative Medicine. 2017;6:19. doi:10.1186/s13741-017-0079-y.

43 Wilson JL, Poulin PA, Sikorski R, et al. Opioid use among same-day surgery patients: prevalence, management and outcomes. Pain Res Management. 2015;20:300–4.

44 Chapman CR, Davis J, Donaldson GW, Naylor J, Winchester D. Postoperative pain trajectories in chronic pain patients undergoing surgery: the effects of chronic opioid pharmacotherapy on acute pain. J Pain. 2011;12:1240–6.

45 Hina N, Fletcher D, Poindessous-Jazat F, Martinez V. Hyperalgesia induced by low-dose opioid treatment before orthopaedic surgery: an observational case-control study. Eur J Anaesthesiol. 2015;32:255–61.

46 VanDenKerkhof EG, Hopman WM, Goldstein DH, et al. Impact of perioperative pain intensity, pain qualities, and opioid use on chronic pain after surgery: a prospective cohort study. Reg Anesth Pain Med. 2012;37:19–27.

47 Armaghani SJ, Lee DS, Bible JE, et al. Preoperative opioid use and its association with perioperative opioid demand and postoperative opioid independence in patients undergoing spine surgery. Spine (Phila Pa 1976). 2014;39(25):E1524–30. https://doi.org/10.1097/BRS. 0000000000000622

48 Hah JM, Sharifzadeh Y, Wang BM, et al. Factors associated with opioid use in a cohort of patients presenting for surgery. Pain Res Treat. 2015;2015:1–8. https://doi.org/10.1155/2015/829696

49 Rapp SE, Ready LB, Nessly ML. Acute pain management in patients with prior opioid consumption: a case-controlled retrospective review. Pain. 1995;61:195–201.

50 Pivec R, Issa K, Naziri Q, Kapadia BH, Bonutti PM, Mont MA. Opioid use prior to total hip arthroplasty leads to worse clinical outcomes. Int Orthop. 2014;38:1159–65.

51 Hoofwijk DM, Fiddelers AA, Emans PJ, et al. Prevalence and predictive factors of chronic postsurgical pain and global surgical recovery 1 year after outpatient knee arthroscopy: a prospective cohort study. Medicine (Baltimore). 2015;94(45):e2017. doi:10.1097/MD.0000000000002017.

52 Martinez V, Üçeyler N, Ben Ammar S, et al. Clinical, histological, and biochemical predictors of postsurgical neuropathic pain. Pain. 2015;156:2390–8.

53 Sing DC, Barry JJ, Cheah JW, Vail TP, Hansen EN. Long-acting opioid use independently predicts perioperative complication in total joint arthroplasty. J Arthroplast. 2016;31(9 Suppl):170–4.

54 Cheah JW, Sing DC, McLaughlin D, Feeley BT, Ma CB, Zhang AL. The perioperative effects of chronic preoperative opioid use on shoulder arthroplasty outcomes. J Shoulder Elb Surg. 2017;26(11):1908–14. doi:10.1016/j.jse.2017.05.016

55 Shanmugam VK, Fernandez S, Evans KK, et al. Postoperative wound dehiscence: predictors and associations. Wound Repair Regen. 2015;23:184–90.

56 Sacerdote P. Opioid-induced immunosuppression. Curr Opin Support Palliat Care. 2008;2(1):14–18. doi: 10.1097/SPC.0b013e3282f5272e.

57 Plein LM, Rittner HL. Opioids and the immune system—friend or foe. Br J Pharmacol. 2018;175:2717–25.

58 Hutchinson MR, Shavit Y, Grace PM, Rice KC, Maier SF, Watkins LR. Exploring the neuroimmunopharmacology of opioids: an integrative review of mechanisms of central immune signaling and their implications for opioid analgesia. Pharmacol Rev. 2011;63:772–810.

59 Gessi S, Borea PA, Bencivenni S, Fazzi D, Varani K, Merighi S. The activation of μ-opioid receptor potentiates LPS-induced NF-kB promoting an inflammatory phenotype in microglia. FEBS Lett. 2016;590:2813–26.

60 Eidson LN, Inoue K, Young LJ, Tansey MG, Murphy AZ. Toll-like receptor 4 mediates morphine-induced neuroinflammation and tolerance via soluble tumor necrosis factor signaling. Neuropsychopharmacology. 2017;42:661–70.

61 Serhan CN, Chiang N. Novel endogenous small molecules as the checkpoint controllers in inflammation and resolution: entrée for resoleomics. Rheum Dis Clin North Am. 2004;30:69–95.

62 Lam CF, Chang PJ, Huang YS, et al. Prolonged use of high-dose morphine impairs angiogenesis and mobilization of endothelial progenitor cells in mice. Anesth Analg. 2008;107:686–92.

63 Rook JM, Hasan W, Mccarson KE. Morphine-induced early delays in wound closure: involvement of sensory neuropeptides and modification of neurokinin receptor expression. Biochem Pharmacol. 2009;77:1747–55.

64 Martin JL, Koodie L, Krishnan AG, Charboneau R, Barke RA, Roy S. Chronic morphine administration delays wound healing by inhibiting immune cell recruitment to the wound site. Am J Pathol. 2010;176:786–99.

65 Martin JL, Charboneau R, Barke RA, Roy S. Chronic morphine treatment inhibits LPS induced angiogenesis: implications in wound healing. Cell Immunol. 2010;265:139–45.

66 Rittner HL, Roewer N, Brack A. The clinical (ir)relevance of opioid-induced immune suppression. Curr Opin Anaesthesiol. 2010;23:588–92.

67 Menendez ME, Ring D, Bateman BT. Preoperative opioid misuse is associated with increased morbidity and mortality after elective orthopaedic surgery. Clin Orthop Relat Res. 2015;473:2402–12.

68 Cron DC, Englesbe MJ, Bolton CJ, et al. Preoperative opioid use is independently associated with increased costs and worse outcomes after major abdominal surgery. Ann Surg. 2017;265:695–701.

69 Zywiel MG, Stroh DA, Lee SY, Bonutti PM, Mont MA. Chronic opioid use prior to total knee arthroplasty. J Bone Joint Surg Am. 2011;93:1988–93.

70 Morris BJ, Laughlin MS, Elkousy HA, Gartsman GM, Edwards TB. Preoperative opioid use and outcomes after reverse shoulder arthroplasty. J Shoulder Elb Surg. 2015;24:11–6.

71 Morris BJ, Sciascia AD, Jacobs CA, Edwards TB. Preoperative opioid use associated with worse outcomes after anatomic shoulder arthroplasty. J Shoulder Elb Surg. 2016;25:619–23.

72 Ben-Ari A, Chansky H, Rozet I. Preoperative opioid use is associated with early revision after total knee arthroplasty: a study of male patients treated in the Veterans Affairs system. J Bone Joint Surg Am. 2017;99:1–9.

73 Bell KL, Shohat N, Goswami K, Tan TL, Kalbian I, Parvizi J. Preoperative opioids increase the risk of periprosthetic joint infection after total joint arthroplasty. J Arthroplasty. 2018;33:3246–51.

74 Waljee JF, Cron DC, Steiger RM, Zhong L, Englesbe MJ, Brummett CM. Effect of preoperative opioid exposure on healthcare utilization and expenditures following elective abdominal surgery. Ann Surg. 2017; 265:715–21.

75 Rozell JC, Courtney PM, Dattilo JR, Wu CH, Lee GC. Preoperative opiate use independently predicts narcotic consumption and complications after total joint arthroplasty. J Arthroplasty. 2017; 32:2658–62.

76 Gupta A, Nizamuddin J, Elmofty D, et al. Opioid abuse or dependence increases 30-day readmission rates after major operating room procedures: a national readmissions database study. Anesthesiology. February 22, 2018. doi: 10.1097/ALN.0000000000002136. [Epub ahead of print] PubMed PMID: 29470180.

77 Lentine KL, Lam NN, Schnitzler MA, et al. Predonation Prescription Opioid Use: A Novel Risk Factor for Readmission After Living Kidney Donation. Am J Transplant. 2017;17:744–53.

78 Jain N, Phillips FM, Weaver T, Khan SN. Pre-operative chronic opioid therapy: a risk factor for complications, readmission, continued opioid use and increased costs after one- and two-level posterior lumbar fusion. Spine (Phila Pa 1976). March 20, 2018. doi: 10.1097/BRS.0000000000002609. [Epub ahead of print] PubMed PMID: 29561298.

79 Raebel MA, Newcomer SR, Reifler LM, et al. Chronic use of opioid medications before and after bariatric surgery. JAMA. 2013;310:1369–76.

80 Zarling BJ, Yokhana SS, Herzog DT, Markel DC. Preoperative and postoperative opiate use by the arthroplasty patient. J Arthroplast. 2016;31:2081–4.

81 Deyo RA, Hallvik SE, Hildebran C, Marino M, Dexter E, Irvine JM, et al. Association between initial opioid prescribing patterns and subsequent long-term use among opioid-naïve patients: a statewide retrospective cohort study. J Gen Intern Med. 2017; 32:21–7.

82 Brat GA, Agniel D, Beam A, et al. Postsurgical prescriptions for opioid naive patients and association with overdose and misuse: retrospective cohort study. BMJ. 2018;360:j5790. doi: 10.1136/bmj.j5790.

83 Lawrence JT, London N, Bohlman HH, Chin KR. Preoperative narcotic use as a predictor of clinical outcome: results following anterior cervical arthrodesis. Spine (Phila Pa 1976). 2008a;(33):2074–8.

84 Anderson PA, Subach BR, Riew KD. Predictors of outcome after anterior cervical discectomy and fusion: a multivariate analysis. Spine (Phila Pa 1976). 2009;34:161–6.

85 Nguyen LC, Sing DC, Bozic KJ. Preoperative reduction of opioid use before total joint arthroplasty. J Arthroplast. 2016;31(9 Suppl):282–7.

86 Faour M, Anderson JT, Haas AR, et al. Neck pain, preoperative opioids, and functionality after cervical fusion. Orthopedics. 2017;40:25–32.

87 Villavicencio AT, Nelson EL, Kantha V, Burneikiene S. Prediction based on preoperative opioid use of clinical outcomes after transforaminal lumbar interbody fusions. J Neurosurg Spine. 2017;26:144–9.

88 Lerman SF, Rudich Z, Brill S, Shalev H, Shahar G. Longitudinal associations between depression, anxiety, pain, and pain-related disability in chronic pain patients. Psychosom Med. 2015;77:333–41.

89 Strøm J, Bjerrum MB, Nielsen CV, et al. Anxiety and depression in spine surgery-a systematic integrative review. Spine J. 2018;18:1272–85.

90 Huffman KL, Sweis GW, Gase A, Scheman J, Covington EC. Opioid use 12 months following interdisciplinary pain rehabilitation with weaning. Pain Med. 2013;14:1908–17.

91 Cunningham JL, Evans MM, King SM, Gehin JM, Loukianova LL. Opioid tapering in fibromyalgia patients: experience from an interdisciplinary pain rehabilitation program. Pain Med. 2016;17:1676–85.

92 Zhou K, Jia P, Bhargava S, Zhang Y, Reza T, Peng YB, Wang GG. Opioid tapering in patients with prescription opioid use disorder: a retrospective study. Scand J Pain. 2017;17:167–73.

93 Hundley L, Spradley S, Donelenko S. Assessment of outcomes following high-dose opioid tapering in a Veterans Healthcare System. J Opioid Manag. 2018;14:89–101.

94 Frank JW, Lovejoy TI, Becker WC, et al. Patient outcomes in dose reduction or discontinuation of long-term opioid therapy: a systematic review. Ann Intern Med. 2017;167:181–91.

95 Kurita GP, Højsted J, Sjøgren P. Tapering off long-term opioid therapy in chronic non-cancer pain patients: A randomized clinical trial. Eur J Pain. May 13, 2018. doi: 10.1002/ejp.1241. [Epub ahead of print] PubMed PMID: 29754428.

96 Westanmo A, Marshall P, Jones E, Burns K, Krebs EE. Opioid dose reduction in a VA health care system—implementation of a primary care population-level initiative. Pain Med. 2015;16:1019–26.

97 McAnally HB. How to Wean Friends and Influence Patients: Biopsychosocial-Spiritual Opioid Replacement. (In submission.)

98 Eccleston C, Fisher E, Thomas KH, et al. Interventions for the reduction of prescribed opioid use in chronic non-cancer pain. Cochrane Database Syst Rev. 2017;11:CD010323. doi:10.1002/14651858.CD010323.pub3.

99 Berna C, Kulich RJ, Rathmell JP. Tapering long-term opioid therapy in chronic noncancer pain: evidence and recommendations for everyday practice. Mayo Clin Proc. 2015;90:828–42.

100 Gowing LR, Ali RL, White JM. The management of opioid withdrawal. Drug Alcohol Rev. 2000;19:309–18.

101 Plunkett A, Kuehn D, Lenart M, Wilkinson I. Opioid maintenance, weaning and detoxification techniques: where we have been, where we are now and what the future holds. Pain Manag. 2013;3:277–84.

102 Darnall BD, Colloca L. Optimizing placebo and minimizing nocebo to reduce pain, catastrophizing, and opioid use: a review of the science and an evidence-informed clinical toolkit. Int Rev Neurobiol. 2018;139:129–57.

103 Darnall BD, Ziadni MS, Stieg RL, Mackey IG, Kao MC, Flood P. Patient-centered prescription opioid tapering in community outpatients with chronic pain. JAMA Intern Med. 2018;178:707–8.
104 Hanna MN, Speed TJ, Shechter R, et al. An innovative perioperative pain program for chronic opioid users: an academic medical center's response to the opioid crisis. Am J Med Qual. 2019 Jan/Feb;34(1):5–13. doi:10.1177/1062860618777298.
105 Manhapra A, Arias AJ, Ballantyne JC. The conundrum of opioid tapering in long-term opioid therapy for chronic pain: A commentary. Subst Abus. 2018;39(2):152–61. doi:10.1080/08897077.2017.1381663.
106 Darnall BD, Ziadni MS, Krishnamurthy P, et al. "My Surgical Success": Impact of a digital behavioral pain medicine intervention on time to opioid cessation after breast cancer surgery. Pain Med. 2019 May 13. pii: pnz094. doi:10.1093/pm/pnz094. PMID: 31087093.
107 Volpe DA, McMahon Tobin GA, et al. Uniform assessment and ranking of opioid μ receptor binding constants for selected opioid drugs. Regul Toxicol Pharmacol. 2011;59:385–90.
108 Macintyre PE, Russell RA, Usher KA, Gaughwin M, Huxtable CA. Pain relief and opioid requirements in the first 24 hours after surgery in patients taking buprenorphine and methadone opioid substitution therapy. Anaesth Intensive Care. 2013;41:222–30.
109 Silva MJ, Rubinstein A. Continuous Perioperative Sublingual Buprenorphine. J Pain Palliat Care Pharmacother. 2016;30:289–93.
110 Childers JW, Arnold RM. Treatment of pain in patients taking buprenorphine for opioid addiction #221. J Palliat Med. 2012;15:613–14.
111 Sen S, Arulkumar S, Cornett EM, et al. New pain management options for the surgical patient on methadone and buprenorphine. Curr Pain Headache Rep. 2016;20(3):16. doi: 10.1007/s11916-016-0549-9.
112 Jonan AB, Kaye AD, Urman RD. Buprenorphine formulations: clinical best practice strategies recommendations for perioperative management of patients undergoing surgical or interventional pain procedures. Pain Physician. 2018;21(1):E1–E12.
113 Bryson EO. The perioperative management of patients maintained on medications used to manage opioid addiction. Curr Opin Anaesthesiol. 2014;27:359–64.
114 Wenzel JT, Schwenk ES, Baratta JL, Viscusi ER. Managing opioid-tolerant patients in the perioperative surgical home. Anesthesiol Clin. 2016;34:287–301.

11

Putting It All Together

Heath B. McAnally, Lyn Freeman, and Beth Darnall

A Preoperative Optimization Plan

Recruitment

While we believe that all patients suffering with chronic pain can benefit from adaptive lifestyle modifications, and that operative outcomes would be improved by such efforts, many patients exhibit varying degrees of resistance (or conversely readiness to change), and intrinsic motivation may be lacking.

System-level changes, beginning with the surgeon are often necessary to provide extrinsic motivation for perioperative health behavioral change. The majority of surgeons favor and encourage such efforts and we've found (see discussion later) that most are more than willing to support and facilitate elective operative delay in order to optimize their patients. As such, we've chosen to target the surgeon and other physician population primarily in terms of program exposure and marketing; without complete perioperative team buy-in the effort doesn't work. Recruitment of patients for the program generally begins in the surgeon's office, although existing pain management practices will certainly contain an appropriate sample.

Motivation

As discussed in chapter 3 at some length, motivation is the heart and soul of preoperative optimization. Education rendering positive health outcomes more salient, and negative consequences of neglect/poor choices more recognizable are a necessary component of such motivation, yet are frequently insufficient to effect change. Per the health belief model (Figure 3.3) perceived threat (a function of both perceived severity and susceptibility) is only one axis of action stimulation, with perceived benefit:barrier ratio and self-efficacy level providing either significant inertia or catalyst.

In the context of limited energy/effort resources (typically especially compromised in the chronic pain state) even a clear understanding of the benefits of change versus the consequences of failure to do so may fail to elevate the pursuit of health in the individual's overall hierarchy of needs. One tactic that has proven effective in facilitating behavioral change is to emphasize the impact of action or lack thereof on others [1]. This phenomenon finds theoretical support in the concept of relatedness as one of the triumvirate of factors undergirding intrinsic motivation (along with autonomy and competence) in Ryan and Deci's self-determination theory [2]. Along those lines, both relatedness and competence may be enhanced and harnessed by encouraging the patient's sense of a supportive community, beginning with the preoperative teams involved.

Finally, while application of extrinsic motivation may not find universal or even general acceptance among many behavioral health theorists and practitioners, the reality of the opportunity for leverage, frankly, conferred by the perioperative period must not be overlooked. It is more frequently construed as "a teachable moment," and surgeons have for decades withheld elective operation for patients who continue to smoke or have dangerously elevated body mass index, and so forth, and it must not be forgotten that elective surgery is exactly that. It may be necessary to remind patients that our first duty is to do no harm, and that proceeding with a nonurgent operation in the face of poor health status (whether that be nonoptimized cardiac disease or chronic pain) is contradictory to that directive.

Goal Setting and Implementation

While we'd like to think in terms of progressing from motivation to habit formation, the realities of our time constraints generally hamper solid habit formation, which seem to require at least 2 months of solid and dedicated activity to cement (see chapter 4). That's not to say we don't discuss habits at great length—especially the critical concept of replacing deleterious habits with beneficial ones (which forms the practical backbone of the program). Habit change (or simple formation), however, is inconvenient and requires considerable expenditure of resources, and the repetition required to form habits requires goal-setting, planning, and anticipating obstacles/forming contingency plans in order to reliably occur.

Goals
Human beings need goals to attempt and to achieve when action is not instinctively nor habitually directed. Goal-setting is a "fundamental component of successful interventions" [3] and the meta-analysis of 141 investigations ($n = 16,523$)

from which that quote is taken revealed that effectiveness is increased when the goal is difficult, formulated as a group goal, set both face to face and publicly, and subject to external monitoring. In our preoperative optimization program, these conditions are readily met (we emphasize the concept of participating in a team activity along with program staff as well as other patients).

Framing goals in terms of positive outcome (e.g., "I will develop the habit of eating healthy food") rather than solely negative ones (e.g., "I will stop eating junk food"), and anticipating specific benchmarks for success (e.g., "I'm looking forward to feeling better about myself, and dropping 2 pounds this month") are also beneficial.

We also support/employ the widely utilized SMART (Specific, Measurable, Achievable, Relevant, Timed) goal-setting construct [4]. The foci and confines of our program direct the specifics and timing of the goals set for the most part (e.g., opioid weaning target, tobacco cessation, specific dietary and sleep and activity modifications) with individual fine-tuning to ensure achievability.

Implementation Intention

Crafting a solid plan is essential in any new endeavor—the old adage "failure to plan is a plan for failure" is as true in health behavior change as it is in business or government. "I will exercise three days a week!" doesn't help improve activity if one doesn't form a concrete mental representation and provide for the physical necessities (e.g., tennis shoes, a bicycle, swimming pool pass). Discrete and simple initial steps for change (e.g., "I will purchase a YMCA membership and go there before work on Mondays, Wednesdays and Fridays") are necessary for success.

Implementation intention [5] describes the critical link in translation of goal into goal-directed behavior, and may be defined loosely as a plan specifying action triggers and means. The practical application of implementation intention revolves around constructing, rehearsing (forming a mental representation), and executing "if-then" plans; an example being "When I feel anxious and crave a cigarette, I will call my QuitCoach." A more complex preventive implementation intention identifying potential obstacles and circumvention might be "If I shop when I'm really hungry or tired I may break down and put things in the shopping cart I don't really want. So I need to not shop when I'm hungry or tired; I will shop on Saturday morning after I've eaten 2 eggs and some fruit, and watched a healthy cooking show on TV first."

A priori identification of the various and sundry temptations to relapse into suboptimal behaviors (e.g., driving by fast food restaurants, encountering others smoking) is critical for success; not least of these is the tremendous distraction and suffering that pain itself confers. Formulating specific implementation intentions addressing pain flare-ups is essential ("When my back starts hurting badly, I'm not going to reflexively go to the pill cabinet. I'm going to lay down on a heating pad for 10 or 15 minutes while I listen to my relaxation CD, and then I'm going to go for a gentle 20 minute walk.")

One of the main goals of motivational interviewing (see chapter 3 for more detail) is eliciting "change talk," whereby the individual expresses their own intent (and ideally rationale) for behavioral change; the experience of hearing oneself vocalize such intent is a powerful predictor of change, and incorporating implementation intentions into the process improves the odds even further [6].

Priming

Priming of behavioral responses may be accomplished by the use of prompts—simple and (ideally) temporary antecedent cues such as putting jogging shoes in plain view at the front door, or putting the fish oil capsule bottle in front of the alarm clock. Incorporation of the desired behavior into existing daily rituals may also be useful, for example, placing an exercise bicycle in front of the television and not allowing oneself to indulge in viewing without pedaling, or implementing a daily 20- to 30-minute walk into a lunch break.

Habit-Breaking

Eliminating maladaptive habits is a fundamental task undergirding this effort. Two basic principles that find ready practical application are:

- Bad habits generally can't simply be removed—they need to be replaced with good ones, and,
- Disrupting the established cue/routine is essential for habit-breaking. For example, if driving by a particular convenience store or fast food restaurant always triggers junk food consumption, altering the normal route is advisable.

Practical Program Issues

Time Requirements

We (HM, LF) have organized a 10-week preoperative optimization course (VALERAS) with weekly visits (see Figure 11.1). The duration of the course is informed by a synthesis of time requirements necessary to reliably achieve the various health goals outlined throughout this book, for example, opioid weaning, adequate tobacco-free state, prehabilitation. The weekly interval provides consistency of encouragement/external reinforcement and facilitates opioid weaning, the practicalities of which are increasingly complicated given various state government regulations, and so forth.

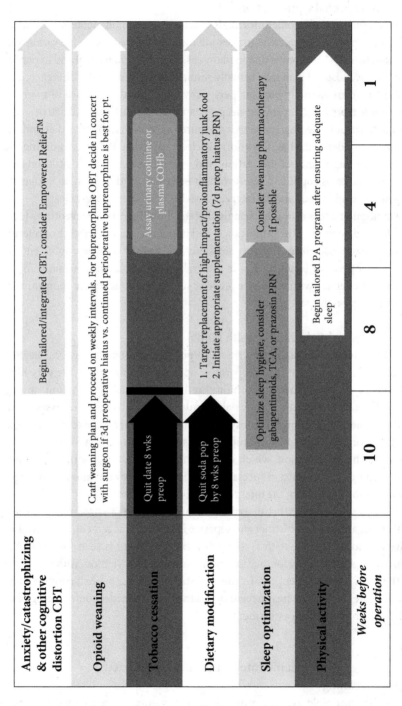

	Weeks before operation			
	10	**8**	**4**	**1**

Figure 11.1. Overview of the VALERAS Preoperative Optimization Program

Multidimensional Optimization

While the argument is sometimes made that too many simultaneous health intervention attempts may overwhelm the individual, both anecdotal observation and the literature [7–11] support that in many cases a multidimensional and in particular, biopsychosocial plan may actually result in improved effort, adherence, and outcome. From a strictly biologic perspective, the interdependence of many of these endeavors (e.g., improving sleep often requires more physical activity, and adequate/sustainable physical activity requires adequate sleep; poor diet and tobacco use hinder both) helps to inform such an approach. When considering the paramount importance of motivation, and overcoming cognitive distortions including pain catastrophizing, fear-avoidant behaviors, and so forth, the exigency of conjoined and simultaneous interventions becomes increasingly clear.

Economic factors also increasingly dictate "bundling" of interventions [12]. While not discounting the importance, and in many cases advisability of referral to specialized disciplines (e.g., physical therapy, dietary services), sufficient focused preoperative optimization is generally achievable and certainly much more cost-effective within a single practice setting, given adequate commitment and training on the part of staff.

Shared Medical-Behavioral Health Model

We do, however, maintain the critical importance of joint behavioral health/ medical management of the preoperative optimization program. The very high prevalence of psychiatric comorbidity and psychosocial dysfunction among individuals suffering with chronic pain requires expert psychological assessment and treatment if meaningful biopsychosocial improvements are to be achieved. Furthermore, as highlighted throughout this book, both motivational enhancement and habit formation, which clearly find their most appropriate guidance and support in the context of specialty behavioral health evaluation and management, are the key to all of the interventions discussed herein.

Various solutions for this shared model are of course possible, ranging from within-organization to distinct and separate entity comanagement; we (HM, LF) have developed a tele-health system whereby the patient is seen weekly in the pain management clinic for medical evaluation and intervention, with half (five) of the visits conducted entirely by medical staff, and the other half conducted by the (off-site) behavioral health team over a live-Internet videoconferencing platform after brief medical assessment.

Specific Interventions Summarized

Opioid Weaning

[Note that the opioid weaning protocol and commentary here are specific to Drs. McAnally and Freeman's VALERAS program.]

Although opioid reduction is likely not the most important factor, we address it nonetheless immediately at our initial visit. Clinical experience supports the association between long-term opioid use and helplessness/lack of self-efficacy, and these factors may impede engagement not only in voluntary opioid weaning but also in other health improvement efforts. A tremendous amount of resistance is invariably encountered, generally disproportionate to withdrawal symptoms, and it takes a great deal of time and attention directed toward education, motivational enhancement, encouragement and support, and so forth, to overcome these barriers.

While complete opioid cessation is ideal, in many cases it is not realistic. Every situation is unique, in our experience complicated more by psychological factors than somatic pathology in most cases. Given that a 50% reduction in preoperative opioid use seems to confer benefit equivalent to an opioid-independent state [13], it is often more realistic to target that endpoint, and many patients find that far easier to accept/less intimidating and paralyzing. Regardless of the individual goal and trajectory, adequate time for weaning is certainly beneficial, and the 10-week structure we've adopted for the VALERAS program seems to facilitate these efforts adequately.

In all cases a graduated and consistent weaning of opioid dose is planned out a priori with a visual roadmap provided to the patient (and revisited at every encounter.) As a matter of practicality we provide a 7-day prescription on a weekly basis. Not all prescription opioids lend themselves easily to 5% or 10% dose reductions on a daily basis; some creativity is generally required. Toward that end, we often find it more beneficial to target a weekly rather than daily total dose reduction. Rationing out opioids at the new weekly reduced baseline (e.g., 10% decrement for the week) will often disrupt the habit of regularly scheduled dosing (frequently advised by practitioners to "stay ahead of the pain"). In our clinical experience over the past several years, this approach of titrating to effect (e.g., withholding a habituated dose on nonexercise days while facilitating exercise with an analgesic dose on training days) provides tremendous empowerment to patients who have become conditioned and dependent.

Multimodal pain management is of the essence in preoperative optimization, as it is in general; a biopsychosocial-spiritual approach is required. From the biologic axis alone, prevention (e.g., sleep optimization, dietary, postural, and exercise improvements), and diversification of analgesia (alternate pharmacotherapeutics, modalities of temperature, topical approaches including transcutaneous electrical nerve stimulation) are of the essence. You can't just take opioids away from someone who's dependent on them; they need to be replaced with something better.

A specific word about oxycodone is in order here; our practice, based on experience and the literature is to discontinue that drug immediately, transitioning to an alternate agent. Oxycodone is by many metrics the most addictive prescription opioid [14], and in our experience also predisposes more strongly to opioid-induced hyperalgesia than any other prescription agent. These phenomena appear to result from both disproportionately high active transport and sequestering across the blood-brain barrier with markedly increased striatal dopaminergic activity attesting to its hedonic reward activity, and also disproportionately increased kappa receptor–mediated withdrawal dysphoria and distress driving pursuit of more oxycodone.

Finally, perioperative management of opioids used in medication-assisted treatment (MAT) of opioid use disorder requires consideration of multiple factors (relapse and overdose risk, legal issues) and early and frequent communication with the surgeon and behavioral health providers. These issues are addressed in somewhat greater detail in chapter 10.

Tobacco Cessation

Four weeks of tobacco cessation is good, but five or six is even better, and the literature seems to indicate that 8 weeks of tobacco cessation is optimal (see chapter 9), so we address this issue early as well.

Whenever nicotine replacement therapy (NRT) is acceptable to both patient and surgeon we administer it. Other MAT (e.g., bupropion or varenicline) is often beneficial, but harm:benefit ratio needs to be carefully assessed of course in every situation. Behavioral counseling (see some examples of tips in chapter 9) is frequently invaluable in helping patients overcome habituated routines of procurement and practice.

We currently employ urinary cotinine assays for compliance monitoring (with the understanding that specificity is poor, as NRT yields positive results. We have not found exhaled carbon monoxide testing to be practical at present given the cost of the equipment balanced against lack of payer reimbursement in our environment; in rare cases we will order serum carboxyhemoglobin if NRT is confounding.

Sleep

Adequate sleep duration and architecture are critical for psychological and physical health and pain management, as discussed in chapter 6. The importance of sleep is magnified when introducing or increasing exercise, which causes tissue microtrauma and damage requiring sufficient restorative sleep and especially slow-wave sleep (SWS) quotient, when reparative mediators (e.g., human growth hormone, insulin-like growth factor 1) are released. On the other hand, healthy sleep is facilitated by and in some cases dependent on adequate exercise.

A careful assessment of both domains must precede a tailored prescription for exercise (discussed in what follows), and thorough investigation of sleep hygiene is necessary. While elimination of afternoon/evening stimulants and other poor habits (volitionally staying awake, watching TV in bed, etc.) in concert with institution of good sleep hygiene practice and a gentle exercise regimen may be sufficient, in many cases we choose to temporarily add or augment existing pharmacotherapy to facilitate SWS. Gabapentinoids or low-dose tricyclic antidepressants have a reasonable risk:benefit ratio and support SWS, in contradistinction to sedative-hypnotics, which favor alpha-wave/superficial sleep planes at the expense of SWS and are also highly addictive.

Diet Plan

As discussed in chapter 8, we focus preoperative dietary intervention on a few key areas, foregoing detailed education regarding specific macro- and micronutrients unless the patient is uniquely interested and motivated. We limit our efforts to discussing:

- Basic principles of caloric intake optimization and macronutrient proportioning (e.g., using the USDA MyPlate template (https://www.choosemyplate.gov/).
- Basic concepts of proinflammatory dietary choices and their contribution to chronic pain.
- Limitation/elimination of processed/convenience foods and simple sugars, especially soda pop/soft drinks, other sweetened beverages, and high-calorie/pro-inflammatory snacks including pastries and chips.
- Supplementation with a multivitamin, additional magnesium (avoiding carbonate, chloride, gluconate, and oxide anions due to increased risk of gastrointestinal upset), and ω-3 polyunsaturated fatty acids.
- Supplementation with curcumin (1,000–2,000mg/day) + piperine; discontinue 7 days preoperatively.
- For anticipated major surgery, supplementation with arginine 5–10 g/day beginning 7–14 days preoperatively (available very economically as a bulk powder).

Beyond such simple information transfer, we have found that the application of two overarching principles is required for effective nutritional optimization: the first is substitution of achievable and palatable healthy alternatives for habituated patterns (e.g., substitution of frozen berries and nonsweetened yogurt for desserts, or nuts for potato chips) and the second has to do with purchasing patterns and preparation.

Two points of vulnerability to poor dietary choices exist for most people; the first is snacking or eating outside the home (e.g., purchasing junk food from vending machines or fast food restaurants) and the second is the domestic pantry and refrigeration/freezer system. Both need to be adequately assessed and discussed (with repetitive evaluation and feedback) and we provide education and a plan for:

- Weekly grocery shopping that ensures healthy/well-balanced nutritional needs with sufficient diversity to reward efforts, and
- Healthy eating patterns throughout the day that not only provide necessary nutrition but also reduce the risk of poor snacking choices.

We employ a simple but attractive handout and documentation/log system to remind and track adherence to these principles as well as specific micronutrient/supplementation instruction on a scheduled basis.

As discussed in chapter 8, we do not routinely address specific issues of overweight/obesity status; however, when we do, a comprehensive assessment and plan evaluating sleep disorders including but not limited to obstructive sleep apnea, nutritional and physical activity, and psychosocial factors is used.

Exercise

The literature shows that even 4 weeks of physical "prehabilitation" is beneficial (see chapter 7). We aim to begin sooner (e.g., 6 to 8 weeks preoperatively) if possible, due to the additive benefits and for the sake of pain management and the facilitation of habit formation. However, as discussed previously, we don't allow initiation of moderate-intensity exercise if the patient is sleep-deprived (with the understanding of the "Catch-22" that sleep often doesn't improve until adequate exercise becomes regular). Furthermore, in the context of chronic pain syndromes, which are often associated with physical limitations and even more frequently kinesiophobia and fear-avoidant behaviors, a slow, gentle, and tailored approach is required. Our philosophy is that while improvements in cardiopulmonary and musculoskeletal fitness are important, improvements in confidence and self-efficacy are far more important among the chronic pain population, and sacrificing some (or much) physical improvement potential for the sake of developing/improving biopsychosocial self-management capacity is strategically sound.

Anxiety/Catastrophizing

As discussed in chapter 5, presurgical anxiety and pain catastrophizing are powerful prognostic indicators for surgical outcomes, including both acute and chronic postsurgical pain, opioid use, and functional recovery. These psychological factors must be assessed prior to surgery, yet remain rarely addressed.

In general, the literature suggests that pain catastrophizing has the highest predictive value, and as such a validated catastrophizing scale (such as those suggested in chapter 5, Table 5.1) should be administered. (The term "pain catastrophizing" is both polarizing and stigmatizing, and it is recommended that healthcare providers discuss the issue with patients using patient-friendly terms, for example, "Your nervous system is doing a good job of trying to protect you, but in the long run that's not helpful for your pain. Humans aren't born knowing how to calm their nervous system, but you can learn to use skills that will help you be more in control of how your pain condition impacts you"). The initial assessment is a rich opportunity to foster engagement in behavioral pain management—a powerful tool to help patients stay more comfortable after surgery with less medication. Chapter 5, Table 5.1 provides a clinical toolkit for healthcare clinicians to use with patients, addressing key components of this assessment including validation of the patient's complaint(s), which is of course vital to establishing rapport and buy-in.

In the VALERAS program, anxiety and catastrophizing are addressed by first assessing patient complaints, fears, and pain perception with the Brief Battery for Health Improvement (BBHI2) and its extended report. This instrument, created specifically for a population suffering with chronic pain, identifies key areas of anxiety and depression as well as pain location and severity. Patient defensiveness is also assessed; together these data give the therapist a "jump start" on what to target in terms of cognitive and functional barriers in the limited time available.

Pain-CBT (cognitive-behavioral therapy for pain) remains the "gold-standard" treatment option for pain-related anxiety and pain catastrophizing, though admittedly, access to this treatment remains poor. Chapter 5, Table 5.1 provides a clinical toolkit for healthcare clinicians to use with patients, including patient resources that may be integrated right away, even in clinics that have no behavioral therapists on staff. Additional scalable resources could include the integration of a single-session, 2-hour pain class into your clinical care pathways, such as Empowered Relief, which allows for increased efficiency by simultaneously treating several patients at once.

Digital/online behavioral pain medicine is the future of expanded access to pain care in the perioperative care pathway. Patients may access such digital/online behavioral pain medicine at home or in the hospital after surgery. While not yet publicly available, My Surgical Success has demonstrated promise as an accessible, low-cost, scalable way to help patients enhance self-regulation skills and reduce catastrophizing. Early research conducted by Dr. Beth Darnall and colleagues has shown that the fully automated, online intervention is associated with reduced time to opioid cessation after surgery relative to controls [15], and Phase II studies are underway at Stanford University. We expect My Surgical Success to be widely available in 2020.

In the VALERAS program (Figure 11.1), depending on patient interest and commitment, a series of anxiety-reducing strategies may be chosen for the individualized plan, including neuroplastic perceptual change education on the "negativity bias" of the brain and how to compete against that bias by using any of the following:

- "Savoring the Good" exercises.
  - Gratitude and appreciation strategies.
  - ANTS (automatic negative thoughts stomping) reduction exercises.
  - Purposeful alteration of thoughts, images, sensation, memories, emotions, and movement to calm the body and mind.
- Free audiofiles of autogenic relaxation.
- Free breathing "apps" to perform when anxiety escalates.
- Free meditation "apps."
- Low-cost biofeedback devices that can be used by the patient. In many instances, local church groups will purchase these devices for the patient if they cannot afford them. In other cases, "loaners" can be used with selected patients.
- Behavioral prescriptions that allow the patient to practice these approaches between sessions and report progress over time.

The approaches most enticing to the patient are individualized into the VALERAS sessions for stress reduction and mood enhancement. All of these approaches are appropriate for populations with limited financial resources.

Remember that the goal is *optimization* of patients versus treating diagnosable "problems," and as such, we recommend a much lower threshold for treatment. In fact, the surgical "event" can gather motivation to engage in self-regulatory skills use as a way to improve the surgical result. In short, even people with relatively low levels of pain catastrophizing and anxiety can benefit from introduction to the concepts and the resources in chapter 5, Table 5.1 as a pathway to an improved surgical result.

Obstacles to Implementation

The Surgical Team

No surgeon desires a poor operative outcome, and most advocate, encourage, and even work toward rendering their patients "fit for surgery." However, not all are willing to delay an elective operation for sufficient length of time to optimize chronic pain–related variables—even tobacco use—as they would be for more well-publicized risk factors such as poorly managed coronary disease or out-of-control diabetes. Nonetheless, we have found that with collegial dialogue most surgeons are supportive of at least a 2- to 3- month delay for preoperative optimization, especially if the patient is well known to them. In a local survey we carried out in 2016, only 21% of surgeons were unwilling to delay the operation by at least 2 months, with 33% happy to support a 2- to 6-month optimization period and 46% vocalizing support for at least 6 months of optimization if required [16].

Institutional

We have not found institutions to be an obstacle—in fact administrators, increasingly recognizing the economic and accreditation pitfalls of poor surgical outcomes, have been eager to provide at least verbal and moral support for our efforts. Coordination of care with existing preoperative assessment clinics is not generally difficult nor unwelcome. Perhaps the main challenge encountered in setting up an outpatient preoperative optimization program is establishing and ensuring collaboration with the anesthesia and acute pain management service, if present; if possible, credentialing at the institution(s) greatly facilitates such efforts.

Patient

Patient refusal to participate is by far the most prevalent obstacle. Absolute unwillingness to participate in the program in toto is obviously an insurmountable barrier. Not uncommonly we will receive referrals for patients who display significant resistance to some (or all) components of the program but are willing to work with us nonetheless—in some cases because their surgeon mandates it and they are unwilling or unable to establish with a different surgeon who isn't requiring them to go through the program. In cases of such resistance we attempt to employ motivational interviewing principles of expressing empathy, developing discrepancy, "rolling with resistance," and supporting self-efficacy until some degree of readiness to change allows for tailored interventions.

Relapse of problematic behaviors is virtually inevitable in some patients, and having a plan in place ahead of time for how to deal with such contingencies is wise. In most cases such a breach does not necessarily derail the whole program nor justify postponing surgery, but in other cases, depending on the issue (e.g., cigarette smoking or illicit opioid use) and the perspective of the surgeon, the operation may indeed be delayed or even aborted.

Cultural

From our perspective, however, the biggest barrier to preoperative optimization of the chronic pain patient is what the US National Pain Strategy [17] recognizes as a failure of the current system to adequately address the complex needs of individuals suffering with chronic pain (and its inevitable bankruptcy if a biopsychosocial-spiritual preventive and self-management-eliciting overhaul doesn't occur). The current mainstream passivity-inducing and frequently opioid-reliant chronic pain management culture (including primary care, surgical disciplines, and pain medicine) doesn't generally encourage health, hope, or proactive solutions, but rather fosters dependence on reactive efforts to blunt symptoms with pharmacotherapy or procedures. Overshadowing that is a society that loudly denounces any discomfort, pain, and suffering as an aberrancy to be intervened on swiftly, aggressively, and as conveniently as possible. It's no wonder patients suffering with chronic pain in this country should for the most part find it far-fetched that anything short of stronger drugs, more procedures, and surgery will benefit them.

As discussed in the introduction and chapter 1, the current elective surgery pathway in the United States shares culpability for this complex problem by allowing patients suffering with antecedent chronic pain (and frequent comorbid opioid dependence) to undergo elective operations without optimization. Passivity and lack of self-management skills, as well as low distress tolerance frequently drive patients to seek a perceived quick fix for their complaint, which all too often results in worsening of their pain syndrome and opioid dependence. Unfortunately the system has traditionally reinforced this phenomenon by incentivizing operating room encounters.

Economic pressures, however, are beginning to exert themselves on this previously relatively shielded arena of medicine, with outcome-based reimbursements and bundled care models sure to alter business as usual. It is incumbent on us to prepare our patients with or without chronic pain for either potential surgery, or perhaps conversely restriction of surgical options and offerings. That preparation should look the same in either case, with the individual's maximally optimized biopsychosocial health as the determinant of "fitness for surgery," or in the best case, obviation of perceived need.

References

1   Rothman AJ, Gollwitzer PM, Grant AM, Neal DT, Sheeran P, Wood W. Hale and hearty policies: how psychological science can create and maintain healthy habits. Perspect Psychol Sci. 2015;10:701–5.

2   Ryan RM, Deci EL. Self-Determination Theory: Basic Psychological Needs in Motivation, Development and Wellness. New York: Guilford Press; 2017.

3   Epton T, Currie S, Armitage CJ. Unique effects of setting goals on behavior change: Systematic review and meta-analysis. J Consult Clin Psychol. 2017;85:1182–98.

4   Bovend'Eerdt TJ, Botell RE, Wade D. Writing SMART rehabilitation goals and achieving goal attainment scaling: a practical guide. Clin Rehab. 2009;23:352–61.

5   Gollwitzer PM. Implementation intentions: Strong effects of simple plans. Am Psychologist. 1999;54: 493–503.

6   Gollwitzer PM, Sheeran P. Implementation intentions and goal achievement: A meta-analysis of effects and processes. Adv Exp Soc Psychol. 2006;38:69–119.

7   Hollis JF, Gullion CM, Stevens VJ, et al. Weight loss during the intensive intervention phase of the weight-loss maintenance trial. Am J Prev Med. 2008;35:118–26.

8   de Wit S, Dickinson A. Associative theories of goal-directed behaviour: a case for animal-human translational models. Psychol Res. 2009;73:463–76.

9   Luther A, Gabriel J, Watson RP, Francis NK. The impact of total body prehabilitation on post-operative outcomes after major abdominal surgery: a systematic review. World J Surg. 2018;42:2781–91.

10   Li C, Carli F, Lee L, et al. Impact of a trimodal prehabilitation program on functional recovery after colorectal cancer surgery: a pilot study. Surg Endosc. 2013;27:1072–82.

11   Gillis C, Li C, Lee L, et al. Prehabilitation versus rehabilitation: a randomized control trial in patients undergoing colorectal resection for cancer. Anesthesiology. 2014;121:937–47.

12   Evans DC, Martindale RG, Kiraly LN, Jones CM. Nutrition optimization prior to surgery. Nutr Clin Pract. 2014;29:10–21.

13   Nguyen LC, Sing DC, Bozic KJ. Preoperative reduction of opioid use before total joint arthroplasty. J Arthroplast. 2016;31(9 Suppl):282–7.

14   Remillard D, Kaye A, McAnally H. Oxycodone's unparalleled addictive potential: IS it time for a moratorium? Curr Pain Headache Rep. 2019 Feb 28;23(2):15. doi:10.1007/s11916-019-0751-7.

15   Darnall BD, Sturgeon JA, Kao MC, Hah JM, Mackey SC. From Catastrophizing to Recovery: a pilot study of a single-session treatment for pain catastrophizing. J Pain Res. 2014;7:219–26.

16   McAnally H. Rationale for and approach to preoperative opioid weaning: a preoperative optimization protocol. Perioper Med (Lond). 2017;6:19. doi: 10.1186/s13741-017-0079-y.

17   Interagency Pain Research Coordinating Committee. National Pain Strategy: A Comprehensive Population Health-Level Strategy for Pain. US Dept. of Health and Human Services. https://iprcc.nih.gov/sites/default/files/HHSNational_Pain_Strategy_508C.pdf. Accessed December 29, 2018.

Index